Family-Oriented Primary Care
Second Edition

Family-Oriented Primary Care

Second Edition

Susan H. McDaniel, PhD

Professor of Psychiatry and Family Medicine, Associate Chair of the Department of Family Medicine, and Director of the Wynne Center for Family Research at the University of Rochester School of Medicine and Dentistry in Rochester, Rochester, New York, USA

Thomas L. Campbell, MD

Professor of Family Medicine and Psychiatry and Chair of the Department of Family Medicine at the University of Rochester School of Medicine and Dentistry in Rochester, Rochester, New York, USA

Jeri Hepworth, PhD

Professor and Vice-Chair of Family Medicine at the University of Connecticut School of Medicine and Saint Francis Hospital and Medical Center in Hartford, Hartford, Connecticut, USA

Alan Lorenz, MD

Associate Professor of Family Medicine and Psychiatry at the University of Rochester School of Medicine and Dentistry in Rochester, Rochester, New York, USA

Foreword by David Satcher, MD, PhD

With 26 Illustrations

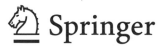 Springer

Susan H. McDaniel, PhD
Professor of Psychiatry and
   Family Medicine
Associate Chair of the Department of
   Family Medicine
and
Director of the Wynne Center for
   Family Research at the University of
   Rochester School of Medicine and
   Dentistry in Rochester
Rochester, New York, USA

Thomas L. Campbell, MD
Professor of Family Medicine and
   Psychiatry and Chair of the
   Department of Family Medicine at
   the University of Rochester School
   of Medicine and Dentistry in
   Rochester
Rochester, New York, USA

Jeri Hepworth, PhD
Professor and Vice-Chair of Family
   Medicine at the University of
   Connecticut School of Medicine
   and Saint Francis Hospital and
   Medical Center in Hartford
Hartford, Connecticut, USA

Alan Lorenz, MD
Associate Professor of Family
   Medicine and Psychiatry at the
   University of Rochester School of
   Medicine and Dentistry in
   Rochester
Rochester, New York, USA

Library of Congress Cataloging-in-Publication Data
Family-oriented primary care / Susan H. McDaniel . . . [et al.].—2nd ed.
   p. ; cm.
   Rev. ed. of: Family-oriented primary care / Susan H. McDaniel, Thomas L. Campbell,
David B. Seaburn, 1990.
   Includes bibliographical references and index.
   ISBN 0-387-98614-6 (softcover : alk paper)
      1. Family medicine.   2. Family.   I. McDaniel, Susan H. Family-oriented primary care.
   II. McDaniel, Susan H.
      [DNLM: 1. Family.   2. Family Practice—methods.   3. Primary Health Care—methods.
   WB 110 F1976 2003]
   R729.5.G4M3735 2003
   610—dc22   2003063348

ISBN 0-387-98614-6   Printed on acid-free paper.

Printed in the United States of America.   (BS/EB)

9 8 7 6 5 4 3 2 1   SPIN 10689369

springeronline.com

To our families:

David, Hanna, and Marisa
Kathy and Megan
Robert, Jon, and Katie
Jenny, Kate, August, Emily, David, Amylark, Rebecca,
and Annalise

Foreword

I was a Medical Student in 1966 when the Millis Report on the training of the generalist physician was published, defining the concept of primary care. According to the Report, the primary provider has four major responsibilities or roles. The first role is that of initial contact care of the undifferentiated patient. The second is to provide comprehensive care based on the belief that the primary provider should be able to manage the overwhelming majority of problems with which patients present. Equally important is the third role—continuity and coordination of care within the health care system. Finally, the primary provider is responsible for demonstrating leadership in the community. This Report's description of a primary provider seems as relevant today as it was when it was written. In 1994, the Institute of Medicine's assessment of primary care added the responsibility of family and community integration of care to the Millis Report description.

Without question there are many challenges to a contemporary implementation of this comprehensive description of primary care, beginning with the level of individual patients who so often suffer from complex problems, such as mental disorders and obesity. Treating these conditions in a brief primary care visit is difficult. At the level of the larger system, reimbursement is often inadequate and can represent policies that are unsupportive of primary care, such as those that compromise payment for preventive services that help patients to quit smoking or lose weight. Perhaps the major policy barrier for comprehensive primary care is the profoundly limited access to care for people who are either uninsured or underinsured. According to a recent Institute of Medicine report, lack of access has been shown to dramatically impact quality of care; at least 18,000 deaths a year are attributed to patients being uninsured. At the community and national levels, when America and many other countries are trying to draw strength from our diversity, major disparities continue to exist in health and health care for different populations. Much of the weakness in our healthcare system is on the frontline with primary care. If people do not get into the healthcare system, with problems clearly defined and strategies for care effectively implemented, then they suffer and the whole system suffers.

At the level of clinical practice, the family represents what may be the most important challenge *and* opportunity for today's primary care provider. As the concept of family continues to evolve, research makes it more and more evident that relationships have a powerful effect on health, for better and for worse. A major contribution of this text is its compelling case for family issues and family dynamics to be recognized in primary care, not only as potential influences on illness, but also as powerfully positive resources in providing quality primary health care. The extent to which families are appropriately valued, respected, educated and involved will increase the opportunity we have to enact the roles described by the Millis Report and to significantly enhance the achievement of early diagnosis, continuity of care, health promotion and disease prevention, and successful treatment, especially of chronic diseases. It is refreshing and useful to have a book that helps us to understand the role of the family in recognizing illness and influencing treatment adherence, and to show us how to establish and maintain a truly family-oriented primary care practice.

The principles described in this book can be applied to many of the clinical challenges facing providers today. For example, the United States has more than 35 million people, ages 65 and older, and this population is projected to double by 2030. The good news, of course, is that life expectancy has increased significantly—by 30 years in the last century. The fastest growing group of people in America today are people more than 85 years of age. The bad news is that quality of life for older adults has not kept pace; today more than half of the people over the age of 80 are incapacitated physically, mentally or both. Primary care has a major role in dealing with the challenges provided by the aging of our population; it is through a partnership between the family and the primary care provider that these issues can be most successfully addressed.

Family-Oriented Primary Care, Second Edition, gives us the insights and tools needed to address some of the many challenges listed above. If we are to achieve the goals of Healthy People 2010, or even Healthy People 2020, it will be not only because we rectify some of the healthcare disparities that threaten our system, but also because of our commitment to treat the whole person with the illness, understanding that the person lives in a family that affects his/her health beliefs, lifestyle, and healthcare. If we as health professionals can partner with families to support and educate them, listen closely to their concerns, and advocate for their health, together we can increase the physical, mental, and social well-being of all our citizens and communities.

David Satcher, MD, PhD
Director, National Center for Primary Care
Morehouse School of Medicine, and
16th Surgeon General of the United States

Preface to the Second Edition

Much has happened since *Family-Oriented Primary Care* first was published in 1990. Many physicians and nurses wrote to us about their experiences with family-oriented care, in the United States as well as in England, Germany, Israel, South Africa, Finland, Spain, Japan, and South Korea, to name just a few countries with strong family-oriented health professionals. We have been influenced by many of these colleagues and by the changes in the healthcare climate and practice. Ours is a time that requires innovation and rethinking of clinical approaches. This second edition of *Family-Oriented Primary Care* represents our current thinking and practice in response to the current healthcare environment.

Primary care is delivered in so many different settings and contexts that we are acutely aware that one approach cannot fit all situations. An intervention can have a variety of meanings across cultures. The examples in this book come from our experiences. The particulars may not fit your context or culture; however, we understand from our contact with others regarding the first edition that the principles of family-oriented primary care hold true regardless. For example, the meaning given by a patient to the symptom of fatigue or fainting may be different in the Rio Grande area of Texas than it is in New York City or outside Capetown, South Africa, but the principle of asking about and understanding the meaning or belief of the patient remains the same.

In addition to belief systems, family-oriented primary care is also very much affected by the economics of the particular healthcare delivery system in which the clinician works. In the United States, with the increasing corporatization of healthcare, clinicians have had to become even more aware of the bottom line. With decreased reimbursement in the face of increased paperwork, clinicians are even more pressured for time. The need to be efficient has never been greater. At the same time, there has been increased emphasis on "customer satisfaction." Primary care has new prominence as a key element of this new delivery system, with primary care clincians sometimes functioning as gatekeepers who decide when and how much to utlize other services.

All this change and turmoil in the delivery of healthcare has been both stressful and exciting. Whereas many professionals worry about patients receiving the appropriate quality of care when decisions are driven by financial considerations, one of the real benefits of attention to cost has been the overdue respect now given to the patient and family as consumers of healthcare. Healthcare systems are suddenly competing openly, and they want to know what their patients want.

Family-oriented approaches have become more, not less, relevant in this environment. With the decreased length of hospital stays and increased use of less-expensive paraprofessionals for a range of services, family members increasingly are care providers for patients with a broad range of problems. It has become essential for primary care clinicians to know how to work with family members, and to understand the family context even when only working with an individual patient as is typical.

Another development that influences this edition is the work of McDaniel and Hepworth, with their colleague Bill Doherty, in the development of an approach for mental health professionals termed "medical family therapy" (2). This biopsychosocial approach to psychotherapy has the same underlying principles as family-oriented primary care, and provides a complementary approach for family-oriented behavioral health clinicians on the primary care team.

New organizations and new journals have sprung up to support these innovations in healthcare. For example, the Collaborative Family HealthCare Association (CFHA)[1].org is a multidisciplinary organization for professionals interested in family-oriented, collaborative approaches to integrated healthcare. Its members include primary care physicians, nurses, a range of behavioral health specialists, and others committed to collaborative care. The journals *Families, Systems & Health* and the *Journal of Family Nursing* both devote themselves to research, literature reviews, and care reports about family-oriented healthcare. The research on the efficacy and effectiveness of family interventions has grown, will be seen in Chapter 2.

These many changes motivated our desire to update the first edition of *Family-Oriented Primary Care*. David Seaburn has turned his considerable talents to training in the area of research and health (thank you, Dave, for all of your important contributions to the first edition), and two new authors joined Susan McDaniel and Thomas Campbell in the revision of this volume: Jeri Hepworth, a family therapist who has taught and practiced in a Family Medicine residency program since 1981, and Alan Lorenz, a family physician who had a rural, family-oriented primary care practice for 10 years before coming to the University of Rochester Department of Family

---

[1] Information about CFHA is available by writing 40 West 12 St, NY, NY 10011, Fax: 212-727-1126, E-mail: staff@cfha.org, Web site: www.cfha.org

Medicine in 2001. Both authors bring a long history of experience and creativity to this project.

For those who know the first edition, you will notice that we have added new chapters on topics that students, residents, and practitioners continuously asked us about: how to conduct a routine, family-oriented visit with an individual; how to work with the difficult (angry, uncooperative, multiproblem) patient and family; and a family-oriented approach to genetic screening. In addition, much of the previous material has been updated and expanded. In the chapter on abuse, for example, we include approaches to partner violence and elder abuse, as well as on child abuse. This manual reflects our rapidly changing field, although we retain material and principles that seem to us to be timeless. We have given more attention in this volume to diversity: the diversity of patients treated in primary care, the diverse family forms that are part of our current cultural fabric, and the diversity of clinicians now working in primary care.

Health professionals today come in a variety of forms. In the first edition, we focused our efforts on family physicians. Part of the purpose of the second edition has been to broaden the focus to include internists, pediatricians, nurse practitioners, physician assistants, obstetrician/gynecologists, and any specialty physicians wishing to bring more of a family focus to their practice.

Many of these changes are the result of feedback that our readers have provided on the first edition. We hope you will do the same, as we continue to try to provide a practical, working guide to the practice of family-oriented primary care.

There are many people to thank in making a project this large and long-standing finally come to fruition, most especially Jeanne Klee, the assistant to Susan McDaniel and Tom Campbell, who supported the revision and development of this book, drew genograms and figures, and performed countless other tasks, always with a smile.

There are also the many professionals who read specific chapters and gave us invaluable feedback. Thank you to: Louise Acheson, Robert Cushman, Laurie Donohue, Steven Eisinger, Kevin Fiscella, Starlene Loader, Robert McCann, June Peters, Peter Rowley, Robert Ryder, Aric Schichor, David Siegel, Linda Sinapi, and the residents and fellows in the Departments of Family Medicine at the University of Connecticut and the University of Rochester.

Thank you to Michelle Schmitt and Laurel Craven at Springer-Verlag who advised and nudged us until the project was complete.

Our patients, of course, taught us the most about family-oriented primary care. Thank you to all of them.

And finally, to our own families, who have loved and supported us throughout this project: David, Hanna, and Marisa Siegel; Kathy Cole-Kelly and Megan Campbell; Robert, Jon, and Katie Ryder; Jenny and Annalise Lorenz, August and Amylark Lorwood, and Kate, Emily, David, and Rebecca Sharp. We love you all.

Susan H. McDaniel, PhD
Thomas L. Campbell, MD
Jeri Hepworth, PhD
Alan Lorenz, MD

References

1. Bakan D: *The Duality of Human Existence.* Chicago: Rand McNally, 1969.
2. McDaniel SH, Hepworth J, & Doherty WJ: *Medical Family Therapy: A Biopsychosocial Approach to Families with Health Problems.* New York: Basic Books, 1992.

Preface to the First Edition

This book is a manual for physicians who want to enhance their skills in working with patients in the context of their families. It has evolved out of our work with physicians, patients, and families in a primary care medical setting, as well as our teaching within the Department of Family Medicine at the University of Rochester School of Medicine and Dentistry. Respected colleagues, such as Medalie, Doherty and Baird, and Christie-Seely, have made contributions to the theory of family systems medicine, but little has yet been written about the practicalities and skills involved in day-to-day family-oriented primary care. Building on this theoretical work, we are taking the step of integrating theory into the daily practice of primary care physicians.

Family-oriented primary care offers the practitioners a useful perspective that will help in caring for both the individual patient and the family. The skills that operationalize this approach enable the physician to utilize the support inherent in most families to the benefit of the patient. The National Heart, Lung, and Blood Institute has recognized the importance of the family in increasing compliance and promoting continuity of care. Based upon research studies and clinical experience with hypertension, they recommend that the physician:

> Enhance support from family members—identifying and involving one influential person, preferably someone living with the patient, who can provide encouragement, help support the behavior change, and, if necessary, remind the patient about specifics of the regimen (1).

In this book, we have extended this basic strategy to apply to all of primary care.

Whereas family-oriented primary care can result in more effective care of a patient, we also feel it is important to note that this perspective can be useful to the physician. Primary care can be a stressful and taxing, albeit rewarding, career. Recognizing the important of the family and utilizing its resources allows the physician to share the responsibility of care and decision making with those who care most about the patient. This approach can help to prevent physician burn-out so that energy can be conserved for the physician's own personal and family life.

We begin the manual with a section that spells out our theory of family systems medicine, reviews the relevant research, and provides a guide for assessing and interviewing families in primary care. This section is called, "The Biopsychosocial Assessment of the Family." We then turn to a section entitled, "Health Care of the Family in Transition," and discuss how to treat specific health-care issues that arise when the patient and his or her family are facing normal developmental challenges. These issues range from the concerns of new couples, pregnancy, and adolescent difficulties, to sexual issues, aging, and death. In the next section, "A Family-Oriented Approach to Specific Medical Problems," we provide guidelines for a family-oriented approach to substance abuse, anxiety and depression, chronic illness, somatic fixation, and sexual and physical abuse. The final section, "Implementing Family-Oriented Primary Care," addresses general issues: the implementation of a family-oriented practice; hospitalization; collaborating and making referrals with family therapist; and managing personal and professional boundaries.

Throughout the book we will use case material to illustrate how to approach specific treatment problems in a family-oriented way. The case examples are actual primary care cases or composites of cases; however, identifying data have been changed and pseudonyms added to protect the confidentiality of our patients. Protocols appear at the end of the each chapter to be used as a quick guide in daily practice.

Many people have helped us in the completion of this project. Our patients have provided us with invaluable opportunities to learn about family-oriented primary care. The residents who we teach and the faculty with whom we work at the University of Rochester Department of Family Medicine have provided important feedback on our ideas and our clinical practice. Our colleagues in the Division of Family Programs in the Department of Psychiatry have also stimulated and informed our work. Particularly, the thinking and teaching of M. Duncan Stanton, The director of the division, and Judith Landau-Stanton have influenced and broadened our perspectives. The administration of the Department of Family Medicine, and Highland Hospital, has provided us with the financial support to work on this project. We would especially like to thank Jay Dickinson, The chairman of the Department of Family Medicine, for his guidance and support.

We would also like to acknowledge the many people who read and reviewed these chapters before publication. Their responses helped us to clarify our theories and sharpen our techniques. We are most grateful to three people who read the entire book in process and provided us with constructive feedback: Kathy Cole-Kelly, Eugene Farley, and Thomas Schwenk. Numerous colleagues read specific chapters along the way and responded from their areas of expertise. Thank you to: Marvin Amstey, Macaran Baird, Richard Botelho, T. Berry Brazelton, Barbara Elliott, Annmarie Groth-Junker, Jeff Harp, Allison Beth Maher, Carl Maskiell, Cathy Morrow, Steve Munson, Elizabeth Naumburg, Paul Rapoza, Deborah Richter, Eric Schaff, Joseph Scherger, Cleveland Shields, Bernard Shore, David Siegel, Earl Siegel, Lucy Siegel, David Stoller, Sarah Grafton, Donald Treat, Michael Weidner, and Lyman Wynne.

Finally, thank you to our families for their understanding support during a project of this size. Thank you to our editor, Shelley Reinhardt, for her helpful support and guidance. Thank you to our colleague, Peter Franks, for his technical assistance. Our thanks to Sally Rousseau for her endless and creative efforts in producing and refining the tables and figures. Any many thanks to our secretary, Jeanne Klee, who helped us with her typing, her editing, and her always present smile.

Susan H. McDaniel, PhD
Thomas L. Campbell, MD
David B. Seaburn

Reference

1. Working Group on Health Education and High Blood Pressure Control: *The physician's guide—improving adherence among hypertensive patients.* Bethesda, MD: U.S. DHHS, PHS, NIH, 1988.

Contents

1
Basic Premises of Family-Oriented Primary Care

There is a tendency for all living things to join up,
establish linkages, live inside each other,
return to earlier arrangements, get along whenever possible.
This is the way of the world.
—Lewis Thomas, The Lives of a Cell, 1974 (1)

Each day, clinicians[1] manage and treat the illnesses of patients who are joined to, linked with, and live within a larger context–the family. In fact, despite the popular attention given to singles living alone or with a non-family roommate, more than 70% of the American population still make their home with other family members (2). The family remains the most basic relational unit in society.

When we speak of the *family*, each of us develops a picture in our minds of what that means. For some, it is Mom, Dad, brother, and sister, as well as the family dog. For others, it may be Mom and stepdad, Grandma, Grandpa, and an aunt or uncle. For still others, the arrangements are less "traditional": single-parent families, gay relationships, adoptive families, remarried families. Beyond that, there are those who feel their truest family is found in a religious community or among a set of friends. All of us have a personal sense of what the family is, but the task becomes difficult when it comes to defining the "typical family."

The television stereotype of the American family in the 1950s, in which the husband is employed and the wife is a homemaker with dependent children, accounted for 28% of all married couples and only 10% of all households in the 1990s (3). More common family forms that have emerged are single-parent families and "nonfamily households," composed of single persons or persons living with nonrelatives. The American family of the late

---

[1] We want to recognize that a variety of family-oriented health professionals provide care, including family physicians, internists, pediatricians, obstetrician-gynecologists, nurse practitioners, and physician assistants. As such, we will vary the term used to denote the clinician in our attempt to recognize and respect this professional diversity.

twentieth and early twenty-first century is a mix of couples (29%), two parents with children (25%), single-parent households (16%), and non-family households (30%) (2, 3) (see Fig. 1.1).

Even with these social changes, it is the family, however constituted, that most often addresses the individual's need for physical and emotional safety, health, and well-being. Research supports the view that the family plays a vital role in the health and illness of its members (see Chap. 2). Because the nature of the family is evolving, our understanding of it also needs to evolve in order to capture its rich diversity.

We define *family as any group of people related either biologically, emotionally, or legally*. That is, the group of people that the patient defines as significant for his or her well-being. The family-oriented practitioner gathers information about these family relationships, patterns of health and illness across generations, emotional connections with deceased and geographically removed members, and life-cycle transitions, in order to understand the patient within his or her larger context. In other words, *the family-oriented clinician mobilizes the patient's natural support system to enhance health and well-being.*

In daily practice, the family-oriented clinician is most often interested in family members who live within the same house or apartment. Even though involvement of nonhousehold family members can be important to a patient's medical care, the household is generally the primary focus in determining a diagnosis and carrying out a treatment plan (4). It is important for the primary care physician to offer and encourage the whole household to register with him or her. In this way the clinician has access to the people who may most influence each other's illness and health.

Without considering the patient in his or her family context, the physician may inadvertently eliminate both a wider understanding of illness and a broader range of solutions as well. "Family-oriented primary care" does not mean the physician or nurse practitioner always sees entire households together. Rather, by *family-oriented* we mean an approach or way of thinking that a clinician can bring to any patient encounter, with or without accompanying family members. A family-oriented approach involves thinking about a symptom or problem in the context of the whole person and the person's significant others. This way of thinking may at times mean the inclusion of other important persons in the assessment and treatment process; at other times, it may not.

We do not advocate family-oriented primary care because we believe that the family alone can cure disease; instead, we believe—and research is beginning to support—that planned and purposeful family participation in healthcare can be useful to the patient, the family, and the clinician. Not including family members, or family information, can at times run the risk of incurring roadblocks or, at least, detours on the road to effective and efficient primary care. Including family members means the clinician has enlisted his or her most potent allies in the treatment of his or her patients.

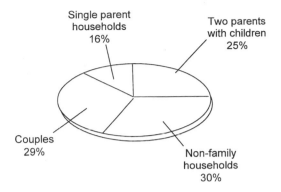

FIGURE 1.1. The American family of the late twentieth–early twenty-first centuries.

Basic Premises of Family-Centered Medical Care

A family-oriented approach to healthcare incorporates and expands upon a biomedical approach. Some of the basic premises are:

Premise 1: Family-Oriented Healthcare Is Based on a Biopsychosocial Systems Approach

An exclusively biomedical model, based on molecular biology, assumes that disease can be reduced to "measurable biological variables" (5). The task of the physician operating strictly from a biomedical approach is to analyze and eliminate all factors in the development of illness until the simplest biological elements are identified. This approach ignores the influence of social and psychological factors. From a biomedical perspective, for example, the cause of tuberculosis is the tubercule bacillus. The dramatic fall in the incidence of the disease, however, has resulted more from public health measures and improvements in social environment than from the introduction of antitubercular drugs (6). Few primary care clinicians now believe an exclusively biomedical approach is effective in primary care; instead, a biopsychosocial systems approach places illness within a larger framework involving multiple systems (7, 8). In his seminal article from 1980, George Engel, MD, first articulated the biopsychosocial approach and rendered a visual representation that illustrates this comprehensive view. To understand illness, the clinician must attend to the biological contributors as well as the person, the clinician–patient interaction, the family, the social setting, and how these factors may be connected in the creation of symptoms (see Fig. 1.2). Note that the relationship between these various factors involves continuous and reciprocal feedback. Each level responds and adjusts to changes in other levels. In that way, stability is maintained through a process

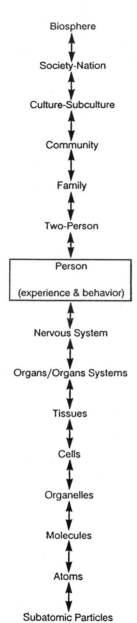

FIGURE 1.2. Systems hierarchy. (From: Engel GL. The clinical application of the biopsychosocial model. *Am J Psychiatry*. Copyright May 1980. The American Psychiatric Association. Reprinted with permission from The American Psychiatric Association.)

of change, much the same as a tightrope walker maintains balance by making frequent shifts and adjustments. Dym (9) illustrates this process with a "simple" case of childhood asthma.

> John is a 33-year-old Russian-American man who is a frequent drinker. When he drinks, his younger partner, Mary, criticizes him. (Mary's Baptist parents never drank.) John and Mary's son, Harry, 14, unable to deal with the stress of the fighting, flees to a friend's house for the night. When the fight continues, George, 11, becomes anxious and has an asthma attack. Mary shifts her focus to George and gives him medicine through an inhaler. She then blames John who feels guilty. He leaves home temporarily, and the fight stops. The next day he drinks again and the cycle continues.

Asthma can represent a complex interaction of multiple factors at different levels of the problem. George may have a genetic predisposition to the illness, and there may be environmental allergens that activate George's symptoms. In addition, the illness is affected by a relational pattern that precipitates the symptom of wheezing. For the family-oriented clinician, understanding and addressing all these variables is necessary for comprehensive treatment (10).

Many clinicians now operate from a "split biopsychosocial" model (11). This means that they work up a problem like asthma at the biomedical level, and then switch to a psychosocial assessment when they have not successfully treated the problem from a purely biomedical point of view. The "split" approach produces resistance in the patient, who believes the clinician feels it is "all in my head." This manual operationalizes an integrated biopsychosocial systems approach in which the patient and the problem are understood at multiple levels in context from the beginning.

Premise 2: The Primary Focus of Healthcare Is the Patient in the Context of the Family

The clinician who operates from a biopsychosocial systems perspective highlights the patient's family context as the primary arena in which health issues typically are addressed. Leaders in the field of family medicine have disagreed on the efficacy of considering the family as the "unit of care" (12–17). There are those who feel the individual is the primary "unit of care," whereas others argue for the family. This argument is specious because it pits two levels of the biopsychosocial model against each other (i.e., the "individual" and the "family") and forces a choice of what will be the "unit of care." Although a clinician might choose to intervene primarily at only one of these levels in any given case, to argue for only one of them to be the sacred "unit of care" results in conceptual confusion (e.g., What does it mean for the family to be the "unit of care"?), and is antithetical to the interrelationships between levels that are fundamental to the original meaning of the biopsychosocial systems model. For that reason, we have chosen to think of the patient in the context of the family as the "focus" rather than the "unit" of medical care. From this perspective, the physician is reminded of the importance of the person as a biological and emotional entity as well as the significance of the family's influence on illness and health.

A balance must be achieved between the goals of agency for the individual, and communion for the group (8, 18). *Agency* is a sense that one can make personal choices in dealing with illness and the healthcare system. For patients with an illness, agency means not remaining passive. It means coming to grips with what they must accept while discovering what action they can take. Agency is a sense of activism about one's own life in the face of all that is uncertain.

The other goal, *communion*, refers to strengthening emotional and spiritual bonds that can be frayed by illness, disability, and contact with the healthcare system. It is the sense of being cared for, loved, and supported by a community of family members, friends, and professionals. Serious illness or disability is an existential crisis that can isolate people from those who care for them, with significant health consequences. Family-oriented primary care is an approach that takes into account the need for communication, connection, and choice, in addition to high-quality biotechnical medicine in the delivery of healthcare today.

Both agency (of the individual) and communion (of the group) are important; not one at the expense of the other. Adolescent healthcare can drive this point home.

> Billy Smith's[2] diabetes was first diagnosed at the age of 13 when he was admitted to the hospital with diabetic ketoacidosis (DKA). He adjusted well while in the hospital and began to manage his own insulin and diet shortly thereafter. An only child in an African-American family, Billy received support from his parents, especially his mother, who did not work outside the home. Billy's diabetes was stable until his senior year in high school; his blood sugars were often in the 300s. Billy claimed to be taking his insulin and sticking to his diet. His diabetes eventually became so out of control that he was admitted to the hospital.

In this, and other situations like it, the family-oriented clinician will explore family issues to see how they may influence or be a resource in a crisis. As part of this process, four major considerations influence family-oriented primary care:

---

[2] All cases in this book are actual primary care cases. Identities have been changed to protect confidentiality. Because of the importance of race and ethnicity to health beliefs, process, and uniqueness, we have included such attributions while acknowledging considerable individual and family variations within subgroups.

The Family Is the Primary Source of Health Beliefs and Behaviors

The initial appraisal of physical symptoms is usually made within the family and is based upon family beliefs about health. Many families have a health expert, often the oldest female. The family health expert, in the preceding case Billy's mother Mrs. Smith, often makes an initial health assessment and treatment plan and decides whether a physician should be consulted. Mrs. Smith made the first contact with Dr. B. She suggested that her son may be "under too much pressure" and wondered if that could affect his illness.

Many health behaviors and risk factors are shared by members of a family. For example, children are more likely to smoke if their parents smoke (19). Most families share the same diet, which along with genetic influences result in elevated cholesterol levels occurring within certain families (20). A family approach to health promotion and risk reduction is therefore likely to be more efficient and cost effective (21, 22).

The Stress of Family Developmental Transitions May Become Manifest in Physical Symptoms

The family-oriented clinician is sensitive to the impact of life cycle changes on the health of family members (see Chap. 3). Marriage, birth of the first child, adolescence, leaving home, midlife, divorce, remarriage, loss of a job, death of a parent, and retirement are all developmental transitions that may occur in the life of a family (23). The health of family members may be more vulnerable due to the stress that can occur during these periods.

The Smiths were going through three significant transitions simultaneously. Mr. Smith had made a career shift at midlife, Mrs. Smith's mother died, and Billy, who was soon to graduate from high school, was facing the issue of leaving home. Each family member was under tremendous strain. The family as a whole was being transformed by the demands these changes were requiring.

Somatic Symptoms Can Serve an Adaptive Function Within the Family and Be Maintained by Family Patterns (24)

Dr. B. learned that Billy had a very close relationship with his mother. Mrs. Smith was protective of her son and Billy depended on his mother's support during his illness. Mr. Smith supported the family primarily through his role as breadwinner and provider. Even though Mr. and Mrs. Smith were not very close, Billy and his father were able to maintain a good relationship. In the year prior to the acceleration of his illness, Mrs. Smith's mother died and Mr. Smith had been traveling more since receiving a promotion. Billy was also making plans to leave home for college. Mrs. Smith's needs for closeness increased due to her loss of her mother. Her neediness coincided with her husband's frequent absence. Billy found himself in the position of having to meet his mother's needs while feeling angry and frustrated over his father's absence. Billy developed symptoms during this time. As Billy's symptoms worsened, Mr. Smith began to curtail his traveling. Mr. and Mrs. Smith also began to pull together to try to help their son.

Billy's symptoms can be understood, in part, as a barometer of the pressure felt within the family. In a sense, the symptoms were both a problem and a solution. They were obviously a problem in that they presented a challenge to his health and well-being, and created great concern for his parents who love him. Billy's symptoms, however, may also be seen as a solution in that they brought Billy's parents together to care for him, thus stabilizing their marital difficulties; the symptoms kept Billy from leaving home too quickly at a time when he was clearly concerned about his parents; in turn, they sounded an alarm for the alert physician that the whole family was in need.

Families Are a Valuable Resource and Source of Support for the Management of Illness

Physicians and nurse practitioners recommend treatment that is usually carried out in the home by the patient and family members. To ignore the family is to invite sabotage and "noncompliance."

In Billy's case, he had taken responsibility for his insulin and diet with the support and supervision of his parents. As Dr. B. addressed this recent crisis he once again engaged the parents in planning for the management of their son's illness. Despite their differences, Mr. and Mrs. Smith's commitment to their son made coordinated planning and treatment possible.

Dr. B.'s approach to Billy's diabetes takes his symptoms into account as well as the family context. It highlights how the family is a factor in both illness and health, and sets the stage for utilizing the family as a resource in developing and carrying out a treatment plan.

Premise 3: The Patient, Family, and Clinician Are Partners in Healthcare

To provide quality healthcare, family-oriented physicians and nurse practitioners use the most basic resources available to them—the patient and his or her family. It is through these people that the physician gains the most significant information for understanding symptoms and planning treatment. In this way, the family is a natural partner in healthcare.

This partnership destroys what Doherty and Baird have called "the illusion of the dyad in medical care" (25, p. 12). The illusion is that medical care only involves a one-to-one relationship between clinician and individual patient. Doherty and Baird point out that except in the most rare situations the family is involved in what takes place between physician or nurse practitioner and patient (see Fig. 1.3). Even when the family is not physically in the room, the patient's role within the family, the family's expectations of medical care, and the family's relational patterns as they pertain to health and illness play a part in what transpires.

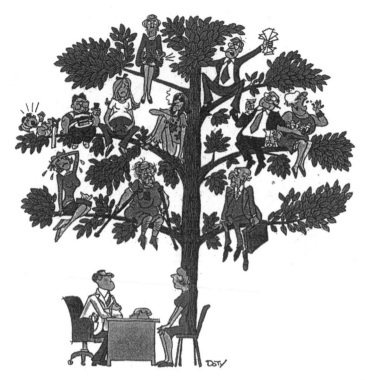

FIGURE 1.3. The patient's family tree. (*Source*: Crouch M., Roberts I., 1987. *The Family in Medical Practice*. New York: Springer-Verlag.)

In place of a dyadic approach, Doherty and Baird propose a "triangular perspective" (see Fig. 1.4). This triangle involves the clinician, patient, and family working together in a medical-care partnership. Together they define what needs to be done. This includes identifying symptoms, establishing a treatment plan, and clarifying responsibilities. Medical treatment can go awry when this partnership is not in place.

A new patient, Mr. Samuel, a 30-year-old Romanian bricklayer, was prescribed medication and a low-salt diet for his hypertension by Dr. L. Mr. Samuel's parents, with whom he had immigrated and now lived, had doubts about the efficacy of medical treatment. They questioned the medication and also felt the diet would mean their lifestyle would have to change as well. Mr. Samuel was caught between opposing expectations from his physician and his parents. He resolved the dilemma by complying with the treatment plan only in part. He took his medication irregularly and followed his diet for a few days. Partial compliance ironically convinced both Dr. L. and the family that each was right. Dr. L. saw it as confirmation that the patient must try harder. The family was convinced that the treatment was not working. Both

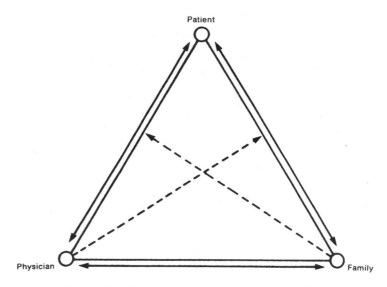

FIGURE 1.4. The therapeutic triangle in medicine.

sides escalated their positions and Mr. Samuel continued his compromise. In the meantime, his blood pressure remained elevated.

Dr. L. soon recognized the situation and invited the patient's parents
to come in with him. He explained their son's hypertension and the
rationale for the treatment plan. He enlisted their help, clearly indicating
that they could bring about some change for their son. Mr. Samuel's
mother was utilized as an expert on diet. The parents gave their
"permission" for their son to take the medication.

The importance of the family in a patient's adherence to medical treatment
is well-documented (see Chap. 2). The family-oriented physician engages
the patient and the family as an ally and a resource in negotiating a treatment plan that all can support.

Premise 4: The Family-Oriented Clinician Reflects on How He or She Is Part of the Treatment System

Physicians who operate from a biopsychosocial systems perspective believe
that "the observer constantly alters what he [or she] observes by the obtru-
sive act of observation" (26, p. 129). Biopsychosocially oriented clinicians
observe the interaction between themselves and their patients and ask
themselves, "How am I part of what is happening?" In that sense they
understand themselves as part of an interactional process in which their
behavior contributes to what transpires. In fact, their interaction with the
patient and family system may unwittingly support rather than relieve the
problem.

Mrs. Jackson brought Mary, an 11, to the doctor's office for the third time in 3 months with symptoms of sore throat. Dr. K., alert to larger, systemic issues in this interesting Latina/British-American family, asked about stress and how the rest of the family was doing. In the course of the visit, she learned that Mrs. Jackson had returned to work for the first time in 12 years. Mr. Jackson was not pleased about the change. He felt it had an adverse effect on Mary, the youngest of three. The Jackson's older children were away at college. Mr. Jackson felt he provided well for his family and believed the income from Mrs. Jackson's job was not needed. Mrs. Jackson wanted to work as an opportunity to grow as well as to help support the family. She felt Mary, who had recently entered sixth grade in a new middle school, did not need her attention as much as before. Mary said she just didn't feel well and that things weren't the way they used to be.

Dr. K. wondered if her exclusive focus on Mary's sore throat in the past 3 months had unintentionally supported the ongoing battle between Mr. and Mrs. Jackson over whether or not Mrs. Jackson should be working. Each time Mary became ill, Mr. Jackson insisted Mrs. Jackson take time off work to bring her to the doctor. He also seemed to use it as an opportunity to underscore his contention that Mary needed her mother at home. The monthly visits to Dr. K. for throat cultures became part of a larger pattern in the life of the family.

If Dr. K. continued to focus only on the sore throat, more fuel would have been added to the fire of Mr. and Mrs. Jackson's disagreement and Mary's resultant distress. By incorporating a family perspective, Dr. K. saw the larger picture and recognized how she fit into it. The next step was to call Mr. Jackson to understand more about his perspective and begin to sort out his differences with his wife.

When treatment falters, a change in our own behavior may help facilitate change throughout the system. In the case of the Jackson family, Dr. K.'s understanding of her role in the family dynamics helped move the couple toward resolving their differences. Left unadvised, Mary would likely come back with a series of escalating complaints.

Multiple vehicles exist to help clinicians attend to our own issues in patient care. These include regular discussion with trusted colleagues, consultation with behavioral health consultants, personal awareness groups, Balint groups that examine problematic clinician–patient encounters (27, 28), and readings about the emotional experience of facing illness, whether as a patient, a family member, or clinician (29).

Developing Skills for Family-Oriented Primary Care

Primary care physicians have a range of skills available to them in practicing family-oriented primary care, depending on the kind of family involvement the clinician thinks would be most useful. Doherty and Baird (30)

TABLE 1.1. Levels of family involvement for primary care clinicians

Level 1: Minimal Contact
Families are dealt with for practical or legal reasons. One-way communication prevails.

Level 2: Information and Collaboration
Communicate information clearly to patients and families. Elicit questions and areas of concern, and generate mutually agreed-upon action plans.

Level 3: Feelings and Support
Demonstrate empathic listening and elicit expressions of feelings and concerns from patients and families. Normalize feelings and emotional reactions to illness.

Level 4: Primary Care Family Assessment/Counseling*
Assess the relationship between the illness problem and the family dynamics. If the problem is not complex or long-standing, work with the family to achieve change. If the problem is entrenched or family counseling is not effective, make a referral and educate the family and therapist about what to expect. Continue to collaborate.

Level 5: Medical Family Therapy
Medical family therapy is intensive specialty care delivered by professionals with advanced psychotherapy training. Primary care clinicians should collaborate closely on those patients with whom they have active involvement.

*See Chapter 25 for a discussion of Levels 4 and 5. *Source*: Doherty WJ, Baird MA. Developmental levels of family-centered medical care. *Family Medicine* 1986;**18**:153–156. Adapted with permission.

describe five levels of physician involvement with families (see Table 1.1). At Level 1, the family is included only when necessary for practical and medical/legal reasons. At Level 2, the clinician is primarily biomedically focused and communicates regularly with the family about medical issues. The clinician functioning at Level 3 both gathers information and also addresses family stress and feelings by actively eliciting family feelings in a supportive way. At Level 4, the clinician gathers information and deals with family affect, and intervenes in ways that may alter the family's interactional patterns. The clinician at this level has an understanding of family systems theory and a grasp of the skills to counsel the families to make constructive changes that increase agency for family members and communion for the family as a whole. Level 5 is family therapy, which addresses more deeply rooted family patterns of dysfunction. Most clinicians will refer families who need this level of intervention to trained family therapists. (Some physicians and nurse practitioners themselves obtain postresidency training and supervision in family therapy.)

This book focuses primarily on developing skills at Levels 2–4. We will mention the importance of Level 2 (i.e., basic communication with the family). We will encourage physicians and nurses to use the skills involved at Level 3 when it is important to elicit family feelings and deal with them in a supportive manner. Many clinicians already operate at Levels 2 and 3. The goal of this book is to increase skills and comfort with Level 4 (i.e., to assess family interaction, utilize family resources, and, when necessary, engage the family in primary care counseling in order to treat illness in the most effective, efficient way).

Given the basic premises just described, our goal is to help clinicians develop the skills necessary to implement family-oriented primary care. We believe family-oriented primary care provides better, more comprehensive care for routine patients, and more effective care for patients with such challenging problems as somatizing, domestic violence, and chronic illness. Once family-oriented primary care skills are learned, *it does not take more time* than traditional care. In fact, it may *save* time because the clinician gains a comprehensive view of the problem early, and the patient and family participate in negotiating and delivering the treatment. Finally, family-oriented primary care involves partnerships among care providers, and between professionals and the patient and family. As such, it is a more interesting, less stressful, and more satisfying way for the clinician to deliver primary care.

References

1. Thomas L: *The Lives of a Cell: Notes of a Biology Watcher*. New York: Bantam Books, Inc., 1974, p. 147.
2. U.S. Bureau of the Census, *Statistical Abstract of the United States: 1996* (116th Edition). Washington DC: U.S. Bureau of the Census, 1996.
3. Family Service America *Family Facts: Families in the 90s*. Grosse Pointe Woods, MI: Center for the Advancement of the Family, 1990.
4. North American Primary Care Research Group (NAPCRG) Committee on Standard Terminology. *A Glossary for Primary Care*. Presented at the Annual Meeting of NAPCRG, Williamsburg, VA, March, 1977.
5. Engel GL: The need for a new medical model: a challenge for biomedicine. *Science* 1977;**196**:129–136.
6. McKeown T: *The Role of Medicine: Dream, Mirage, or Nemesis*. Princeton, NH: Princeton University Press, 1979.
7. Engel GL: The clinical application of the biopsychosocial model, *Am J Psychiatr* 1980;**137**:535–544.
8. McDaniel SH, Hepworth J, & Doherty WJ: *Medical Family Therapy: A Biopsychosocial Approach for Families with Health Problems*. New York: Basic Books, 1992.
9. Dym B: The cybernetics of physical illness. *Fam Process* 1987;**26**:35–48.
10. Campbell T, McDaniel S: Applying a systems approach to common medical problems, in Crouch M, Roberts L (Eds). *The Family in Medical Practice: A Family Systems Primer*. New York: Springer-Verlag, 1987, 112–139.
11. Doherty WJ, Baird M, & Becker L: Family medicine and the biopsychosocial model: the road toward integration, *Marriage Fam Rev* 1987;**10**:51–70.
12. Schmidt DD: The family as the unit of medical care. *J Fam Prac* 1978;**7**(2):303–313.
13. Carmichael LP: Forty families—a search for the family in family medicine. *Fam Sys Med* 1983;**1**(1):12–16.

14. Christiansen CE: Making the family the unit of care: what does it mean? *Fam Med* 1983;**15**(6):207–209.
15. Ransom DC: On why it is useful to say "the family is the unit of care" in family medicine: Comment on Carmichael's essay. *Fam Sys Med* 1983;**1**(1):17–22.
16. Schwenk TC, Hughes CC: The family as patient in family medicine: rhetoric or reality? *Soc Sci Med* 1983;**17**:1–16.
17. Franks SH: The unit of care revisited. *J Fam Prac* 1985;**21**(2):145–148.
18. Bakan D: *The Duality of Human Existence* Chicago: Rand McNally, 1969.
19. Bewley RB, Bland JM: Academic performance and social factors related to cigarette smoking by school children. *Br J Prevent Soc Med* 1977;**31**:18–24.
20. Hartz A, Giefer E, & Rimm AA: Relative importance of the effect of family environment and heredity on obesity. *Ann Hum Genet* 1977;**41**:185–193.
21. Campbell TL, Patterson J: *J Marriage Fam Ther* 1995.
22. Doherty WJ, Campbell TL: *Fam Health* Beverly Hills, CA: Sage, 1988.
23. Carter EA, McGoldrick M (Eds): *The Changing Family Life Cycle: A Framework for Family Therapy*. New York: Gardner Press, 1988.
24. Watzlawick P, Weakland J, & Fisch C: *Change: Principles of Problem Formation and Problem Resolution*. New York: W.W. Norton, 1974.
25. Doherty WJ, Baird M: *Family Therapy and Family Medicine* New York: Guilford Press, 1983.
26. Keeney B: *The Aesthetics of Change* New York: Guilford Press, 1983.
27. Balint M: *The Doctor, His Patient & His Illness*. New York: International Press, 1957.
28. Botelho R, McDaniel SH, & Jones JE: A family systems approach to a Balint-style group: a report on a CME demonstration project for primary care physicians. *Fam Med* 1990;**22**:4:293–295.
29. McDaniel SH, Hepworth J, & Doherty WJ: *The Shared Experience of Illness: Stories of Patients, Families & their Therapists*. New York, Basic Books, 1997.
30. Doherty WJ, Baird MA: Developmental levels in family-centered medical care. *Fam Med* 1986;**18**(3):153–156.

Protocol: Basic Premises of Family-Oriented Primary Care

We define *family* as any group of people related either biologically, emotionally, or legally. Although involvement of nonhousehold family members can be important to a patient's healthcare, the household is more often than not the primary focus of the family-oriented clinician's care.

1. Family-oriented healthcare is conceptualized within a biopsychosocial framework.
2. The primary focus of healthcare is the patient in the context of the family:
   a. The family is the primary source of many health beliefs and behaviors.
   b. The stress of family developmental transitions may become manifest in physical symptoms.
   c. Somatic symptoms can serve an adaptive function within the family and be maintained by family patterns.
   d. Families are a valuable resource and source of support for the management of illness.
3. The patient, family, and clinician are partners in medical care.
4. The clinician is part of the treatment system.

2
How Families Affect Illness: Research on the Family's Influence on Health

Clinical experience holds that families influence and are influenced by the health of their members, and that family-oriented primary care can lead to improved health for both the individual and the family as a whole. Assumptions and experiences that point toward a new approach to medical care, however, should be scientifically validated through empirical research (i.e., they should be evidence-based). This chapter will examine some important lines of research on families and health, especially the family's impact on physical health. There is now a body of well-designed studies and randomized controlled trials that demonstrate that family interventions can improve health outcomes (1). This research supports the contention that a partnership between physician, patient, and family may provide the most effective and efficient form of medical care. The clinical implications of this research are presented in the Protocol section of the chapter.

The Family Health and Illness Cycle

The family health and illness cycle developed by Doherty and Campbell can help organize research on families and health because it provides a sequence of families' experiences with health and illness (2) (See Fig. 2.1). The two-way arrows between the family and the healthcare system emphasize the importance of families' ongoing interactions with healthcare professionals. Starting at the top of the cycle with health promotion and risk reduction, research in each of the six categories will be reviewed.

Family Health Promotion and Risk Reduction

Much of the current suffering and mortality from physical illness now results from chronic, degenerative diseases that result from our own unhealthy behaviors. For example, cardiovascular disease and cancer, which currently account for 75% of all deaths in the United States, are largely the result of unhealthy lifestyles (3). As a result, the Federal government has

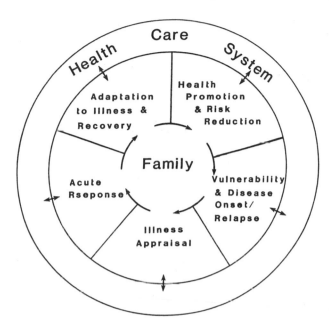

FIGURE 2.1. Family health and illness cycle.

initiated a major program entitled "Healthy People 2000" to help promote health and reduce health risks (4).

The World Health Organization has characterized the family as the "primary social agent in the promotion of health and well being" (5). A healthy lifestyle is usually developed, maintained, or changed within the family setting. Behavioral health-risk factors cluster within families because family members tend to share similar diets, physical activities, and use of substances (e.g., tobacco, alcohol, and illicit drugs) (2). Parents' health-related behaviors strongly influence whether a child or adolescent will adopt a healthy behavior, and family support is an important determinant of an individual's ability to change an unhealthy lifestyle. In a 1985 Gallup survey of health related behaviors, more than 1000 adults reported that the spouse or significant other was more likely to influence a person's health habits than anyone else, including the family doctor.

Almost every important health behavior is a family activity or is strongly influenced by the family. An emphasis on physical activity and fitness is usually a shared family value. Parents' exercise habits and attitudes have a strong influence on their children's level of physical activity (6). Individuals with or at high risk for cardiac disease are more likely to participate in a cardiac rehabilitation or exercise program if their spouses are supportive or attend with them (7).

Smoking remains the number one health problem in the United States today. Like other health behaviors, the initiation, maintenance, and cessation of smoking is strongly influenced by the family. A teenager who has a parent and older sibling who smokes is five times more likely to smoke than a teenager from a nonsmoking family. Smokers are much more likely to marry other smokers, to smoke the same number of cigarettes as do their spouses, and to quit at the same time (8). Although some of this is explained by assortative mating (smokers marry smokers), studies also show smoking behaviors of spouses become more similar with longer marriages, suggesting that spouses have a strong influence on each other's smoking behavior.

The spouse also plays an important role in smoking cessation. Smokers who are married to nonsmokers or ex-smokers are more likely to quit and to remain abstinent than are smokers who are married to smokers. Supportive behaviors involving cooperative participation (e.g., talking the smoker out of smoking a cigarette) and reinforcement (e.g., expressing pleasure at the smoker's efforts to quit) predict successful quitting. Negative behaviors (e.g., nagging the smoker and complaining about the smoking) predict relapse (9). Randomized trials of partner support in smoking cessation, however, have not been able to improve long-term abstinence rates, in part because they have failed to consider the marital dynamics involved in addiction (1).

Nutrition is an obvious family activity. Family members usually share the same diet and ingest similar amounts of salt, calories, cholesterol, and saturated fats (10). Eating behaviors and obesity can play important homeostatic functions within families, and the family plays an important role in the development and treatment of the major eating disorders (i.e., anorexia nervosa and bulimia). Parents often use food as a reward or punishment for their children. Parents' encouragement of children to eat has been shown to correlate with childhood obesity (11).

Dietary interventions directed at an individual in the family often influence the nutrition of other family members. School-based child nutrition programs have resulted in improvements in the parent's diet, and the wives of men in cardiac risk reduction programs tend to improve their nutrition as well. Several family focused cardiac risk factor trials have resulted in healthier lifestyles across the entire family (12–14).

In the treatment of obesity, spousal support has been shown to predict successful weight loss, whereas criticism and nagging are associated with poor outcomes. Several randomized controlled trials have shown how the involvement of the spouse significantly improves long-term weight loss.

This research demonstrates that families influence most health-related behaviors and suggests that interventions involving the family are effective and efficient. This research should encourage clinicians to move beyond thinking just about healthy individuals, to promoting healthy families, and directing our prevention efforts at families as well as individuals.

Vulnerability and Disease Onset/Relapse

There is now ample evidence that psychosocial factors can affect an individual's susceptibility to disease, whether it is the common cold or cancer. Studies of stress and social support have shown the most convincing evidence that the family is often the most important source of stress or support and has a potent influence on health.

One successful method for studying stress and its impact on health has been to examine the relationship of stressful life events to illness. Many retrospective and prospective studies have used the Holmes and Rahe scale to demonstrate that stressful life events precedes the development of a wide range of different diseases (15).

Most of the events on the Holmes and Rahe scale occur within the family, and 10 of the 15 most stressful events are family events. Because children are likely to be affected by family stress, a number of studies have looked at the relationship of family life events and child health. In an early study, Meyer and Haggerty (16) found that chronic stress was associated with higher rates of streptococcal pharyngitis, and that 30% of the strep infections were preceded by a stressful family event. Children in a day care setting who experienced more stressful life events had longer but not more frequent episodes of respiratory illness (17). A prospective study of more than 1000 preschoolers found that family life events were strongly correlated with subsequent visits to the physician and hospital admissions for a wide range of conditions. Children from families with more than 12 life events during the 4-year study period were six times more likely to be hospitalized (18).

The death of a spouse is the most stressful common life event, and the health consequences of bereavement have been extensively studied. Large, well-controlled epidemiological studies have confirmed that the death of a spouse is associated with an increased mortality in the surviving spouse, especially within the first 6 months (19). The effect is greater on surviving men than women, probably because women usually have better social networks and supports.

Divorce or marital separation is also an extremely stressful event, and is ranked second on the Holmes and Rahe scale. Cross-sectional studies reveal that divorcees have a higher death rate from all diseases than do single, widowed, or married persons (20). Chronic physical illness, however, can have an adverse effect on marital satisfaction and may eventually lead to divorce. Prospective studies of divorce and health are needed to understand these relationships.

Research in psychoimmunology has demonstrated that stress can lead to immunosuppression and an increase in illness (21). Two well-controlled studies demonstrated a decrease in cellular immunity (T-lymphocyte stimulation) during bereavement (22, 23). Divorced or separated women have significantly poorer immune function than sociodemographically matched married women (24). Among the married women, poor marital quality correlated with both depression and decreased immunity. Immune function is also impaired in major depression, and researchers have suggested that changes occurring in the central nervous system during depression may be a final common pathway.

Although family stress can have harmful effects on health, family support can be beneficial. An extensive body of research has demonstrated that social networks and supports can directly improve health, as well as buffer the adverse effects of stress. Furthermore, the family has been found to be the most important source of social support.

Several large epidemiological studies have demonstrated that social isolation is highly predictive of mortality and that family support, particularly marriage and contact with relatives, is protective. In an article in the journal *Science*, sociologist James House (25) reviewed the research on social support and health and concluded:

> The evidence regarding social relationships and health increasingly approximates the evidence in the 1964 surgeon general's report that established cigarette smoking as a cause or risk factor for mortality and morbidity from a range of diseases. The age-adjusted relative risk ratios are stronger than the relative risks for all causes of mortality reported for cigarette smoking.

The relative importance of different aspects of family support may change over the lifespan. Elderly persons with impaired social supports have two- to threefold the death rate of those with good supports (26, 27), but widowhood is not associated with mortality. The presence and number of living children are the most powerful predictors of survival in the elderly. This finding suggests that adult children become the most important source of social support in older populations.

Family support and family stress, especially bereavement, can have a powerful influence on health and mortality. An understanding of the family and potential sources of stress and support can provide health care professionals with ways to reduce family stress, bolster family supports, and improve health.

Family Illness Appraisal

Most individuals who experience physical symptoms never consult health professionals, but handle these problems at home with family and friends. It is estimated that only 10–30% of all health problems are brought to professional attention. Little is known about what factors influence whether an individual consults a physician or other health professional under these circumstances. Most research in this area has focused exclusively on such individual factors as the severity of the symptoms, individual's health beliefs, and access to health care services. There is considerable evidence, however, that health-care utilization and health appraisal is influenced by family factors and that there are distinct family patterns of healthcare utilization.

When an individual develops symptoms, he or she usually discusses the problem with those closest to that individual (i.e., other family members). The decision-making process may involve the entire family and be affected by the family's history with other health problems. One study of middle age couples found that when a decision was made to consult a physician about a symptom, it was usually initiated by the spouse. If the decision was made to wait or delay medical consultation, it was usually the symptomatic person who made the decision, sometimes against the spouse's advice or wishes. Prior experiences with similar symptoms often influenced the decision making (28).

Older couples are often more dependent upon each other and seem to have different patterns of decision making. One study found that elderly couples made their health-care decisions jointly, but that the wife usually had a more influential voice in the final decision. This is consistent with the concept that many families have a "family health expert" (29) who has been assigned and assumes the role as the expert in health matters. This role is traditionally played by a woman, often the wife or mother, but it can also be assumed by family members who are health professionals.

The appraisal of a child's symptom and decision to consult a physician is strongly influenced by the parents' health beliefs and levels of stress. A child may serve as a surrogate patient who directly or indirectly expresses the stress and dysfunction within the family. A study of 500 families (30) found that family stress dramatically increased utilization of health services, and that there was no evidence of any physical symptoms in one third of visits. Others have found that a family history of a similar symptom or problem was the strongest predictor of healthcare treatment for children's symptoms.

Families often have distinct patterns of healthcare behavior and utilization. Several studies have shown a strong association among families in their use of medication and health-care services. For example, mother's health-care utilization is a better predictor of the number of medical visits by the child than the child's own health status (31). An individual's use of medications is more strongly related to other family members' medication use than the individual's severity of symptoms or illness. Because many of the barriers to health-care access (e.g., lack of health insurance, money, transportation, or identified source of healthcare) are usually shared by family members, efforts to improve access to healthcare are likely to be more effective and cost efficient if they are directed at families versus individuals.

This research documents the important role of the family in healthcare decision making. It highlights the need for clinicians to inquire about other family members' concerns or opinions about the presenting symptoms. Learning more about the family decision-making process will help the clinician to understand better the reason for the patient's visit and underlying fears or concerns of the patient and family.

Family's Acute Response to Illness

The diagnosis of a serious or life-threatening illness is one of the most feared threats to family life. Illness in the family ranks near the top of the Holmes and Rahe's Stressful Life Events Scale (15). Many family members can remember the moment that they learned of a serious illness in their family.

A family's initial response to the diagnosis of a serious illness often follows a predictable course. There may be a period of denial or disbelief about the diagnosis, followed by a rapid mobilization of resources and support within the family. During this crisis phase, most families pull together and rally around the patient, even when there is a history of major conflicts, separation, or disengagement.

Most research on the spouses of acutely ill patients have shown that they experience as high or higher levels of stress and anxiety than the patients (32). This effect is strongest for the wives of male patients. Some men recovering from a myocardial infarction (MI) may seem relatively unconcerned, whereas their wives are extremely anxious. Many male cardiac patients report feeling overprotected by their wives, and some studies suggest that this interaction predicts poor functional outcomes. A large body of research, largely from the nursing field, has demonstrated that the family's greatest need during this acute period is for information about the patient's health problems. Family members often report feeling left out and uninformed. Providing information to family members helps to reduce their anxiety and feelings of helplessness. One study of post-MI couples found that the best predictor of the patient's recovery was whether the wife was provided with information at the time of discharge (33).

Many hospitals still allow only limited family contact with seriously ill patients, often for 5–10 minutes every hour in intensive care units (ICUs). These policies are based on the unproved belief that family members will either interfere with ongoing medical treatments or tire the patient. Studies have shown that even the presence of a loved one can have beneficial physiologic effects, especially in the ICU (34). There is some evidence that more collaborative, family-centered inpatient programs speed up the patient's recovery, reduce hospital stays, and improve patient and family satisfaction. Some hospitals [e.g., the New York University (NYU) Cooperative Care Program] have developed innovative programs that allow family members to remain with the patient throughout the hospitalization and provide physical care and emotional support (35).

Research on the family's response to the acute phase of illness suggests that providing medical information to the family (Level 2—see Chap. 3) may be the most beneficial level of involvement by healthcare providers. If the illness progresses to a chronic phase, families may experience more difficulties and need more intensive involvement (Level 3 or 4).

Family Adaptation to Illness and Recovery

Families, not healthcare providers, are the primary caretakers for patients with chronic illness. They are the ones who help most with the physical demands of an illness, including the preparation of special meals, administering medication, and helping with bathing and dressing. In addition, families are usually the major source of emotional and social support: someone to share the frustrations, discouragement, and despair of living with chronic illness.

A substantial amount of research has addressed family caregiving and the impact of chronic disease on the family. Chronic illness affects all aspects of family life. Old and familiar patterns of family life are changed forever, shared activities are given up, and family roles and responsibilities must often change. Most patients and their families cope well with the stresses and demands of chronic illness, and tend to pull together and become closer. Some families may become too close or enmeshed; by assuming too much responsibility and care for the ill member, they may inhibit his or her autonomy and independence. Other families may come apart under the stress of chronic illness, and separate or divorce.

The quality of family life and functioning has a strong impact on how well the patient copes with the illness and on long-term health outcomes. The impact of the family on chronic illness has been best studied in children. Adequate control of diabetes and asthma is strongly correlated with healthy family functioning (2). Chronic family conflict, parental indifference, and low cohesion have all been associated with poor metabolic control in diabetes, whereas clear family organization and high parental self-esteem correlate with good control (1).

In a series of seminal studies, Salvador Minuchin and his colleagues at the Philadelphia Child Guidance Clinic (36, 37) studied poorly controlled diabetic children and their families. These children had recurrent episodes of diabetic ketoacidosis, but when hospitalized, their diabetes was easily managed. It appeared that stress and emotional arousal within the family directly affected the child's blood sugar. In these families, Minuchin discovered a specific pattern of interaction, characterized by enmeshment (high cohesion), overprotectiveness, rigidity, and conflict avoidance. He called these families "psychosomatic families."

To determine how these family patterns can affect diabetes, Minuchin (37) studied the physiologic responses of diabetic children to a stressful family interview. During the family interview, the children from psychosomatic families had a rapid rise in free fatty acids (FFA) (a precursor to diabetic ketoacidosis) that persisted beyond the interview. The parents of these children exhibited an initial rise in FFA levels, which fell to normal when the diabetic child entered the room. Minuchin hypothesized that parental conflict is detoured or defused through the chronically ill child in psychosomatic families, and the resulting stress leads to exacerbation of the illness. Minuchin was the first investigator to demonstrate a link between family and physiologic processes.

In general, the family can influence a disease process by one of two pathways. As Minuchin demonstrated, the family can have direct psychophysiologic effects, or they can influence health-related behaviors (e.g., compliance with medical treatments). In diabetes, it appears that both pathways are important. In emotionally distant or disengaged families, inadequate supervision and parental support can lead to noncompliance with treatment and poor diabetic control. In enmeshed families, family conflict may lead to emotional arousal and hormonal changes that disrupt diabetic control.

Several different family interventions have been shown to have a beneficial effect on childhood illness outcomes. Minuchin and his colleagues (36) successfully treated psychosomatic families using structural family therapy to help disengage the diabetic and establish more appropriate family boundaries. In 15 cases, the pattern of recurrent ketoacidosis ceased and insulin doses were reduced. He reported similar success with asthma and anorexia nervosa occurring in psychosomatic families.

Two randomized controlled trials of family therapy in severe childhood asthma have reported improved health outcomes (38, 39). The therapy was designed to change the family's strong emotional response to the child's symptoms. The children who received family therapy had reduced symptoms, medication use, and school absences. Their lung function improved as well.

The most successful and widely used family interventions for chronic illnesses have been family psychoeducation programs. Family psychoeducation provides information, support, and problem-solving skills to help families cope with a chronic illness. Unlike traditional family therapy, the focus of family psychoeducation is on the illness rather than on the family. Family dysfunction is generally viewed as inadequate coping with the illness. Family psychoeducation has been shown to improve outcomes in childhood diabetes, asthma, recurrent abdominal pain, and developmental disabilities (1), and is one of the most promising areas for family interventions.

Two different types of family interventions have been effective in the treatment of hypertension. Couples-communication training can lower blood pressure in couples where one member has hypertension (40). In one large study, providing family support to assist with compliance with blood pressure medication resulted in improved compliance, reduced blood pressure, and a 50% reduction in cardiac mortality (41). Based upon this and similar compliance research, the National Heart, Lung, and Blood Institute (42) recommends that to increase compliance with antihypertensive regimens, physicians should enhance support from family members by identifying and involving one influential person, preferably someone living with the patient, who can provide encouragement, help support the behavior change, and, if necessary, remind the patient about the specifics of the regimen.

With the aging of the population, an increasing number of elderly must rely on family members for care. Most elderly people with Alzheimer's Disease or some other incapacitating illnesses are cared for at home by adult children and are never institutionalized. Family caregivers experience a tremendous burden and strain in caring for their impaired elders. These caregivers, usually spouses or children, suffer poorer physical and emotional health and have high rates of anxiety and depression (43). Several family psychoeducational programs for caregivers have reduced caregivers' distress and depression, improved caregivers' physical health, and have reduced or delayed nursing home admissions (1, 43). These interventions appear to be very cost effective.

Conclusion

Research on families and health demonstrates the powerful influence of the family on health and illness and the benefits of family interventions. It supports the importance of a family-oriented approach to clinical practice; however, we are just beginning to understand the relationship between families and health, and much more research is needed. Effective family interventions for a wide range of illnesses need to be developed and tested. Studies of the process of family-oriented medical care are also needed and should include research on different methods of family assessment and the impact of family conferences on patient and family satisfaction and health outcomes.

References

1. Campbell TL, Patterson JM: The effectiveness of family interventions in the treatment of physical illness. *J Marital Fam Ther* 1995;**21**:545–584.
2. Doherty WA, Campbell TL: *Families and Health*. Beverly Hill, CA: Sage, 1988.
3. McGinnis JM, Foege WH: Actual causes of death in the United States [see comments]. *JAMA* 1993;**270**:2207–2212.
4. Posner BM, Cupples LA, Gagnon D, Wilson PW, Chetwynd K, & Felix D: Healthy people 2000. The rationale and potential efficacy of preventive nutrition in heart disease: the Framingham offspring-spouse study. *Arch Intern Med* 1993;**153**:1549–1556.
5. World Health Organization: Statistical Indices of Family Health 1991;**589**:17.
6. Sallis JF, Nader PR: Family determinants of health behaviors. In: Gochman DS (Ed). *Health Behavior*. New York: Plenum Publishing, 1988.

7. Heinzelmann F, Bagley RW: Response to physical activity programs and their effects on health behavior. *Publ Health Rep* 1970;**85**:905–911.

8. Venters MH, Jacobs DR, Jr, Luepker RV, Maiman LA, & Gillum RF: Spouse concordance of smoking patterns: the Minnesota Heart survey. *Am J Epidemiol* 1984;**120**:608–616.

9. Coppotelli HC, Orleans CT: Partner support and other determinants of smoking cessation maintenance among women. *J Consult Clin Psychol* 1985;**53**:455–460.

10. Venters MH: Family life and cardiovascular risk: implications for the prevention of chronic disease. *Soc Sci Med* 1986;**22**:1076–1074.

11. Klesges RC, Coates TJ, Brown G, Sturgeon-Tillisch J, Moldenhauer-Klesges LM, Holzer B, et al.: Parental influences on children's eating behavior and relative weight. *J Appl Behav Anal* 1983;**16**:371–378.

12. Mitchell BD, Kammerer CM, Blangero J, Mahaney MC, Rainwater DL, Dyke B, et al.: Genetic and environmental contributions to cardiovascular risk factors in Mexican Americans. The San Antonio Family Heart Study. *Circulation* 1996; **94**:2159–2170.

13. Hollis JF, Sexton G, Connor SL, Calvin L, Pereira C, & Matarazzo JD: The family heart dietary intervention program: community response and characteristics of joining and nonjoining families. *Prevent Med* 1984;**13**:276–285.

14. Anonymous: Randomised controlled trial evaluating cardiovascular screening and intervention in general practice: principal results of British family heart study. Family Heart Study Group [see comments]. *Br Med J* 1994;**308**:313–320.

15. Holmes TH, Rahe RH: The social readjustment rating scale. *J Psychosom Res* 1967;**11**:213–218.

16. Meyer RJ, Haggerty RJ: Streptococcal infections in families: factors altering individual susceptibility. *Pediatrics* 1962;**29**:539–549.

17. Boyce WT, Chesterman E: Life events, social support, and cardiovascular reactivity in adolescence. *J Devel Behav Pediatr* 1990;**11**:105–111.

18. Beautrais AL, Fergusson DM, & Shannon FT: Life events and childhood morbidity: a prospective study. *Pediatrics* 1982;**70**:935–940.

19. Martikainen P, Valkonen T: Mortality after death of spouse in relation to duration of bereavement in Finland. *J Epidemiol Comm Health* 1996;**50**:264–268.

20. Burman B, Margolin G: Analysis of the association between marital relationships and health problems: an interactional perspective. *Psychol Bull* 1992; **112**:39–63.

21. Calabrese JR, Kling MA, & Gold PW: Alterations in immunocompetence during stress, bereavement, and depression: focus on neuroendocrine regulation. *Am J Psychiatr* 1987;**144**:1123–1134.

22. Bartrop RW, Luckhurst E, Lazarus L, Kiloh LG, & Penny R: Depressed lymphocyte function after bereavement. *Lancet* 1977;**1**:834–836.

23. Schleifer SJ, Keller SE, Bond RN, Cohen J, & Stein M: Major depressive disorder and immunity. Role of age, sex, severity, and hospitalization. *Arch Gen Psychiatr* 1989;**46**:81–87.

24. Kiecolt-Glaser JK, Fisher LD, Ogrocki P, Stout JC, Speicher CE, & Glaser R: Marital quality, marital disruption, and immune function. *Psychosom Med* 1987; **49**:13–34.

25. House JS, Landis KR, & Umberson D: Social relationships and health. *Science* 1988;**241**:540–545.

26. Blazer D, Burchett B, Service C, & George LK: The association of age and depression among the elderly: an epidemiologic exploration. *J Gerontol* 1991; **46**:M210–M215.

27. Zuckerman DM, Kasl SV, & Ostfeld AM: Psychosocial predictors of mortality among the elderly poor. The role of religion, well-being, and social contacts. *Am J Epidemiol* 1984;**119**:410–423.

28. Dowds BN, Bibace R: Entry into the health care system: the family's decision-making process. *Fam Med* 1996;**28**:114–118.

29. Doherty WJ, Baird MA: *Family Therapy and Family Medicine: Toward the Primary Care of Families*. New York: Guilford Press, 1983.

30. Roghmann KJ, Haggerty RJ: Daily stress, illness, and use of health service in young families. *Pediatr Res* 1973;**7**:520–526.

31. Newacheck PW, Halfon N: The association between mother's and children's use of physician services. *Med Care* 1986;**24**:30–38.

32. Oberst MT, James RH: Going home: patient and spouse adjustment following cancer surgery. *Top Clin Nursing* 1985;**7**:46–57.

33. Fiske V, Coyne J, & Smith D: Couples coping with myocardial infarction: an empirical reconsideration of the role of overprotectiveness. *J Fam Psychol.*

34. Lynch JJ: *The Broken Heart*. Baltimore: Bancroft Press, 1998.

35. Grieco AJ, Garnett SA, Glassman KS, Valoon PL, & McClure ML: New York University Medical Center's Cooperative Care Unit: patient education and family participation during hospitalization—the first ten years. *Pat Ed Counsel* 1990;**15**:3–15.

36. Minuchin S, Baker L, Rosman BL, Liebman R, Milman L, & Todd TC: A conceptual model of psychosomatic illness in children. Family organization and family therapy. *Arch Gen Psychiatr* 1975;**32**:1031–1038.

37. Minuchin S, Rosman BL, & Baker L: *Psychosomatic Families: Anorexia Nervosa in Context*. Cambridge, MA: Harvard University Press, 1978.

38. Gustafsson PA, Kjellman NI, & Cederblad M: Family therapy in the treatment of severe childhood asthma. *J Psychosom Res* 1986;**30**:369–374.

39. Lask B, Matthew D: Childhood asthma. A controlled trial of family psychotherapy. *Arch Dis Childhood* 1979;**54**:116–119.

40. Ewart CK, Burnett KF, & Taylor CB: Communication behaviors that affect blood pressure. An A-B-A-B analysis of marital interaction. *Behav Mod* 1983; **7**:331–344.

41. Morisky DE, Levine DM, Green LW, Shapiro S, Russell RP, & Smith CR: Five-year blood pressure control and mortality following health education for hypertensive patients. *Am J Pub Health* 1983;**73**:153–162.

42. National Heart LaBI. Management of patient compliance in the treatment of hypertension. *Hypertension* 1982;4:415–423.

43. Biegel DE, Sales E, & Schulz R: *Family Caregiving in Chronic Illness*. Newbury Park, CA: Sage, 1991.

3
Family Systems Concepts: Tools for Assessing Families in Primary Care

The book title, *Every Person's Life is Worth a Novel*, is also a clinical truism. Each person lives among an exciting cast of characters who inspire them, support them, and also criticize and fight with them. To know a person is to know the people in their lives. Imagine the difficulties of setting up a discharge plan without knowing whether families can carry out the needed tasks. A clinician who knows who the players are, and how they function together, has a far easier time of negotiating their patient's care. Knowledge of patients and their families is not just good public relations, it is an efficient and responsible way to provide health care.

Most of us get our ideas about "proper" family functioning from our own families. Our families of origin serve as the yardstick by which we compare other families, expecting them to "measure up" or function better than what we experienced. We also have ideas about family functioning based on television shows, movies, or novels we admire. All of these assumptions and emotions come with us when we meet families professionally, requiring us to monitor our personal and cultural biases as we consider a family's response to an illness or new challenge.

Family assessment begins with the first visit and is a continuous process. As in any medical assessment, clinicians can assess the "anatomy," the development, and the functioning of a family. The anatomy of a family is the membership, which is easily obtained through a genogram. Family development is noted by the family member's ages and developmental stages, and functioning is assessed through history and observation of family process. Even at routine appointments, one notices whether a parent or spouse is comforting to the patient, and whether family members seem to be supportive of one another. Over time and with more complicated medical problems, patients inevitably describe their family functioning as they discuss stresses and coping strategies. At critical junctures, these impressions may lead to a family conference (see Chap. 5) to assess a situation in greater depth (1, 2).

The Genogram (Family Anatomy)

The family genogram (family anatomy) is an essential tool for busy practitioners to recall information about family member's names, relationships, and overall structure (3–5). A visual map of connections among family members, the genogram extends the geneticists' pedigree to indicate the quality of those relationships.

A basic genogram can be completed when initial family history is obtained, and it can be updated at subsequent visits (see Appendix 3.1 for a summary of standard genogram symbols). Genograms can have a biomedical focus, as a way of organizing family medical and genetic information, and still set a biopsychosocial tone to the encounter and the overall practice. For established patients, a physician might explain that "I reviewed your chart, and want to fill in some details about your background." Patients generally appreciate the clinician's interest, and usually expect to provide this information.

Genogram information should include names, ages, marital status, former marriages, children, households, significant illnesses, dates of such traumatic events as deaths, and occupations. It can also include emotional closeness, distance, or conflict between members, significant relationships with other professionals, and other relevant information. Genogram construction may reveal transgenerational family patterns of loss, dysfunctional emotional patterns, or common medical problems. A quick glance at the genogram prior to a visit is a reminder of names and family relationships.

The Family Life Cycle

The family life cycle (family development) provides a template to quickly assess a patient and family's developmental concerns. Developed by family sociologists Hill (6) and Duvall (7), the family life cycle identifies stages of family development that reflect the biological functions of raising children. Multiple family forms, and ethnic and cultural variations in family development, result in no single "normal" family life cycle, but all families with children go through predictable periods of forming adult relationships, bearing and raising young children, and launching children to begin the cycle anew.

The family life cycle, described by family therapists Carter and McGoldrick (8), is useful for primary care. This adaptation begins with young adults leaving home and includes those who choose to marry, or live together in heterosexual or same-sex relationships, and those who may adopt or postpone childbearing. The developmental tasks of raising an infant are somewhat independent of the couples' ages, gender, or social class, and a clinician can easily ask any couple with young children about the stresses of balancing couple relationships with child care responsibilities. Additional stages of the changing family life cycle include families with adolescents, launching children, and families in later life. General tasks for families at these stages are described in Table 3.1 and are expanded throughout this book.

As a family system moves together through time, parents become grandparents, and are still part of an extended relational system. The individual life cycles of each family member intertwines with the life cycles of other family members, represented by the Family Life Spiral (9) (see Fig. 3.1). This representation of the connections among generations depicts the oscillation of the family system from developmental periods of family closeness, based on the care of young children or elder relatives, to periods of relative distance, reflecting greater independence of individuals within the system. Combrinck-Graham describes these shifting periods as *centripetal*, indicating forces that pull the family together, or *centrifugal*, reflecting the forces that pull family members more apart from one another. When illness occurs during a centripetal period, like infancy, the family may be more easily mobilized to care for the ill member than it is during a centrifugal period like adolescence, when the individuals are moving toward increased independence from one another. Parents of teenagers with diabetes, for example, are notorious for having difficulty helping their children balance their need for autonomy with the demands of the illness.

Family Assessment

Family assessment is a continuous activity based on theoretical concepts and tools that easily can be integrated into daily practice. Doherty and Baird (1) first described primary care family assessment in their landmark volume, *Family Therapy and Family Medicine*, in 1983. Based on the long history of family assessment in family therapy and family sociology, they suggested that there are no simple tests for family functioning that lead to clear treatment decisions. Most valid instruments, used for research or family therapy interventions, are too lengthy or require extensive coding. Although some primary care clinicians have developed screening instruments and assessment methods useful in primary care, we concur that no single test can replace a practitioner's thoughtful gathering of information about a family over time.

Some practitioners may choose to use brief assessment tools in comprehensive health assessments, as part of regular patient interviews, or as screening instruments. The Family APGAR (10), a five-item questionnaire, assesses patient satisfaction with family support, communication, and sharing of activities. The Family Circle (11), is a technique in which patients draw circles to identify the important people and contexts in their lives. PRACTICE (2) is an acronym to guide interviews of patients or families. PRACTICE stands for Presenting problem, Roles, Affect, Communication

TABLE 3.1. The stages of the family life cycle

Family life cycle stage	Emotional process of transition: Key principles	Second-order changes in family status required to proceed developmentally
1. Leaving home: Single young adults	Accepting emotional and financial responsibility for self	a. Differentiation of self in relation to family of origin b. Development of intimate peer relationships c. Establishment of self re work and financial independence
2. The joining of families through marriage: The new couple	Commitment to new system	a. Formation of marital system b. Realignment of relationships with extended families and friends to include spouse
3. Families with young children	Accepting new members into the system	a. Adjusting marital system to make space for child(ren) b. Joining in childrearing, financial, and household tasks c. Realignment of relationships with extended family to include parenting and grandparenting roles
4. Families with adolescents	Increasing flexibility of family boundaries to include children's independence and grandparents' frailties	a. Shifting of parent child relationships to permit adolescent to move in and out of system b. Refocus on midlife marital and career issues c. Beginning shift toward joint caring for older generation
5. Launching children and moving on	Accepting a multitude of exits from and entries into the family system	a. Renegotiation of marital system as a dyad b. Development of adult to adult relationships between grown children and their parents. c. Realignment of relationships to include in-laws and grandchildren d. Dealing with disabilities and death of parents (grandparents)
6. Families in later life	Accepting the shifting of generational roles	a. Maintaining own and/or couple functioning and interests in face of physiological decline; exploration of new familial and social role options b. Support for a more central role of middle generation. c. Making room in the system for the wisdom and experience of the elderly, supporting the older generation without overfunctioning for them d. Dealing with loss of spouse, siblings, and other peers and preparation for own death. Life review and integration

Source: Carter B, McGoldrick M, 1989. Reprinted with permission.

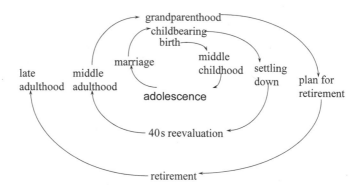

FIGURE 3.1. Family life spiral. (From Combrinck-Graham L, 1985. Reprinted with permission.)

patterns, Time in family life cycle, Illness history, Coping with stress, and Ecology and culture. The form, which is also identified as the McGill Family Assessment Tool, is fairly lengthy for standard screening use, but identifies concepts useful for interviewers. These questions and measures provide opportunities for patients to tell their physicians about the support and stress they receive in their daily interactions that may affect their health.

Family Systems Concepts in Primary Care

This section describes family systems concepts used throughout this book. Our general definition of families, as a group of people related by blood or choice who move together through time, allows for a range of intimate family structures we see. Following discussion of each family systems concept are examples of questions that will enhance the family-oriented care of any patient.

Family Characteristics

The Family as a System

Systems theory teaches that the human body is more than organ systems operating next to one another. Attention to the relationships among those organ systems is one difference between primary and specialty care. The family system is similarly also more than just the sum of its individual members. Family groups have unique characteristics, and are organized by interpersonal structures and processes that enable them to be both stable and adaptable over time.

- Who are the members of your family?
- When it comes to daily support, who do you consider as family?

Family Stability

Family stability, or homeostasis, is the interpersonal process by which the family strives to maintain emotional balance in the system (e.g., a grandmother, who picks up parenting duties to help a significantly disabled mother care for her children).

- With all of the changes, how are you able to make sure that there is a good family balance so everyone feels cared for?
- If the illness progresses too quickly, what do you think might happen to your family?

Family Transition

Family transition is the interpersonal process by which the family adapts to developmental growth in members, and varying expectations and roles in the community.

- How have things changed now that your mother-in-law has moved in with you?
- How are you as a family making adjustments to Emily's starting high school?

Family World View

Based on culture (12), previous history, and individual perspectives, families have general views of themselves as either competent or ineffective, cohesive or fragmented. The family's sense of efficacy can be enhanced when they feel that they have coped with a crisis well, or when the healthcare provider recognizes their efforts and affirms their strengths.

- Do you folks generally feel that you are able to help each other out in crises?
- How has it worked when you've had to "fill in" for one another before?
- How do family members let one another know when they need help?

Relational Context of the Symptom

The presenting symptom is part of a large family and psychosocial context that can influence and be influenced by that symptom. For some acute, self-limited illnesses, a primarily biomedical intervention may be sufficient treatment for a symptom. For many medical problems, however, the relational context becomes central to treatment.

- How do Kyla's symptoms influence everyone else in the family?
- Have you noticed if there are things that you as parents do that make Marvin take more or less responsibility for his medications?

Understanding family characteristics is one of the outcomes of a comprehensive patient or family interview. In the following example, family characteristics are obtained during a medical history. Without adding much time to the interview, questions about family functioning allow a clinician to feel more comfortable with a working diagnosis.

> Mr. Purcell, a 42-year-old Jamaican factory worker, had been experiencing more frequent chest pains over the prior 2 months. Mr. Purcell had a history of chronic stable angina that had previously been well controlled with medication. Medical evaluation revealed that Mr. Purcell's blood pressure, physical exam, and electrocardiogram had not changed. Dr. M. increased Mr. Purcell's medication, ordered an exercise stress test, and scheduled him to return in 1 week.
>
> At follow up, Mr. Purcell reported that his chest pains were less frequent, but still troublesome. Dr. M. explained that the stress test was mildly abnormal, but was unchanged from his previous test, and recommended that he start taking a new medication. Mr. Purcell was agreeable to Dr. M.'s plan, but still appeared distressed. Dr. M. asked about stress in Mr. Purcell's life. She learned that Mr. Purcell's wife had started cleaning houses in the last 6 months to earn some extra income. Mr. Purcell's son, Bob, 17, a high-school senior, worked with his mother after school. Mr. Purcell seemed irritated by how busy his wife was and how little time he had with his son. Mr. Purcell felt his main support was his 21-year-old daughter, Mary, who lived and worked in a nearby town, but visited on weekends. Three months ago Mary announced she was engaged. Although Mr. Purcell liked Mary's fiancee, he felt she was making a decision to marry prematurely and was worried about her future.
>
> Dr. M. acknowledged the many changes that were occurring in the family, and how hard it is for all of us to accept change, especially when things had been going well before. Dr. M. also noted how impressed she was that members so readily helped one another. She invited the family to come in together to talk about all the changes, the stresses and excitement, and the effects on everyone, including Mr. Purcell's increasing angina.

Dr. M.'s discussion of Mr. Purcell's family helped place the *symptom in a larger relational context*. The family's emotional balance (*family stability*) had been disrupted by the numerous changes of Mrs. Purcell's new job, Bob's upcoming graduation, and Mary's engagement. Mr. Purcell was experiencing the stress of all these transitions and his symptoms may have been a signal that the family was also having difficulty navigating the changes (*family transition*). Dr. M. acknowledged the family's strengths and caring for one another (*world view*) and invited the family in to explore how the family's functioning as a whole might play a part in Mr. Purcell's symptoms and their alleviation (*family as a system*) (Fig. 3.2).

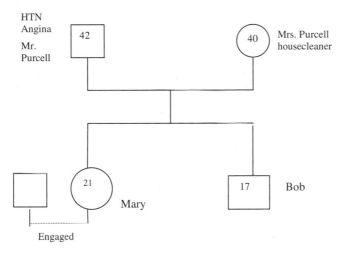

FIGURE 3.2. The Purcell family.

Family Structure

Hierarchy

Hierarchy reflects how power or authority is distributed within the family (13). General cultural consensus places parents above children in the family hierarchy. Single parents are encouraged to recognize that they have greater authority than their children, and parents, even when separated, are encouraged to share authority for decision making with each other.

- Who is overtly and covertly in charge in the family system?
- Is the family's hierarchy clear and appropriate (parents in charge of their children) or reversed (i.e., parents controlled by children)?

A *parentified child*, often the oldest, performs parental functions when one or both parents have abdicated the role (e.g., an oldest daughter does the cooking and child care because of her mother's chronic disabilities, or a son in a single-parent home feels responsible for helping his dad financially support his siblings). These roles can sometimes be functional, helping children feel responsible and competent; however, they can often lead to feelings of resentment among the individuals when parents, out of choice or necessity, continue to abdicate their roles.

- Does a child in the family function as a parent?
- Have one or both parents abdicated their role?

Boundaries

Boundaries help define different functional subgroups in the family, (e.g., the marital subgroup, the sibling subgroup, the grandparents, etc.). In respectful interactions, families recognize the boundaries around subgroups, allowing, for example, parents to have a private relationship that is not undermined by children or grandparents.

- What are the subgroups in the family?
- Are the boundaries between subgroups (i.e., parents and children) clear and appropriate, or confused and problematic?
- How does the family deal with emotional closeness and distance?

Family Role Selection

Family role selection is the conscious or unconscious assignment of complementary roles to members of a family. These roles function to maintain the family system (e.g., mother is the breadwinner and the problem solver; grandmother is the nurturer). During health crises, family members seem to adopt identifiable roles (e.g., caretaker, or the one who "can't handle bad news").

- What roles do family members play, and how do these roles relate to each other?
- Who fills the role of the family's expert on illness and health?
- Who is most often the "sick" member of the family?

A common family role is the *scapegoat* or *noble symptom bearer*, who is identified by the family as the source of problems, accepts the family's blame, and distracts from other individual or family problems, and also reflects the dysfunction of the family as a whole.

- Does the family have a scapegoat or noble symptom bearer?
- How do his or her symptoms reflect problems for the family as a whole?

Alliance

An alliance is a positive relationship between any two members of a system (e.g., a mother and father cooperating together).

- What are the important alliances in the family?
- How are alliances between family members viewed by other family members?

Coalition

A coalition is a relationship between at least three people in which two collude against a third (e.g., a parent and a child siding against another parent).

- What coalitions exist in the family?
- Who is siding against whom?

> Mr. and Mrs. Purcell, Mary, 21, and Bob, 17, came to the family meeting suggested by Dr. M. After Dr. M. shared her findings, Mary spoke first and expressed concern about her father's "long-standing" health problems. She blamed her mother for "not taking better care of him." Bob quickly defended his mother, saying she had been working very hard and had "a lot on her mind." Bob became upset with Mary for "attacking" their mother. Mrs. Purcell told Dr. M. that her husband had health complaints for as long as she had known him. Mr. Purcell then said that his chest pains were worse since the last doctor's appointment.

Dr. M. could see that the *hierarchy* within the Purcell family was reversed. Mary took charge of the family interaction (*parentified child*). She acted in a *coalition* with her father against her mother, much as Bob was in a *coalition* with Mrs. Purcell against Mary during the meeting. (These relationships can easily be noted in an evolving genogram, as in Fig. 3.3.) A good working relationship (*alliance*) did not exist between Mr. and Mrs. Purcell regarding Mr. Purcell's health. This was due in part to the confused generational *boundaries* in the family which contributed to the distance between Mr. and Mrs. Purcell. Instead of strong marital and sibling subsystems, both children

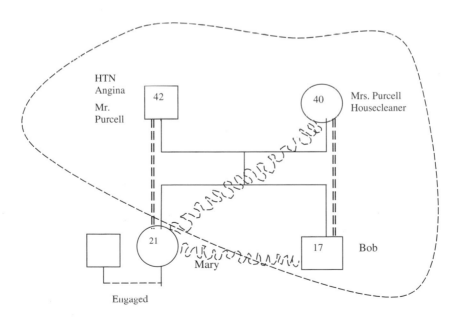

FIGURE 3.3. The Purcell family.

functioned as protectors of their parents. Mr. Purcell was the family's "sick" member; Mary acted as the expert on his health; Mrs. Purcell was cast as the uncaring spouse; and Bob was her defender (*family role selection*). Mr. Purcell drew attention away from the family's conflicts by focusing on his chest pains (*noble symptom bearer*).

Family Process

Enmeshment

Enmeshment characterizes a system in which members have few interpersonal boundaries, limited individual autonomy, and a high degree of emotional reactivity. When families are caring for young children, it is appropriate for them to be highly responsive, and to appear very enmeshed with one another. At later stages of the life cycle, enmeshment can inhibit individual development and growth (e.g., when a mother insists on remaining with her adolescent son during his physical and answers questions for him).

- Are family members involved or overinvolved with each other?
- Do family members "feel each others' feelings"?
- Do family members seldom act independently?

Disengagement

Disengagement characterizes a family system in which members are emotionally distant and unresponsive to each other (e.g., a husband who does not tell his wife or children about any of his health problems). Like enmeshment, disengagement can be viewed along a continuum, in which families with adolescents may appear to be more disengaged than do families with young children, and still be caring well for one another.

- Do family members have little emotional response to each other?
- Are family members distant or isolated from each other?
- Is the degree of emotional separation developmentally appropriate?

Triangulation

Triangulation occurs when a third person is drawn into a two-person system in order to diffuse anxiety or intimacy conflicts in the two-person system (e.g., rather than arguing with each other about personal issues, a mother and father express their marital discontent by arguing over parenting their son). This process differs from family coalitions, in which family members "side" with one another without diverting their attention to a third party.

- Do family members talk directly to each other about personal matters?

- When emotional issues arise between two members do they focus on a third person?

Family Patterns

Family patterns are the ordered sequences of interaction that typify how a family functions, particularly when under stress. In some families, when one spouse pursues, the partner withdraws. Along those lines, when father gets depressed, the family tries to cheer him up; he gets more depressed, and they become frustrated. Instead of responding to each new situation, family members make assumptions based on prior patterns, and the routine communication pattern reoccurs.

- What sequence of behaviors is typically seen when the family becomes stressed?
- Does this pattern make the situation better or worse?
- If worse, what other behaviors might interrupt the sequence or pattern?

> After commenting on his health problems, Mr. Purcell told his wife how upset he was that she had shown so little interest in their daughter's marriage. Mr. Purcell told Dr. M. he discussed his wife's apparent disinterest frequently with his daughter, who was also quite "hurt."
>
> Mr. Purcell had developed a very close relationship with his daughter (*enmeshment*), which at times substituted for the emotional support he felt was missing from his wife. Rather than discussing his own feelings of "neglect," Mr. Purcell became angry at Mrs. Purcell about her "lack of interest" in their daughter's plans to marry (*triangulation*). Dr. M. recognized that the focus of attention shifted to health issues or a third family member when family members became upset with each other (*family pattern*).

The Family Across Time

Family Developmental Stage

Based on the family life cycle, family processes and interactions vary according to whether the family has young children, or whether the household includes an older couple who are grandparents and also are caring for the wife's very elderly mother. Identifying the life cycle stage helps clinicians to tailor their family-oriented questions.

- In what developmental stage is the family?
- What are the important tasks that need to be accomplished in this stage?
- What anticipatory guidance issues are helpful for this developmental stage?
- Are the health concerns occurring when the family is experiencing centripetal or centrifugal pressures? How does this affect the ability of the family to respond to the crisis?

Family Projection Process

Family projection process is the transmission of unresolved conflicts, issues, roles, and tasks from one generation to another, (e.g., the men in each generation never go to physicians for health problems).

- What unresolved issues from past generations may be affecting the family in the present?

Intergenerational Coalition

Intergenerational coalitions involve two members from different generations against a third member of the family (e.g., a grandmother and granddaughter against a mother).

- Is there evidence of family members from two different generations colluding against a third member?

> Dr. M. commented on the many important changes that the Purcell family was facing: their son graduating, their daughter planning to marry, and the mother starting to work. Mr. and Mrs. Purcell both agreed that these changes were affecting them. They were hopeful about their children's future, but anxious, as well, about their leaving. When asked about how they saw their future, Mr. Purcell said, "the future looks bleak." He talked about how he sometimes thought of death, especially after his mother's death 5 years ago. Mrs. Purcell said her husband had never gotten over the loss and he never discussed it with her.

The Purcell family was facing the "launching children" stage in their development (*family life cycle*). Both children were leaving in the near future, one for college and one to marry. This placed increased pressure on the marital relationship as they faced an "empty nest." The anticipation of these changes or losses also reawakened Mr. Purcell's unresolved grief over his mother's death (*family projection process*). Mrs. Purcell's comments about her husband's grief and her own lack of attachment to her mother-in-law led Dr. M. to hypothesize that perhaps Mrs. Purcell had felt excluded from the close relationship between her husband and his mother (*intergenerational coalition*).

The Purcell family illustrates how family systems concepts can be used to understand the interplay between a patient's symptoms and his or her family better. Without an assessment template a family's interactions can seem confusing at best and frustrating at worst. Although not all of the concepts apply to every family, they do help clinicians organize their thinking about any family. The information gathered by assessing a family as a system, its structure, process, and development across time, can be used to ask questions and arrive at an effective treatment plan in collaboration with the patient and family.

References

1. Doherty W, Baird M: *Family Therapy and Family Medicine*. New York: Guilford Press, 1983.
2. Christie-Seeley J: *Working With the Family in Primary Care*. New York: Praeger, 1984.
3. Bowen M: Family therapy in clinical practice. New York: Jason Aronson, 1978.
4. McGoldrick M, Gerson R, & Shellenberger S: *Genograms Assessment and Intervention* (2nd Edition). New York: WW Norton, 1999.
5. Jolly W, Froom J, & Rosen M: The genogram. *J Fam Prac* 1980;**2**:251–255.
6. Hill R: *Family Development in Three Generations*. Cambridge, MA: Schenkman, 1970.
7. Duvall EM: Marriage and Family Development. Philadelphia: Lippincott, 1977.
8. Carter B, McGoldrick M: *The Changing Family Life Cycle: A Framework for Family Therapy*. Needham Heights, MA: Allyn and Bacon, 1989.
9. Combrinck-Graham L: A developmental model for family systems. *Fam Proc* 1985;**24**:139.
10. Smilkstein G: The family APGAR: a proposal for a family function test and its use by physicians. *J Fam Prac* 1978;**6**:1234.
11. Thrower SM, Bruce WE, & Welton RF: The family circle method for integrating family systems concepts in family medicine. *J Fam Prac* 1982;**15**:451.
12. McGoldrick M, Giordano J, & Pearce J: *Ethnicity and Family Therapy*. New York, Guilford Press, 1996.
13. Simon F, Stierlin H, Wynne L: *The Language of Family Therapy: A Systemic Vocabulary and Sourcebook*. New York: Family Process Press, 1985.

Appendix 3.1: Standard Symbols for Genograms

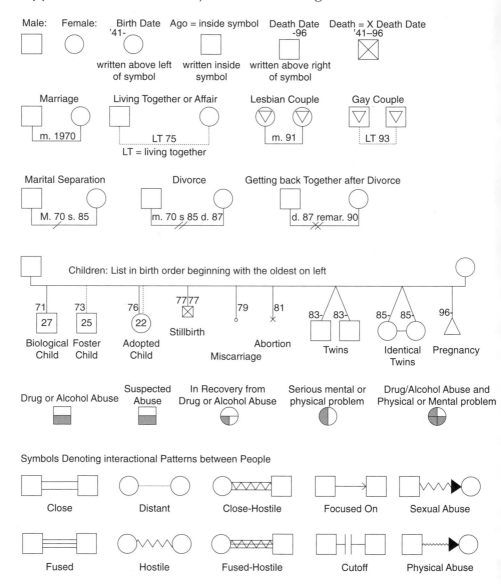

(*Source*: McGoldrick M, Gerson R, and Shellenberger S, 1999. Reprinted with permission.)

4
A Family-Oriented Approach to Individual Patients

With Kathleen Cole-Kelly* and David B. Seaburn†

Rebecca Saunders annoyed the physicians and nurse who encountered her. She stopped taking medication for her seizure disorder because of side effects. She was coming in for other medications after a seizure had landed her in the emergency department (ED). She was angry and demanding with the physicians and nurses. One physician took some time to learn more about her current family and family of origin. With a few family-oriented questions, a story emerged about Rebecca that transformed her from being a very "difficult patient" to a patient who was terrified about being abandoned by her boyfriend, John. Rebecca had recently found out that she most likely could not conceive any more children. At 34, she had a 20-year-old daughter and a 3-year-old grandchild. She had been in two abusive relationships, but now believed she had a really good relationship with her boyfriend; however, John was very clear with her: "You give me children or I'm out of here." Rebecca's family of origin history was as sad as her current situation. Once the physician understood this information about Rebecca, very different treatment priorities emerged. In addition to adjusting her medication for her seizures, a follow-up appointment was scheduled to help Rebecca sort out how to cope with this situation.

A family orientation has more to do with how one thinks about the patient than it does with how many people are in the exam room. A family-oriented approach does not always require the clinician to meet with families in their practice. In fact, most of the time primary care clinicians meet with individuals rather than with families in their clinical practice. As in the situation with Rebecca, it may be as simple as asking a few questions about the patient's family or home situation or inquiring about a family history. The physician with Rebecca brought information about other family

---

* Kathleen Cole-Kelly, MS, MSW, Professor of Family Medicine, Metrohealth Medical Center, Department of Family Medicine, Case Western Reserve School of Medicine, Cleveland, OH, USA.
† David B. Seaburn, PhD, Assistant Professor of Psychiatry, University of Rochester School of Medicine and Dentistry, Rochester, NY, USA.

members into the interview through questions. Broadening the lens to understand Rebecca's anger revealed more of a frightened, sad, and despairing patient rather than a "difficult" or "angry" patient. Once the context of her situation was understood, the picture of Rebecca softened.

In this chapter, we will present a family-oriented approach to interviewing an individual patient during routine medical visits. These visits may range from brief 15-minute visits for an acute medical problem to complete physical examinations or an inpatient evaluation. This approach offers the clinician a way to assess and understand the relational context of each patient's life. Research has demonstrated that many primary care physicians are using a family-oriented approach when seeing individuals in their practices. As part of the Direct Observation of Primary Care study, Medalie and his colleagues (1) examined the extent to which 138 community family physicians focused on the family in clinical practice. Approximately 10% of patient-care time was devoted to addressing family issues. Another family member's health problems were discussed in 18% of visits. Family histories were obtained in 51% of visits for new patients and 22% of visits with established patients; however, genograms or family trees were present in only 11% of charts. Overall, they concluded that the family is alive and well in family practice (1)."

In a qualitative study, Cole-Kelly and colleagues (2) examined how exemplary family physicians integrate a family-oriented approach into the routine care of individual patients. 19% of visits to these physicians were rated as having a high intensity of family orientation. The average length of visits was 13 minutes, with the high family-intense visits lasting a few minutes longer. The visits that were higher in family intensity had several family components that defined a family orientation. Physicians asked both global (e.g., How's everyone at home?) and focused (e.g., How's your wife doing after that bad fall?) family-oriented questions. These questions gathered information about past and present family health history, life cycle adjustment, sources of stress and support, and potential family health collaborators.

In addition to the family-oriented questions, there were some other characteristics that distinguished the high intensity of a family-oriented approach. The physicians were adept at gathering relevant family information while managing time efficiently in the visit. Physicians are often inhibited by concerns about time, driving them to pursue minimally family and other social/contextual information. The exemplars, however, seemed to manage these family-oriented questions adeptly in several ways. They would acknowledge the patient's response (e.g., "Sounds like you all have been through a lot with that recent move"), offer reassurance (e.g., "But knowing you, I am confident you can make it through this"), offer follow up (e.g., "When you come back for your follow-up appointment I'll be eager to hear more"), and then switch smoothly to another topic (e.g., "So, did you find taking the ibuprofen helped the achiness?") or another action, such as an exam or procedure (e.g., "How about if I take a look at that shoulder?").

The family-oriented exemplars were able to store family details that were routinely carried into each patient encounter and using in different ways. A frequent forum for integrating family details was using a family closing ritual.

> Dr. DeChristafaro: "Judy, you take a sticker for yourself and your brother Sammy at home"
>
> Dr. Antenucci: "Steve, I'll see you at the next baby's visit and meanwhile tell Lois hi for me."

These closing rituals solidified a sense of the physician really knowing the patient's family. In addition, to further the clinician's understanding of the patient and other benefits of gathering family, it optimized the sense of a clinician–patient–family relationship.

A risk in the family-oriented interview, with or without family members, is the potential for the clinician to get trapped or triangulated between family members. These exemplar physicians were adept at avoiding getting triangulated when dealing with multiple family members. If other family members were talked about or inquired about, it was done in a way that could not be interpreted as colluding with the patient to the detriment of the family member. Rather, family members were brought in to support or collaborate with the patient rather than to sabotage the patient or family member.

A family-oriented approach to an individual patient builds upon a patient-centered model of clinical practice(3) in which the clinician explores the patient's experience of their illness, an experience that occurs in a family or relational context. A key component of the patient-centered approach is understanding the whole person. We add to this including the patient's family and the family context of the illness. Rebecca's story is a poignant example of this. Once the physician asked Rebecca about her belief about the cause of her infertility (which was of much greater concern to her than her seizure disorder), Rebecca responded without hesitation:

> I'm sure that there are two things that have caused this. One was my getting pregnant at 14 with my daughter and the other was my first husband beat me terrible, and hit my stomach and organs a lot.

The patient's presenting complaint can be thought of as an entrance or window into understanding the patient in the context of the family. By exploring the patient's symptoms and illness, the clinician can learn more about the patient's family, their relationship to the presenting complaint, and how they can be a resource in treatment. A key is to choose appropriate questions about psychosocial and family-related issues without the patient feeling that the clinician is intruding or suggesting that the problem is "all in your head" or "all in your family." Biomedical and psychosocial questions should be integrated throughout the interview to obtain the patient's story of his or her illness. It is helpful to begin with family-oriented questions that relate to the presenting complaint, rather than leaving family and psychosocial questions to the end.

Dr. J.: Hello, Mrs. Reyes. How can I help you today?

Mrs. Reyes: I've been having these terrible headaches for the past month.

Dr. J.: Tell me more about your headaches.

Mrs. Reyes: Well, they feel like my head is being squeezed by a vise. All around the top of my head. It throbs constantly.

Dr. J.: When do you get these headaches?

Mrs. Reyes: Usually in the afternoon. They come on gradually during the day and by 5 o'clock, it's unbearable.

Dr. J.: What happens during the afternoon as these get worse?

Mrs. Reyes: Not much. I'm usually preparing dinner for my husband and daughter. My daughter gets home from school around 3 P.M.

Dr. J.: And how are things going at home?

Mrs. Reyes: Okay with my husband, but my daughter and I have been arguing a lot since she got pregnant.

Dr. J.: I see. Can you tell me more about that?

Mrs. Reyes: Well, she's been going out with this older guy for the past few months and we don't think it's a good thing. Sure enough, she goes and gets pregnant, and now wants to keep the baby. I don't want to be raising her baby. So we argue a lot.

Dr. J.: When did you learn about the pregnancy?

Mrs. Reyes: Several weeks ago.

Dr. J.: Do you think your arguments with your daughter and your concerns about her could be making your headaches worse?

Mrs. Reyes: Perhaps.

With a presenting complaint such as headache or any chronic pain, the clinician's index of suspicion regarding the potential contribution of psychosocial or family factors is high. Even when the clinical problem appears to be "purely" biomedical, learning about the family context can be important to ensure better management of the problem. In the following example, a "red flag" alerted the clinician to the possible role of a family issue in the presenting complaint.

Mr. Janis, a Hungarian-American man, brought in his 6-month-old son with a low-grade fever and upper respiratory symptoms.

Dr. C.: (after inquiring about the infant's current symptoms) I'm glad to see you, but curious how you happened to be the one to bring your child in to see me today?

Mr. Janis: You mean instead of his mother?

Dr. C.: Yes.

Mr. Janis: Well, my wife and I separated a few months ago and have been living apart. My son stays with me every other weekend.

Dr. C.: How is that going for all of you.

Mr. Janis: Not very well. We are having a lot of conflict. I'm worried that my wife is going to ask for sole custody of our son.

Dr. C.: So you want to be sure that you don't overlook any health problems.

Mr. Janis: Yes.

Dr. C.: Do you think the two of you would be able to come in together to talk about the medical care of your son?

Mr. Janis: Well, I know she is concerned about our son's health, so she might be willing to come in with me, but I'm not sure that she'd do it.

Dr. C.: I think it could be very helpful to discuss how you can continue to be co-parents, regardless of what you decide about your marriage.

Gathering family information can let the clinician know who else in the family might have had the same illness or presentation and what was done about it. Gathering this information can go beyond the basic family history and can help the clinician recognize family factors that may influence the patient's attitudes and actions regarding the illness. The family genogram (see Chap. 3) can be an easy way to organize this information. Learning about the family from the patient's perspective can help the clinician know who:

- the potential collaborators are in the family and who could sabotage the patient's adherence with a new medical regimen.
- is contributing to the patient's explanatory belief about his or her illness.
- might be rallied for support while the patient copes with a difficult medical situation.
- could be contributing stress that is playing a role in the patient's current situation.

In this chapter, we suggest five key questions that can be used in any patient interview (4). The questions bring the patient's family metaphorically into the room in a relevant and timely way. In addition to the use of the genogram, there are some additional basic family-oriented questions that can enhance care of the individual patient. These questions are designed with a 15-minute interview in mind. Any or all of them can provide information that will be useful in understanding the patient's illness experience better. We will apply these questions to clinical examples. Finally, we will propose a decision tree for what to do with family information that is gathered from the individual.

Five Family-Oriented Questions

Family History

1. Has anyone else in the family had this problem?

This question provides two important domains of information. It will reveal:

1. whether or not there is a family history of the illness.
2. how the family has responded to this problem in the past.

The treatment used in one generation, or with one member of the family, will be often guide for the patient's approach to his or her illness. For example, George Fagan was recently diagnosed with Type 2 diabetes. His clinician inquired who else in the family had diabetes and learns about how his aunt took care of her diabetes and how that seemed to work. The physician then took this history into consideration when making his or her treatment plan for George's diabetes.

Similarly, when the clinician is confused as to why Jenny Frank is so upset about her sore throat, the family-oriented question could shed important light on the intensity of her worry. Jenny relates a story of her uncle who just died of throat cancer. In response to the question, "Has anyone else in the family had this problem?" She is concerned because her uncle's problem started with similar symptoms. The clinician is much better equipped to respond to Jenny's concerns now that he knows the association she is making. Addressing and allaying Jenny's fears could reduce both her anxiety and her unnecessary return visits to either urgent care, an emergency room, or an outpatient clinic.

Explanatory Models and Health Beliefs

2. What do family members believe caused the problem and how should it be treated?

Patients often have a family explanatory model for their illness (5, 6):

> All my husband's family is blaming me for the baby having cystic fibrosis because there are a lot of people with asthma in my family. I feel so guilty about that.

Had the family clinician not inquired about the family's belief about the baby's cystic fibrosis, the mother of the new baby might have been carrying around unfounded guilt for a long time. It was only as a result of this family-oriented question that the clinician could allay her guilt and explain to the new mother that a history of asthma is unrelated and it takes genetic contributions from both sides of the family to create cystic fibrosis.

In addition to family members having explanations for causes or exacerbation of illness, they also may have beliefs about what constitutes appropriate treatment. Family members may have competing beliefs for either the cause or the cure. This can create confusion and other deleterious effects for the patient and the medical care.

Family members with competing explanatory models can create other dilemmas for patients that are important for the clinician to understand. When Dr. Schaffer asked the mother of a baby, recently hospitalized for failure to thrive, what she and her family thought had caused the baby's weight loss, she tearfully replied:

> My mother told me there could not be anything wrong with the baby
> when I said I thought I should take her to the doctor. She said if there
> was anything seriously wrong, she would probably have a heart attack.
> My mother couldn't take another problem in the family. My mother-in-
> law said that my husband was just as skinny when he was a baby. She
> said I was crazy if I took the baby in, because the worst thing in the
> world is to have a fat baby.

These contradictory messages from the mother and mother-in-law gave the clinician a much richer understanding of the reasons the mother had not brought the baby in sooner. Instead of feeling angry with the mother, the clinician now can empathize with the mother's dilemma and understand the ambivalence and complexity of explanatory beliefs involved.

Understanding the Relational Context of Concern

3. Who in the family is most concerned about the problem?

The clinician may find important clues as to who is most concerned about the problem. The patient in the office is sometimes not the most concerned family member. This can help the clinician to understand:

- why the patient seems to be relaxed about the situation despite its seriousness.
- why the patient may not be an adequate reporter about the problem.
- why a patient might make frequent unwarranted return visits.
- who the important collaborators are for treatment.

Adolescent problems often present in this way. An adolescent female may appear to be unconcerned about her health problem, whether it is an exacerbation of her diabetes or related to her sexual behavior. Her parent continues to bring her in to see the doctor, however, hoping the doctor will "make" her take care of her diabetes or "make" her get on the pill. It is always useful for the clinician to identify who the "customer" is for his or her services (see Chap. 3).

Family Stress and Change

4. Along with your illness, have there been any other recent changes or stresses in your life?

Family-oriented questions about stresses or change can include finding out about other health problems in the family and how they are affecting the patient. Additional sources of stress or change could include recent immigration or household move, death of a family member, violence, remarriage, job loss, and such common life cycle transitions as a first child going to school or leaving home, separation, or divorce. These questions can help the family-oriented practitioner learn important information that might provide a key to previously elusive illness problems, as happened in this situation:

> Edith, an Irish-American woman, was in the hospital for an exacerbation of her congestive heart failure. She also had diabetes and a prosthesis for an amputated leg. When the physician asked Edith if she knew what medications she took, she clearly named all her medications. When asked if she was actually taking her medications, Edith said: "Sometimes." The family physician asked her why she answered "sometimes," and she responded blandly that she did not know why. The physician remembered Edith's husband's health had been failing when she was last in for a visit. "Edith, how is your husband doing?" Edith became tearful and answered he was doing terribly. The physician searched for any connection between the health of the patient's husband and the patient's inconsistency regarding taking her medication. Edith stated: "My husband spoiled me. He brought my medicines to me every day on a tray." Once the physician understood Edith's husband's role, a new plan could be considered. The physician could mobilize Edith's sister, who was at the bedside during this conversation, and lived next door. A plan was made for the sister and Edith's adult children to monitor her medicine intake. The physician also explored the impact of Edith's husband's failing health on her emotional life. Edith revealed how depressed she was and was interested in some counseling to help her cope with her feelings.

Family Support

5. How can your family or friends be helpful to you in dealing with this problem?

The literature on social support makes a clear link between health and social connectedness (see Chap. 2). The most important social support for most patients is their family. In contrast to Question 4, this family-oriented question seeks to expose sources of support that can be used to help the patient with either a new medical regimen, a new nutritional program, appropriate therapy, or additional information that the patient could not recall. The response to this question can also identify other family members who could be invaluable supports in facilitating the patient's healing or coping.

> Mr. Jackson, an African-American man, talked frequently with Dr. Stein about his desire to stop smoking. On several occasions he tried but did not quit for longer than 2 days before starting smoking again. Mr. Jackson was concerned because his father had died at the age of 49 of lung cancer. Like his father, Mr. Jackson, now 41, was a life-long smoker. Dr. Stein suggested that the desire to quit was a significant step that called for as much support from others as possible. She asked Mr.

Jackson if there was anyone who could help him get started. Mr. Jackson said his girlfriend of 5 years might be helpful, but he was not sure she would come in. Dr. Stein got Mr. Jackson's permission to call his girlfriend, and invited her to the next appointment.

Mr. Jackson returned with his girlfriend. During the interview, Dr. Stein learned that Mr. Jackson's girlfriend also smoked. She wanted to quit as well, which surprised Mr. Jackson. Together, they developed a plan to gradually stop smoking with each other's and the doctor's support.

Managing Family Information

The skills required to integrate family systems concepts in the 15-minute visit with the patient can be developed over time. As with so many questions posed by a clinician, one of the most important skills is the ability to "open the window and be able to close it (7)." Branch and Malik (7) describe an important skill needed by clinicians treating individual patients to ensure their confidence in opening up discussions: the complementary skill of closing conversations in ways that patients do not feel cut off or abandoned. Clinicians need to feel confident that the responses will not make the clinician regret his or her systemic inclinations after asking a family-oriented question. Rather than fearing that family-oriented questions will open the lid on Pandora's box, the systemically oriented clinician will therefore think of it as a controlled exploration that can be postponed or closed when necessary (2).

A Decision Protocol

As the clinician listens to the patient's responses to family-oriented questions, he or she will face decisions about how to use the family stories that are elicited. A decision tree can be helpful at this time as a guide for the family-oriented clinician to choose how to use this information. Doherty and Baird's "Levels of involvement in working with families" (8) can be a very helpful guide that compliments the decision tree. The following guidelines can be useful in helping the clinician decide how to use the family-oriented information that he or she has gathered.

1. Keep this family information in mind and make a note of it in the chart.

When the information adds to the overall understanding of the patient's concerns and reveals family stress or support regarding the problem, but does not call for the clinician to take action, the clinician can note it and consider it for the future. Examples of this include family health history, recent changes in the family life (e.g., a move, job change), or life cycle transitions (e.g., a child leaving home). This may involve updating or adding to the family's genogram so the new information is readily available and visible during a subsequent visit.

The information alone may help the clinician shape his or her interaction with the patient. Knowing that a noncompliant diabetic patient comes from a family with many diabetic members who all have resisted treatment may help the clinician manage his or her own expectations and pace the interventions, including deciding when the patient may be open to involving other family members.

2. Explore whether the individual can talk to other family members about the problem.

Through just a brief exploration of a situation, the clinician can sometimes help the patient devise a family-oriented intervention that the patient might want to try out as a first step to change. For instance, a patient may be frustrated that his or her family only makes and serves sweet, sugar-filled desserts. The patient could be coached on how to approach other family members to talk about the dilemmas this creates and what compromises could be arranged to satisfy both their taste needs and the patient's health needs. Other issues in need of family discussion might include additional lifestyle changes or compliance with a treatment regimen.

3. Invite another family member in for the routine office visit.

This action would be taken for purposes of gathering richer information, garnering support for the patient, and clarifying the medical situation for a family member. The "patient" has occasionally come to the physician in an effort to motivate another family member to get health care. The invitation to the other family member can be a mechanism for trying to involve this other family member in health care. (See Chap. 5 for a discussion of how to invite a family member to come to a routine office visit.) Involving a family member is also necessary to gather information about the patient's functioning that the patient may not be able to provide (e.g., memory loss, severe symptoms of depression, etc.). This step can also be taken when the patient tried Step 2 and comes back reporting to the clinician that the patient's own efforts to talk to other family members about support failed to produce the desired outcome.

4. Convene a family conference.

Family conferences are valuable for patients whose health difficulties are embedded in family processes that are problematic to the patient's health care. In a variety of situations the clinician may benefit from convening a family meeting: airing disagreements of treatment recommendations; learning how a patient's illness seems to organize family life; exploring issues about managing a complex problem; delivering a new diagnosis of an illness; when the patient and clinician feel "stuck" in treatment; or when a psychosocial problem is identified as the primary concern of the patient.

(See Chap. 5 for more discussion about how to convene a family conference and Chap. 7 for how to conduct a family conference.)

Refer to a Family-Oriented Mental Health Professional

When the patient or family reports psychosocial or mental health problems that are chronic (greater than 6 months) or multiple in nature, then the clinician should consider consultation with and referral to a family-oriented mental health provider. Common problems requiring consultation and/or referral include most marital problems, substance abuse, suicidality, psychosis, physical and/or sexual abuse, and prolonged grief reaction. See Chapter 25 for a discussion of when and how to refer a patient or family to a mental health professional. In each case it is important that the clinician develop and maintain collaborative relationships with mental health colleagues (9). When the clinician has implemented medication treatment that has been ineffective or is unsure about psychotropic medication for a patient, a referral to a psychiatrist for assessment, diagnosis, and medication is also warranted.

These broad guidelines can help clinicians titrate their involvement with family issues and with family members. They enable clinicians to assess when the best intervention is to collaborate with a psychosocial specialist much the same as they would collaborate with medical specialists regarding any number of biomedical problems. A family-oriented approach to the individual patient has multiple benefits: it puts the presenting complaint in context, enriches the clinician patient relationship, and ensures that diagnostic and treatment decisions consider the role of the family.

References

1. Medalie JH, Zyzanski SJ, Langa D, & Stange KC: The family in family practice: is it a reality? *J Fam Pract* 1998;**46**(5):390–396.
2. Cole-Kelly K, Yanoshik MK, Campbell J, & Flynn SP: Integrating the family into routine patient care: a qualitative study. *J Fam Pract* 1998;**47**(6):440–445.
3. Stewart M, Belle Brown J, Weston WW, McWhinney IR, McWilliam CL, & Freeman TR: *Patient-Centered Medicine: Transforming the Clinical Method.* Thousand Oaks, CA: Sage, 1995.
4. Cole-Kelly K, Seaburn D: Five areas of questioning to promote a family-oriented approach in primary care. *Fam Syst Health* 1999;**17**(3):340–348.
5. Wright LM, Watson WL, & Bell JM: *Beliefs: The Heart of Healing in Families and Illness.* New York: Basic Books, 1996.
6. Rolland J: *Families, Illness and Disability.* New York: Harpercollins, 1998.
7. Branch WT, Malik TK: Using "Windows of opportunities" in brief interviews to understand patients" concerns *JAMA* 1993;**269**(13):1667–1668.
8. Doherty WJ, Baird MA: Developmental levels in family-centered medical care. *Fam Med* 1986;**18**:153–156.

5
Involving the Family in Daily Practice

Walking into an exam room filled with a patient's family can be both daunting and rewarding. Every clinician will have contact with scores of family members in the course of his or her career. We obviously believe that the family is a tremendous resource in the welfare of our patients, and most patients seem to think so, too. Utilizing this resource effectively and efficiently takes practice, involves a particular set of skills, and may produce new norms in the office routine. We will outline the skills in this chapter.

Clinicians can be family-oriented with an individual patient, but there are times when it is helpful actually to meet with the patient's family, either during a routine office visit or in an extended family conference. Meeting with family members can help the clinician obtain a more thorough assessment of a problem, determine the impact of the illness on the family, negotiate a treatment plan and obtain the family's assistance in carrying out that plan. By asking other family members to come in, the clinician implicitly recognizes that the problem affects more than just the patient. This may be the first time for some family members anyone has acknowledged that they are suffering as well as the identified patient. A family conference also provides an opportunity for the patient to receive support and validation from family members.

Families can be important allies to the clinician in the evaluation and treatment process. The clinician usually sees the patient for less than 1 hour every few weeks or months, whereas the family lives with the patient full time. Family members can provide valuable information about the problem, offer their own diagnoses and treatment plans, and assist the patient in carrying out a specific plan and improving compliance, as in the following case:

> Despite suffering a recent heart attack, Mr. Jones found it very difficult to follow his physician's recommendations to stop smoking and reduce the cholesterol in his diet. During a family conference Mr. Jones' physician explained the importance of these recommendations and asked for the family's assistance. Mrs. Jones agreed to eliminate eggs

from her cooking, and serve a low-cholesterol menu to the entire family. Mr. Jones' adolescent son and daughter decided to cut down their smoking, and the family established a rule that cigarettes were not allowed in the house.

The clinician can check to see that there is agreement within the family as to the nature of the problem and the most appropriate treatment. If this is not done, family members may undermine, sabotage, or just not understand the clinician's plan.

When to Meet with Families

Incorporating new techniques and procedures (e.g., family conferences) into clinical practice requires a change in routine and the development of new skills. For physicians in training or those in practice who are developing a family approach to care, it is useful to establish the circumstances when family members are routinely consulted. A family conference becomes the rule rather than the exception at these designated times. Like other practice routines (e.g., measuring blood pressures, Pap smears during pelvic exams), the family conference comes to be expected by patients, staff, and other healthcare providers.

We have found it useful to distinguish among three types of family involvement (see Table 5.1). For most problems it is useful to obtain information about the family, assess family patterns, and encourage family involvement. A family-oriented approach with an individual patient was addressed in the previous chapter and can occur during every visit. Depending upon the type and seriousness of the problem, it may be helpful to consult with one or two relevant family members during a regularly scheduled office visit or to convene a family conference to discuss the problem with the extended family.

TABLE 5.1. Types of family involvement

	Family-oriented interview with individual patient	Family interview in a routine office visit	Family conference
Common Medical Situations	Acute medical problems Self limiting problems	Well child & prenatal care Diagnosis of a chronic illness Non-compliance Somatization	Hospitalization Terminal illness Institutionalization Serious family Problem/conflict
Percent of time used by MD	60–75%	25–40%	2–5%
Length of Visit	10–15 minutes	15–20 minutes	30–40 minutes
How scheduled	Routine care	May need to request family member attendance	Special scheduling & planning

As already described, being family-oriented with all routine individual patient visits is the backbone of family-oriented primary care. This approach involves gathering basic family information with the genogram, inquiring about family health beliefs, and exploring the impact of health problems on the family. The clinician may inquire about who will be giving the medication at home or who else at home is ill for a problem such as an acute otitis media in a child.

Family Involvement During a Routine Office Visit

Routine visits, in which one or more family members are present, are common and may be initiated by the patient, family members, or the clinician. These visits allow clinicians to obtain the family member's perspective on the problem or the treatment plan, as well as to answer the family member's questions. Consulting with family members can be incorporated into a routine 15-minute visit, and will rarely take much extra time for the experienced clinician. Several studies have demonstrated that office visits involving other family members last just a few minutes longer than other visits (1). In some situations, they may be more efficient than a visit with an individual patient because a family member can provide important information about the health problem.

Research has shown that family members often accompany the patient to the medical office, either remaining in the waiting room or joining the patient in the exam room. In the Direct Observation of Primary Care study, Medalie and colleagues studied the content of more than 4000 office visits to 138 family physicians (2). They found that another family member was present in the exam room during 32% of visits (2). This was most common when the patient was a child under 13 (97%) or was elderly (25%), but also occurred 12% of the time with adult patients. Overall, another family member's health problem was discussed in 18% of these visits. In a separate study, Botelho et al. (3) found that 39% of patients came to a family medicine center with a family member or friend and that two thirds of these accompanied the patient into the examination room.

In a study of family practices in Ontario (4), one third of patients were accompanied by a family member or friend, who was usually described as an advocate for the patient. Most companions who accompanied patients to a medical visit are family members. They served various roles for the patients, including helping to communicate patient concerns to the doctor, helping patients remember clinician recommendations, expressing concerns regarding the patient, and assisting patients in making decisions. The patients, companions, and clinicians all agreed that the companion's presence was helpful. The clinicians specifically felt that the family member improved their understanding of the patient's problem and the patient's understanding of the diagnosis and treatment.

Consulting with family members during a routine visit is advised whenever the health problem is likely to have a significant impact on other family members or when family members can be a resource in the treatment plan. There are several situations when involving another family member should be routine.

1. Routine obstetrical and well-child care.

Fathers and other significant support persons should be encouraged to come to all prenatal and well-child care. We urge fathers to attend at least one prenatal visit during the first half of the pregnancy to discuss the pregnancy, one visit toward the end of the pregnancy to discuss labor, delivery and their newborn, and one well-child visit during the first 6 months to discuss their baby and how the family is adjusting to the transitions. When the father is absent, it is especially important to bring in other significant family members (especially the mother's mother) and supportive friends (see Chap. 10 for a discussion of family-oriented pregnancy care).

2. Diagnosis of a serious chronic illness.

The diagnosis of a serious chronic illness (e.g., cancer, diabetes, or ischemic heart disease) can be a time of crisis for patients and families. Both patients and families must gradually accept the new diagnosis and learn to cope with it. This may lead to healthy adaptation (e.g., improved communication, commitment, and intimacy) or family dysfunction (e.g., over- or underinvolvement with the ill family member, overprotectiveness). It is usually helpful to include the patient's spouse or partner at the time of diagnosis or shortly thereafter. The family member can be a source of support for the patient and may be able to help the patient cope with the illness and adapt to the treatment regimen (see Chap. 18).

3. Noncompliance with treatment recommendations.

Some patients are unable or unwilling to follow the clinician's recommendations for medical care, especially when it involves complicated medication regimens or lifestyle changes (e.g., diet, exercise, or smoking cessation). Studies have demonstrated that when family members, especially the patient's partner, support the clinician's recommendations, then the patient is more likely to comply with the treatment (5). Noncompliance is much more common when family members are not supportive and criticize or otherwise undermine the patient's efforts. By meeting with the patient's partner, the clinician can enlist his or her support for the treatment recommendations.

In some cases, it may be unclear whether or why a patient is not following treatment recommendations. Including the patient's spouse or partner in these visits may clarify these issues.

> Dr. C. had been unable to help Mrs. Carroll get her blood pressure under control for several years despite multiple different medications, which she insisted that she took as prescribed. Finally, Dr. C. asked

Mr. Carroll to accompany his wife to her next medical visit. When asked about his wife's medication, he explained that she stored her pills mixed together with other medication in a large glass bowl and took one when she felt her blood pressure was high. Working with the couple, Dr. C. was able to set up a plan in which Mr. Carroll assisted his wife in complying with her medication.

4. Somatization or unexplained medical symptoms.

Patients who present with unexplained physical symptoms are common in primary care and frustrating to clinicians. Many of these patients have underlying psychosocial distress or mental health problems, but are resistant to addressing these issues. Involving a family member, usually the spouse or partner, in visits with these patients can be very helpful. It is often easier to expand beyond a focus on the somatic symptom and obtain a broader biopsychosocial assessment of the problem with the spouse present. Family members may be more willing to address psychosocial issues and provide valuable information about the problem (see Chap. 18).

After numerous visits by Cheryl for chronic abdominal pain, Dr. B. invited her boyfriend to accompany her for her next visit. Her boyfriend described how her abdominal pain seemed to worsen after she argued with her parents. With prompting, she described her conflicts with her parents and how it affected her physically and emotionally. Dr. B. asked them to keep a diary of her pain and how it was related to conflict with her parents and other stresses.

5. Health problems that have a significant interpersonal component.

More than one quarter of patients in primary care have a mental health disorder and a higher percentage experience significant psychosocial distress. Most of these psychosocial problems have a significant interpersonal component. They may result in part from relationship problems, or they have a significant impact on a family relationship. In these situations, it is very helpful and often essential to meet with other family members. For some problems, this can be done during a routine office visit; however, a family conference may be necessary for more complicated problems (see later).

Many psychosocial problems (e.g., marital or sexual problems, and child behavior or parenting) are relationship problems and require meeting with family members. As will be discussed in Chapter 14, meeting with one member of the couple in which there is a marital or sexual problem provides the clinician with only half of the picture and limits options for treatment.

The family-oriented clinician may encourage family members to participate in as many patient visits as possible. With time, patients and families realize that family members are welcome at office visits and find it helpful. For example, many elderly patients may decide to come routinely as a couple for their medical care. It can be useful to have a sign in the waiting room stating that family members are welcome to accompany patients during their medical visits.

Family Conference

In some situations, it is helpful to have a more extended conference to address the patient's illness or family problems. A family conference usually includes all immediate family, relevant extended family, significant friends, and members of the patient's support network. Family conferences may take longer and require some special arrangements. Whether to convene a family conference versus consulting with family members during a routine visit will usually depend upon the seriousness of the problem and its impact on the family. We believe that there are several situations when a family conference should be routinely held.

1. Hospitalization.

This is often a time of crisis for a family. Admission to the hospital may have resulted from an acute and unexpected problem (e.g., myocardial infarction), an exacerbation of a chronic illness (e.g., asthma), or the downward course of a terminal illness (e.g., cancer). In any case, families are usually anxious, stressed, and want information and support. We recommend that the clinician meet with the family as soon as possible after admission to the hospital to explain what has happened, discuss the proposed treatment plan, describe the patient's prognosis, and answer questions.

For most medical problems, treatment continues after the hospitalization, and a second meeting with the family and the inpatient treatment team toward the end of the hospitalization is useful to discuss discharge planning. Such a meeting would include the discussion of medication, physical and sexual activity, home services and treatments, and follow-up care (see Chap. 24). It can be relatively easy to organize a family conference around a hospitalization because family members typically come to the hospital to visit the patient anyway. Hospital social workers can help set up family discharge conference and coordinate home services.

2. End of life care.

It is essential to meet with the family when both the diagnosis of a terminal illness is made and when a patient dies. Families are usually in a state of shock and grief, and they need information and support. Because of the strong emotions surrounding death in the family and in healthcare providers, there is often a high degree of denial that can interfere with effective communication and the sharing of feelings. Decisions must often be made with the family about end-of-life care and decisions about resuscitation (DNR orders). At the same time, death is often viewed as failure by the clinician and may be accompanied by guilt. This may result in the clinician avoiding the family at a time when it is most important for him or her to have contact (see Chap. 16 for further discussion of working with death and grieving families.)

3. Institutionalization of an elderly patient.

The decision to place an elderly patient into a nursing home is one of the most difficult decisions that a family must make. Family members are usually ambivalent about such a decision, and disagreements or overt conflict among family members is common (see Chap. 15 for further discussion of nursing home placement). It can be very helpful in these situations to invite the entire family for a meeting to discuss the patient's condition and plans for the future. These meetings often occur in the setting of an acute hospitalization as part of discharge planning. When an elderly patient is planning to move from home directly to a nursing home, the family conference may occur in the home or the medical office.

4. Family conflict or dysfunction that interferes with patient care.

When families experience conflict or problems that begin to interfere with patient care, meeting with the entire family becomes extremely important.

> Mrs E. lived in her own home with her son, Tim, and daughter-in-law, Laurie. Laurie assumed responsibility for Mrs. E.'s medical care, supervising her medications and helping her with her daily care. As Mrs. E.'s dementia worsened, she began having more conflicts with Laurie over her care. Mrs E.'s other sons and daughters sided with their mother in these conflicts until they forced Tim and Laurie out of the house and one of the sons moved in to care for Mrs. E.

It is usually not adequate in these situations to just consult with the family members who accompany the patient to the visit. One needs to hear each family member's perspective of the problem and do a more complete family systems assessment. Meeting with a few family members may inadvertently draw the clinician into existing family coalitions and reduce one's effectiveness (see Chap. 8).

After the clinician has incorporated family conferences in the routine management of the situations listed earlier, he or she will find it useful to convene the family in other situations, or to conduct mini-family conferences during regular office visits. In addition, it can be very helpful and efficient to invite the family in for a meeting when they first register as patients. Such a meeting lets the family know of the clinician's family orientation and that he or she values the family's involvement in the health of each member. Time can be saved by obtaining a genogram and family history from the entire family rather than from each individual family member.

When Not to Convene Family Members

The only circumstance in which a meeting with other family members is contraindicated is when there is a risk of violence directed toward the patient, a family member, or a clinician. When the patient is a victim of physical abuse or family violence, the clinician should not involve the abusive family member unless he or she can be certain that the patient will remain physically safe after the session, especially if there is a history of serious injury or threats. The clinician should be very cautious about conducting a family conference when the patient or a family member has a history of violence or aggressive outbursts, or the relationships are very toxic. Finally, there may be circumstances in which the level of family conflict is so great, even without violence, that bringing family members together may not be productive, especially without the assistance of a family therapist. This may occur during or shortly after a marital separation or divorce (see Chap. 14).

Who Should Attend?

The patient and clinician together should decide who should attend a family conference. When family members accompany a patient to an office visit, they are usually, but not always, the most important family member involved in the medical problem. To arrange a family conference during a routine office visit, it is usually sufficient to ask the patient to invite whoever is most involved or has helped them most with the health problem. This will be the patient's partner or spouse for most adults. It may in some circumstances be a parent (usually the patient's mother) or a sibling. Involving the father of the baby is particularly important for prenatal and well-child visits.

All the members of the patient's immediate household as well as family members, friends, and professionals involved with the illness should be invited for an initial family conference. This makes it most likely the family health expert and other important figures will be on hand. The clinician can always elect to invite a subsystem of the family for future meetings if that seems appropriate, but it is more difficult to bring in family members who have been excluded from early sessions: Not to invite a family member is to actively exclude that person from the family conference. A patient or family will sometimes try to exclude or protect a certain family member, such as an aged grandparent, by claiming they are not involved in the presenting problem. From a broad perspective, this is rarely true; in fact, at times they may be the most powerful member of the family and little will be accomplished without their support.

> Despite several family conferences, Dr. J. was unable to get the Harriet family to eliminate milk products from the diet of their 5-year-old daughter, who was lactose intolerant. Finally, when asked about other

members of the family, it was revealed that the girl's grandmother had grown up on a dairy farm and now lived with the family. She insisted that her granddaughter drink a glass of milk at each meal. Dr. J. persuaded the grandmother to add Lactaid to her granddaughter's milk.

Children's Involvement in Family Conferences

Children should be specifically invited to family conferences. Parents may otherwise exclude them because of a belief that "they won't understand" or will be confused or upset. If there is a problem or concern about a child, direct observation of the child's behavior within the family is obviously essential. It is equally important, however, that the other children attend to observe the family as a whole and prevent one child from being labeled as having the only problem. Children also offer important and useful information about a problem, either verbally or nonverbally. When inviting children, it is important to have age-appropriate toys or crayons and coloring paper for them. It can be informative to have the children draw pictures of their family and describe the pictures.

> Mr. and Mrs. Simons and their two teenage daughters met with their family physician to discuss Mrs. Simons' depression. When asked about his perceptions of his wife's moods, Mr. Simons was interrupted by his 14-year-old daughter, Jill, who announced, "How would he know? Dad's never home. He's always at the bar." Further discussion revealed that the father's alcoholism was a major contributing factor in the mother's depression.

An exception to this recommendation to invite children to a family conference is when the problem deals with a specific marital or sexual problem. In such cases, the clinician should first meet with the couple alone to assess the problem. It may be useful in later sessions to meet with the children and the couple's parents as well.

How to Convene the Family

Family members are usually eager to attend family conferences to learn more about the patient's problems and how they can help. Research has demonstrated that patients and families desire these conferences and in particular request them for serious medical problems and behavioral or psychosocial problems (6–8). In a survey of patients with hypertension at the Johns Hopkins medical clinics, 70% of patients with hypertension wanted members of their families to learn more about hypertension. An intervention consisting of family education and support was designed and resulted in a significant reduction in blood pressure and mortality. Because of this success, the family intervention has been incorporated into the routine care of hypertensive patients at John Hopkins (9).

The following guidelines will help to insure that all the appropriate family members attend. It may not be necessary to use all of these approaches each time the family is convened; rather, these are guidelines that can be adapted as necessary to particular circumstances during a clinical encounter. They are derived from our clinical experience working with families and the writings of others in family medicine (10, 11) and family therapy (12).

1. *Involve the family early:* Start involving family members as early as possible in the management of a serious health problem, preferably during the first visit. Family members are often sitting in the waiting room and are eager to participate. Routinely ask if any family members came with the patient and if so consider inviting them in. At a minimum take a minute to greet the family member at the end of the interview.

AVOID listening extensively to a patient's complaint about other family members before you have convened the family. Listen empathetically, but say something such as, "I am interested in helping you with this problem. In order to get a proper start, we need your family here to accomplish this." If the patient wishes to continue, gently suggest, "These issues may be better discussed at a later time."

2. *Be positive and direct* about your need to see the family: Expect the family to come in. "I need to meet with the father of your baby. Can he come in for your next prenatal visit?" A family conference is like any other diagnostic test or therapeutic procedure. If the patient and the family are not convinced that the clinician thinks it is important, they are unlikely to follow through. Explain that this is a routine procedure for this type of problem. "This is the way I like to work" or "I often find it useful to meet with other family members for at least a one session evaluation."

AVOID being ambivalent or giving mixed messages about the importance of a family conference. "Do you think it would be possible (or worthwhile) for your family to come in? I understand if they can't all come in." Patients pick up your confidence, or lack thereof, in any procedure you recommend.

3. *Emphasize the importance of the family* in caring for the patient: Tell the family that you need their help or opinion regarding the problem. "When one member of the family is having a problem, I find it helps to get the perspectives of other family members. People who know and care about each other often have a lot to contribute to each other," or, "As a normal part of my work with patients I like to involve family members as a resource." As a clinician you can only observe the patient at a few points in time, whereas family members see the patient every day.

If the problem is described only in individual terms (e.g., "I have chronic low back pain"), ask how others in the family have responded to it (e.g.,

"What does your wife do when your back pain is severe?"). This inquiry enlarges the context of the problem and puts it in interactional terms. Other family members are often involved in some fashion, either influencing or being influenced by the symptom. They may be in pain because of the problem or trying in an unproductive way to help the patient.

AVOID accepting the patient's word that another family member is unwilling to come in. This is often a projection of their own reluctance or protectiveness. First, insist that the patient extend the invitation. Give the patient support and role-play with the patient asking the family to come in. If that fails, or appears it will fail, call them yourself.

4. *Stress the benefits* of a family meeting to the patient and the family. Acknowledge that the problem affects other family members. "When one member is in pain, I often find that other family members are in pain as well. Bringing everyone in can result in more people receiving benefit from treatment."

AVOID blaming the family in any way. Do not imply that there is a "family problem" or that the family is in need of therapy, even if you think there is a family problem and they do need therapy. The family may or may not be at a point where they agree with you. Recommending therapy or counseling can emerge in the family meeting or meetings when it is clear the family is ready and willing to negotiate about referral. These recommendations should not be used prematurely or in any way that they can be construed as blaming. Many families equate "therapy" with "crazy" and will not want to participate if that is the implication.

5. Call the session a *family meeting or conference*, not family assessment, counseling, or therapy. Focus the purpose of the meeting on what the family identifies as the problem, not on your assessment of the problem: "I'd like the whole family to come in to discuss how best to manage Billy's bedwetting," not, "I'd like to assess how family stresses (or problems) might be affecting Billy."

6. *Give specific instructions* for convening the family. Discuss exactly what the patient will say to the other family members. If there is a question or anxiety, role-play the invitation. The patient may otherwise return home and announce to his or her spouse, "The doctor wants you to come in for my next visit because he thinks you are making me depressed." Instruct the patient to say, "The doctor would like to hear your thoughts and ideas about my depression."

Offer to call other family members yourself if needed. This may be necessary if the patient insists that family members will not come in, regardless of what he or she says to them. It is best to call the family members while the patient is in the office and knows what will be said.

Acknowledge the sacrifice that other family members will have to make to come in, and that you would not ask them to do this unless you thought it was important. Specify exactly who you want to come and when you want them to come. Send a postcard to *remind the family* of the meeting, or have your secretary call the day before the meeting.

Circumstances That Promote Reluctance and Resistance to Attending a Family Conference

Families usually want to attend family conferences, particularly when they feel that they can be helpful and will not be blamed. A family occasionally resists coming in. The resistance may be overt (i.e., family members refuse to attend) or covert (i.e., they agree to come but do not show). Resistance can usually be predicted prior to the family conference and is often diagnostic of dynamic difficulties in the family or between the family and the treatment system (see Chap. 6). This most commonly occurs when there is a serious psychosocial problem (e.g., alcoholism, drug abuse, child or sexual abuse, or sexual dysfunction) and one of a number of dynamics may help to explain their resistance:

1. *Significant marital or family conflict* is present, and the presenting problem is part of the conflict. For example, the wife may be angry at her husband, believe that he drinks too much, and want their family physician to get him to stop.

2. *Blame* has been felt by family members for the problem in the past, and they are worried that they will be blamed again. For example, the father of a child with behavior problems may have been told previously that he has been too strict in his discipline. If the clinician fails to get the permission or collaboration of the patient for a conference, or implies any blame for the problem, other family members may be very resistant to coming in.

3. *An exclusive relationship* has been established by one member of the family with the clinician, and other family members may feel excluded. For example, Mr. J. had been followed by his physician for his diabetes for years. At the time he developed impotence, his physician asked his wife to come in for the first time. She refused because she blamed herself for her husband's problem and was afraid his physician would also blame her.

In each situation, family members assume that the physician has heard the patient's version of the problem and has accepted it as the truth.

Dealing with Resistance

When resistance to a family conference is apparent, the following approaches can be helpful.

1. *Do not accept the patient's initial response* that his or her family refuses to come in. The patient may be nervous and want to protect and exclude other family members, but with support be willing to do what is actually needed. (This circumstance is much like the cancer patient who initially refuses chemotherapy out of both fear and denial but slowly accepts his fate and requests treatment.) Inquire how the patient made the request. After getting the patient's permission, call the other family members directly.

2. Sometimes the patient fears how other family members will respond to the request to discuss a problem. *Listen openly* to the realistic difficulty of taking this step.

> PT.: This problem doesn't involve my husband. He would never come in. He doesn't believe in counseling.
>
> MD.: Your husband can help me to understand your problem better. I suspect that he cares for you enough to be willing to come in to help you.
>
> PT.: My parents would be mortified if they knew about all of this. I don't want them to know.
>
> MD.: Most parents appreciate the opportunity to help one of their children. They may be quite worried about you and benefit by discussing their concerns.
>
> PT.: My children are too young to understand any of this. It would only frighten them.
>
> MD.: It can be frightening to discuss these problems openly with your children; however, I am certain that your children are aware that something is wrong. It is more frightening for them when they are left in the dark and are allowed to imagine the worst.

3. *State that you are "stuck"* and cannot help the patient without seeing the rest of the family (11). Firmly request that they come in. "There is simply no way I can help your daughter unless I have your husband's help. He needs to come in for the next appointment."

4. *Do not argue*, when trying to persuade a resisting family member to come in. Agree with him or her as much as possible and try to use the explanations for refusing to come as reasons to come. Note that if the family member is in conflict with the patient, you should stress how important it is for you to get the other side of the story and that his or her viewpoint needs to be heard.

> Husband: Listen, Doc! My wife doesn't listen to anything I have to say, and I certainly don't want to come in and hear her blame me again for all of her problems.
>
> Physician: I don't want you to listen to her blame you either, but I do want to hear your side of the story. I have discussed some of this problem with your wife, but I am certain that the situation is more complicated than she sees it. Your perspective of her problems would be very helpful to my efforts to try to help her.

On the other hand, if family members claim that they are not involved in the problem or that it is none of their business, explain how important it is to have a neutral family member to help you out with the problem.

Mother: My daughter is an adult now, and I try to stay out of her affairs. This is her problem and it doesn't involve me.

Physician: I can see that you have helped your daughter to be independent and allowed her to deal with these problems on her own. To help your daughter cope with her difficulties, I need the help of someone who knows and cares about her, but has not gotten overinvolved in her problems. Do you think you could help me with this?

Finally, if the family member says that the problem is with the patient and not with the family, state you need the family to consult with you to assist in helping the patient.

Sister: This is not a family problem. My brother has been drinking for years, and we did everything we could to help him. He has to stop blaming others for his problems and face up to them himself.

Nurse Practitioner: I agree that your brother needs to confront his alcoholism and get treatment for it. I would like to help him get treatment, but I need you and the rest of the family to help me. At least you can fill me in on what tricks he uses to deny and hide his drinking, and what hasn't worked in the past, so I don't waste my time trying them again.

5. *Make a home visit.* This is a very powerful and effective maneuver to get reluctant family members in. It demonstrates a genuine and serious concern for the family and willingness to meet them on their own turf. After such a visit and appropriate joining, the family will rarely refuse to reciprocate by coming in for a family conference. In addition, a home visit allows the clinician to evaluate the home situation and observe the family in their own environment. This can provide a more comprehensive and valid overall assessment of the family.

When the Family Does Not Come in

Meet with the family members who have come for the family session. Thank them for their time and interest, but express the importance of consulting with the missing family members before proceeding.

Assess why all the invited family members did not come in for the family session. Be wary of such excuses as, "My husband couldn't get time off from work today," or, "Jimmy can't miss any more school than he has already." These explanations may be quite legitimate, but if the family really believes that meeting is important, they can usually get time off or be excused from work or school to attend.

Find out specifically which family members the patient invited, how they were asked, and what they responded. Ask those that have come why the missing family members did not want to attend, and what it would take to get them to come.

Plan how to proceed with the family. This will depend upon the nature and urgency of the problem, and on which and how many of the important family members have come for the family conference. The options for this include the following possibilities.

Reschedule the family conference. If key members of the family are not present for the family conference (e.g., the father in a parent–child problem), or the problem is thought to result in part from dysfunctional family dynamics (e.g., substance abuse or psychosomatic illness), it is usually preferable to reschedule the session than meet without these family members. For example, if the clinician meets only with the mother and child with a behavior problem, the message to the father is that he does not need to take part, and that his involvement is unimportant. If the father is distancing from the family and there are marital problems, as there can be in parent–child problems, meeting with the mother without the father will only make matters worse.

When crucial family members do not come to the session, meet briefly with those present to obtain their advice in getting the other members of the family in to the meeting. *Call* missing family members directly by phone during the session to assess why they did not come in and to help get their cooperation for a meeting.

Meet with the family that has come. In some circumstances (e.g., at the time of hospitalization or immediately after a death), the clinician must meet with whichever family members are present. It is important to determine which family members are not present so that they can be contacted if necessary at a later time. Again it may be useful to call some missing family members directly during the session.

An essential component of family-oriented healthcare is meeting with entire families or subgroups of families when indicated. These meetings may be for routine care, discussion of a new diagnosis, discharge from the hospital, treatment planning, dealing with noncompliance, or assisting with psychosocial problems. Despite the emphasis on the importance of the family in family medicine, many physicians lack the conviction or the skill to convene families effectively. This difficulty can be addressed by routinely meeting with families in the preceding circumstances. Following a protocol will improve success in convening families so that the physician becomes more comfortable with family conferences and uses them more frequently.

References

1. Cole-Kelly K, Yanoshik MK, Campbell J, & Flynn SP: Integrating the family into routine patient care: a qualitative study. *J Fam Pract* 1998;**47**:440–445.
2. Medalie JH, Zyzanski SJ, Langa D, & Stange KC: The family in family practice: is it a reality? [see comments]. *J Fam Pract* 1998;**46**:390–396.

3. Botelho RJ, Lue B, & Fiscella K: Family involvement in routine health care: a survey of patients' behaviors and preferences. *J Fam Pract* 1996;**42**:572–576.

4. Brown JB, Brett P, Stewart M, & Marshall JN: Roles and influence of people who accompany patients on visits to the doctor. *Can Fam Physician* 1998;**44**: 1644–1650.

5. Campbell TL, Patterson JM: The effectiveness of family interventions in the treatment of physical illness. *J Marital Fam Ther* 1995;**21**:545–584.

6. Kushner K, Meyer D: Family physicians' perceptions of the family conference. *J Fam Pract* 1989;**28**:65–68.

7. Kushner K, Meyer D, & Hansen JP: Patients' attitudes toward physician involvement in family conferences. *J Fam Pract* 1989;**28**:73–78.

8. Kushner K, Meyer D, Hansen M, Bobula J, Hansen J, & Pridham K: The family conference: what do patients want? *J Fam Pract* 1986;**23**(5):463–467.

9. Morisky DE, Levine DM, Green LW, Shapiro S, Russell RP, & Smith CR: Five-year blood pressure control and mortality following health education for hypertensive patients. *Am J Pub Health* 1983;**73**:153–162.

10. Christie-Seely J: *Working with the Family in Primary Care: A Systems Approach to Health and Illness*. New York: Praeger Press, 1984.

11. Doherty WJ, Baird MA: *Family Therapy and Family Medicine: Toward the Primary Care of Families*. New York: Guilford Press, 1983.

12. Rolland J: *Families, Illness and Disability*. New York: Harpercollins, 1994.

Protocol for Involving the Family in Daily Practice

A. Family involvement in routine office visits: Include a family member during medical visits in the following situations:

1. Routine obstetrical and well-child care.
2. Diagnosis of a serious or life-threatening illness.
3. Noncompliance with treatment recommendations.
4. Unexplained physical symptoms or somatization.
5. Health problems that have a significant interpersonal component, including mental health disorders.

B. Family conferences: Routinely convene the family in the following circumstances:

1. Hospitalization (at admission and discharge).
2. End-of-life care (diagnosis of terminal illness and time of death).
3. Nursing home placement (during planning and at the time of).
4. Family conflict or dysfunction that is affecting medical care.

How to Convene the Family

1. Involve the family in the patient's medical care as early as possible. Ask patients routinely if any family members came with them and invite those family members in for part of the visit.
2. Be positive and direct about your need to see the family. Expect them to come in for the family conference. Explain that it is a routine procedure.
3. Emphasize the importance of the family as a resource in caring for the patient. Tell the family that you need their help or opinion.
4. Stress the benefits of a family conference to the patient and family. Acknowledge that the problem affects all members of the family.
5. Give specific instructions to the patient on who to invite, and how to invite them.

You must avoid:

1. Being ambivalent or uncertain about the importance of a family conference.
2. Accepting the patient's word that family members are unwilling or unable to come in for a consult.
3. Blaming the family in any way.
4. Suggesting that there is a family problem or that the family needs help in the form of therapy.

Dealing with Resistance to a Family Conference

1. Do not accept the patient's initial response that his or her family refuses to come in for a consult. Inquire how the patient made the request.

2. Elicit the patient's fears concerning how family members will respond to the request to discuss the problem.
3. State that you are "stuck" and cannot help the patient without seeing the rest of the family.
4. Do not argue. Try to use the patient's explanations for the family refusing to come as reasons for the importance of the meeting.
5. Make a home visit.

When the Family Does Not Come in for a Consult

1. Meet the family members who have come and assess why all those invited did not come into the conference.
2. Plan with the family how to proceed, and whether to:
   a. reschedule the family conference, if crucial family members are missing.
   b. have the conference with the family members who are present.
3. Call the missing family members directly.

6
Building Partnerships: Promoting Working Alliances and Motivation for Change

Family-oriented primary care is built upon the relationship between a clinician and the patient and family. The quality of this relationship affects the way all parties exchange information, determine diagnoses, and negotiate treatment of health problems. The relationship is ideally imbued with the features of a partnership: mutual respect, understanding, compromise, and common goals. The clinician has a professional responsibility to cultivate these relationships. In fact, the relationship between clinician, patient, and family may be the single most important treatment variable in fostering a patient's positive health behaviors (1–4). These relationships also directly affect the clinician's job satisfaction (i.e., the better the relationships, the happier the clinician).

Clinicians can develop specific skills that promote a constructive working alliance (i.e., a partnership) with patients and family members. We will assume all clinicians to some degree possess skill at interviewing an individual patient. We will focus here on what is specific to family-oriented primary care, which encompasses building relationships with family members and others involved with the patient. Three interviewing skills enhance the potential for an effective partnership to develop between clinician, patient, and family: building rapport, organizing the interview, and converting resistance into cooperation.

Building Rapport

Clinicians, patients, and their families evaluate each other early in an interview. Clinicians look for whether a patient or family member will be a clear and reliable source of information about the presenting problem. We also look for a spirit of collaboration: Can we easily understand each other and work together; can we easily agree on diagnoses and treatment plans; or will this alliance require more attention to succeed? While clinicians scrutinize patients and their families, patients, of course, assess us as clinicians. They initially wonder: Can I trust you? Will you understand me, my strengths, my weaknesses, my problems, my pain, and my unique situation? Do you ask the right questions, provide adequate information, explore the various possibilities? Are you competent?

During this initial phase of the interview, clinicians are often in a rush to get into the medical data-gathering; however, it is important instead to focus, almost exclusively, on building rapport. The term used by family therapists to characterize this phase is *joining* (5). Joining with each individual patient and family member is like oiling an important piece of machinery. If well-oiled, the machine will run smoothly and effectively when needed. If not, the machine will grind, make a lot of noise, and run inefficiently or sometimes not at all. Joining, like oiling, is a maintenance task that in and of itself will not produce the desired outcome, but when absent threatens any positive end. Multiple people in an exam room complicates the joining process.

Joining most consciously occurs in the socializing phase of an interview or conference. It begins with greeting, making contact, and establishing rapport with each person. This process involves searching for a common wavelength or language with which to communicate. When patients, families, and their clinicians differ significantly in terms of gender, race, class, ethnicity, or age, joining may require extra energy on the part of the clinician to reach for a point of meaningful connectedness. Psychoanalyst Harry Stack Sullivan said, "We are all more human than otherwise" (6). Clinicians have an opportunity to discover this human connection between themselves and every patient. To begin by searching for commonality may involve just commenting on the weather, on a common heritage, or a common interest. The goal is to find a respectful way to make a connection, person to person, before beginning the primary business of the interview. This is especially important if joining with a family member when one already has a well-established connection with the patient. In these beginning interactions, the clinician maintains an earlier alliance with the patient and begins to build an additional alliance with the family member.

> Nurse Practitioner: Thank you very much for taking the time to come in today with your girlfriend, Mr. Hargrove.
> Mr. Hargrove: I want to be part of this pregnancy. I am the father.
> Nurse Practitioner: That's wonderful, Mr. Hargrove. Your baby will benefit, and I look forward to getting to know you. Tell me something about yourself. How do you spend your days?

In these early interactions, a clinician may consciously or unconsciously use different parts of his or her own history or personality to connect with a given patient or family member. In the preceding case, both nurse practitioner and patient were African-Americans in their thirties. This similarity made the connection somewhat easier than when age and ethnicity are different. In addition, joining may be done at the level of content, and it may be done at a process or nonverbal level. For example, with a depressed woman, the clinician may speak in a low, soothing voice; with a loud, anxious man who just had a myocardial infarction, the clinician may speak with strong, comforting conviction. With a particularly difficult patient or family member, part of establishing rapport may involve matching behavior (e.g., sitting in the same position, using similar speech cadence, or mirroring some of that person's gestures until the person has relaxed enough to engage in a productive exchange).

Once these preliminary connections have been formed, joining involves carefully listening to the patient's concerns, without interruption, for a period of time. Research has demonstrated that the average length of time for a clinician to listen to a patient's initial concerns is 23 seconds (7). The inability of some health professionals to listen attentively to their patients is associated with patient dissatisfaction and an increase in malpractice suits (8). Once rapport is established, clinicians must listen carefully to the patient's and family's health beliefs, their cultural explanations for illness, and, especially, their personal diagnoses of the problem. Understanding the patient's and family's assessment provides a starting point for making a diagnosis and collaborating on an effective treatment plan.

> Patient: I think I feel some lumps in my neck, Doctor. I want you to check them for me.
>
> Dr: Of course, but let me ask a few questions first. Is there anything particular you are concerned about?
>
> Patient: Well, my brother died of Hodgkin's Disease several years ago and he started with lumps in his neck too. I have to admit I watch myself like a hawk, and worry constantly that I will meet the same fate.
>
> Spouse: I've told my husband he worries too much, doctor, but he insists on asking you.
>
> Dr: I'm glad you both said something. I need to know about all these things: your family history, your diagnosis, and the general concern about Hodgkin's disease. I'll evaluate the lumps carefully, and then we can decide where to go from here.

This straightforward connection with a patient's agenda and diagnosis, and hearing the spouse's reaction, elicits important information and lays the groundwork for a treatment plan that is understood and approved by all participants. The clinician may choose to enhance this partnership further later in the interview by gathering more information, giving advice, or facilitating an open-ended discussion, depending on the needs of the patient and family.

When interacting with more than one person at a time (e.g., in a family conference), joining also involves being wary of emotional triangles and family coalitions (see Chap. 3 for an explanation of these concepts). To be effective, it is important for the clinician to *develop positive working alliances with both the patient and other family members* rather than being drawn into coalitions with the patient against family members, or vice versa.

> Dr: Thank you, Mr. Howell, for coming in to help me understand your wife's recent sleeping problems.
> Mr. Howell: I don't see how I can contribute. I'm sure my wife has already told you I snore and that's why she can't sleep. But, I've been snoring for years and it never bothered her before. Maybe if you just gave her sleeping pills we could all get some rest.
> Dr: That is certainly one solution, but sleeping pills can have some pretty significant side effects and usually only work in the short term. I would like to see if together we can come up with a solution for the long term.

In this example, Mr. Howell assumed that the doctor had already taken sides with his wife against him. This assumption is frequently made when a patient has a long-standing relationship with a clinician that has not included other family members. For this reason alone, it is useful to *meet routinely with family members early on when seeing a new patient.* The clinician can then put faces to names when a patient talks about family, and you will also have made connections that will facilitate future interactions. It can be awkward during an emergency, or in the midst of a serious problem, to have to join with unknown family members who may be distraught. In the preceding example, the clinician focused on Mr. Howell early in the interaction and elicited his view of the problem. The physician let him know his views would be heard, that he would not be blamed, and that he might contribute to alleviating rather than to worsening the problem. The clinician then turned to give Mrs. Howell the same opportunity to be heard without blaming or taking sides.

In the next example, the clinician again maintains a position that enables her to empathize with and support each person in turn.

> Clinician: Mr. Depko and Ms. Scott, I appreciate you both taking the time to come in and discuss your son's recent difficulty keeping his sugars under control. As I've told Ralph, diabetes can be difficult to manage, and we need all the help we can get.
> Mr. Depko: Well, I think if Ralph's mother would feed the kid the right foods, we probably wouldn't have a problem. I tell her this, but she won't listen to me.
> Ms. Scott: Why should I listen to you? Since you left the house, you don't even know what he eats.
> Clinician: It's clear you both have a perspective that will be important to hear. Each of you is obviously concerned about your son or you wouldn't be here today. Let's begin with Ralph and hear his ideas about why he's having problems sticking to his diet.

If the clinician can maintain an alliance with each member of this family, it might result in a productive conversation in which the parents pull together to help their son stick to his diabetic diet. If Ms. Scott and Ralph consistently berate Mr. Depko, however, then this mother–son coalition might signal a need to the clinician either to consult with or to refer to a family therapist. A new approach is necessary when triangles or coalitions persistently interfere with treatment, as can happen when parents are separated. Being able to negotiate difficult triangles or coalitions and develop constructive working alliances builds both the patient's and family members' confidence in the competence of the clinician; not to do so can result in "noncompliance" due to family members fighting over the treatment plan and in recurring headaches for the clinician, as demonstrated by the next case.

> Dr. C., a middle-aged English-American physician, enjoyed working over the years with Mr. Bell, an older Irish-American gentleman. In the last year, Mr. Bell's daughter moved to town, partly to be near her aging father. Mr. Bell was mildly obese with moderate hypertension. His daughter began bringing him to his medical visits and was soon demanding that Dr. C. reduce her father's medication and give him a "complete physical." Even though his daughter was a quite demanding and difficult person with whom to deal, Mr. Bell remained content with his medical care: He did not see additional tests as being important, and he defended his doctor to his daughter. Because Mr. Bell was "the patient," Dr. C. continued treatment as before and tried to minimize or ignore the daughter's demands and protests.
>
> Several months later Mr. Bell unfortunately had a severe stroke, leaving him comatose until he eventually died. Before the stroke, Mr. Bell's daughter had thought Dr. C. was colluding with her father's tendency to minimize his health problems, so she was furious and blamed Dr. C. after the stroke occurred. This difficult relationship between the clinician and the patient's family made decisions regarding care complex and unpleasant, and made grieving after the patient's death complicated for both the daughter and the clinician.
>
> After this experience, Dr. C. vowed to spend more time and energy forming an alliance with patients' families and recognized that discounting or minimizing their concerns can have grave repercussions in the long run.

Organizing the Interview

A well-organized interview provides a safe and secure structure for the patient and family to express their concerns within the time constraints of a busy clinician's schedule. Rapport promotes honest expression. A well-organized interview builds patient confidence in the clinician's competence, while providing the clinician with the necessary information to arrive efficiently at an accurate diagnosis. Organizing the interview also means having goals for the interview, a structure and method to accomplish these goals, and a clear sense of the responsibilities inherent in both the clinician's and the patient's roles. With regard to these roles, Whitaker, a family therapist, conceptualized the early stages of a psychotherapeutic relationship as involving struggles around structuring the interview and the initiative for change (9). His view was that the clinician must take responsibility for structuring the interview, but also recognize that the patient is in control of any initiative for change. Whitaker believed that many therapeutic impasses are the result of confusion over who is in charge of treatment and who is in charge of change. Adapting these concepts to the primary care context, the clinician should be in charge of the interview and treatment plan, while recognizing that it is patients who are in charge of their own health and recovery.

Guidelines for organizing an interview can help the clinician maintain focus and remain attentive, prevent a family member from dominating the discussion, and make the most effective use of time. The clinician needs to *direct traffic* in a group interview, which is a task that requires skills significantly different from those needed in an individual interview. The following are general guidelines to help the clinician conduct an effective interview:

1. Encourage only one person to speak at a time.

The clinician needs to establish leadership during the interview or conference in order to protect each person's right to be heard (as in the example of the couple who were separated and bringing their child into see the doctor).

2. Encourage each person to use "I" statements.

Ask that each person in the group speak only for himself or herself in order to prevent any discussion from degenerating into blaming and accusations.

> Patient (to Boyfriend): You're always on my back about my weight. No one could lose weight with your nagging.
> Clinician: Let me interrupt for a moment. I've found that we all are able to listen to each other better when we each speak for ourselves. Begin your sentences with "I" and try not to blame one another. (To the patient:) Try it again.
> Patient: Well, I'm having a hard time sticking to the diet we previously agreed to.
> Clinician (to Boyfriend): Dieting is often a challenge for the strongest of us. Maybe you could give us your perspective on when you see your partner doing well with her diet?

In this example the patient quickly moved to blame her boyfriend for her difficulties. By invoking a rule about "I" statements, the clinician was able to shift the interview back to a nonblaming and more constructive path.

3. Emphasize strengths.

Some resource or strength can be noted and used in treatment, even in the most difficult interactions or with the sickest of patients. This approach boosts self-esteem, recognizes positive gains, minimizes conflict, and encourages the family to take as much responsibility as possible for the health of their loved ones.

> Patient: Well, I'm having a hard time sticking to the diet we previously agreed to.
>
> Clinician (to Boyfriend): Dieting is often a challenge for the strongest of us. Maybe you could give us your perspective on when it is that your partner seems to be doing well with her diet?
>
> Boyfriend: Well, I notice that she seems to do quite well when I'm on the road as part of my trucking business.
>
> Patient: I didn't realize you noticed. It's easier to eat well when you aren't here.
>
> Clinician: I'm very impressed, first, that you, Mr. Jones, were so observant. And then, Ms. Van Zandt, it is clear that you're able to make some progress eating well when you are on your own. That is a time many people find the hardest. Perhaps you'd like to talk together now about how you could each use these strengths to your advantage when you are both at home.

4. Model this behavior yourself.

As the interviewer or conference facilitator, the clinician sets the tone for the discussion in the way he or she speaks. Using "I" statements, speaking respectfully to each person, and maintaining a belief in the patient and family's ability to mobilize resources to take care of the illness or problem are all behaviors that can be contagious.

Converting Resistance into Collaboration

Collaboration and resistance are interpersonal phenomena. Both are two-way streets. It is difficult to collaborate with someone who is uninterested or belligerent. It is also difficult to resist someone who refuses to fight. In a primary care context, this means that both collaboration and resistance are measures of the goodness of fit between the clinician and the patient or family. We prefer the term *collaboration* over the term *compliance* because collaboration implies the cooperative, interpersonal nature of the relationship. Compliance, on the other hand, implies that the clinician gives orders that the patient and family should obey. This authoritarian mind-set can lead to situations in which patients either lie or omit information to protect themselves, or they maintain the appearance of compliance to protect their relationship with a valued clinician. (In either case, they may come to be known as "resistant" patients.) Collaboration implies an effort by the doctor, the patient, and the family to express their own and understand each others' points of view.

Collaboration results from an established connection between the clinician and the patient and family (see Chap. 2 and Campbell and Patterson, 10, for a review of the research that supports family involvement in treatment). When disagreements occur, or a patient has difficulty carrying out a treatment plan, it is often useful to involve other family members in discussion of the problem. What Doherty and Baird termed "family-oriented compliance counseling" (11) (i.e., counseling to arrive at mutually agreed upon treatment plans) should be routine in the treatment of stress-related disorders, psychosocial problems, and such serious acute illnesses as myocardial infarctions, strokes, and bleeding ulcers. A new diagnosis of a chronic illness (e.g., diabetes) warrants family involvement and negotiation to achieve the changes necessary for healthy behavior by the patient.

> Patient: I understand I am to reduce my meal portions and avoid all sweet desserts to bring my diabetes under control.
> Husband: Do you recommend that all of us in the family change our diets?
> Clinician (to Husband): How do you feel about that?
> Husband: I feel I should, to support my wife, but I'm also afraid I'll end up resenting that I have to give up foods I really like.
> Patient: I don't expect you to do that.
> Clinician: Many aspects of your wife's diet are part of good nutrition, so you may want to use this as an opportunity to change some of your family's eating habits. But, it is very important that family members not sacrifice too much or, you're right, resentments will build. You and your wife can be creative and find alternative foods for her to eat when the rest of the family wants dessert.
> Husband: I understand. We'll work on this together. Her well-being is important to all of us.

Community support groups (e.g., Alcoholics Anonymous or Weight Watchers) also can be effective in maintaining patient motivation for healthy behaviors.

Resistance occurs when the clinician and the patient or family become involved in a struggle over treatment. This struggle may be obvious, with explicit disagreement over the treatment plan, or the struggle may be covert (i.e., the patient may not be improving and the clinician may be unaware that the patient or family disagrees with the treatment plan and is not fully implementing it). In the following example, there are hints from the husband that he is not fully supportive of the treatment plan and will leave its implementation solely to his wife.

> Patient: I understand I am to reduce my meal portions and avoid all sweet desserts to bring my diabetes under control.
> Clinician (to Husband): How do you feel about that?

> Husband: I don't like it, but I guess she has to do what the doctor says.
>
> Clinician: It is very important to get your wife's diabetes under better control. Losing weight is the most important thing she can do for her health.
>
> Husband: That's up to her.

When working with resistant patients or family members, there is a strong tendency to believe that lack of collaboration results from lack of information or misunderstanding. As a result, when a patient does not do as we ask, we may talk louder and longer, going over and over the same information about the same treatment plan.

> Patient: Well, Doc, I've been trying to watch my sweets, but my sugar just keeps going up and up.
>
> Clinician: Perhaps you should meet with the dietician again to review your diet.
>
> Patient: I've already seen her three times. I'm not sure it's helping.

When the patient education has clearly been discussed and seemingly agreed upon, it is reasonable to assume that "more of the same" is unlikely to be helpful, and that the patient or family may now be showing a lack of agreement or willingness to participate in the treatment plan as it is currently constructed (12).

> Patient: Well, Doc, I've been trying to watch my sweets, but my sugar just keeps going up and up.
>
> Clinician: Has it been difficult trying to watch your sweets?
>
> Patient: Well, to tell you the truth, Doc, my mother had diabetes. She had an occasional dessert on the side and she lived to a ripe old age. I'm her daughter, so I assume I can do that too. I just can't give up everything I enjoy.
>
> Clinician: I certainly wouldn't want that, either. Let's study your diabetes to see how much it is like your mother's and in what ways it is different. Because your sugars are up, we have to be concerned that you can't get away with this as easily as your mother did. I'd like you to keep a diary for the next 2 weeks. Record what you eat every day, including the occasional sweets, and record your sugars. That way we can tell just how much you can treat your diabetes as your mother did. If there is a problem, then we'll need to talk about how we can help you enjoy yourself and give yourself special treats that aren't sweet. Maybe we could have your family come in and help us on that one.
>
> Patient: I hope it doesn't come to that, Doc, but I guess I have to "face the music."

One common scenario that results in mysterious patient resistance occurs when the "customer" (i.e., the person most motivated and interested in treatment) is not the patient (12). For example, the customer in a well-child check is most commonly a parent or grandparent. When a middle-aged man comes in for a complete physical, the customer may be the man, but it is often his wife, who may be concerned that he is "working too hard." An adolescent with vague complaints may only be in the office because of parental pressure. In general, collaboration is easiest when the customer is directly involved in treatment. Resistance may occur when the patient and the customer are not the same person, and the clinician is unaware of that.

> Dr: How may I help you today?
> Patient: I've come in for a physical.
> Dr: Has something particular prompted you to get a physical at this time?
> Patient: Oh, my wife's father died of a heart attack when he was about my age. My wife wants me to get my "ticker" checked out.
> Dr: What do you think about this?
> Patient: I think my wife's a worry-wart. My heart's just fine. I run a mile every day.
> Dr: Why don't we go ahead and check you out, and maybe your wife could join us for the discussion of the results.
> Patient: That's a good idea, doc. She won't necessarily believe what I say.

In this case, the customer was the patient's wife. Both she and the patient are likely to benefit from direct contact with the clinician to discuss the results of the patient's evaluation.

Another common source of resistance occurs when the clinician has not assessed the patient's motivation for change, and his or her family's motivation to support that change. A clinician frequently may view change as desirable (e.g., smoking cessation), but the patient is not motivated to make the change. These different points of view can result in actively negative, or passively aggressive, struggles between clinician and patient. As we have seen in previous vignettes, family members can play significant roles in either supporting or undermining healthy behaviors or compliance with a difficult treatment plan.

Prochaska's stages of change (13, 14) (i.e., precontemplation, contemplation, preparation, and action) provide a model for assessing a patient's motivation to change health behaviors (see Table 6.1 for a description of these stages). The goal for a clinician is to elicit the patient's and family's motivation to change risky health behaviors. This involves assessing their current motivation for change, and collaborating with them to see if they want to move to the next stage. The assumption that the patient is in charge of any change, and that the clinician functions as coach when the patient is motivated to change his or her behavior, is fundamental to this approach. For a clinician to try and motivate a patient to action (e.g., Clinician: "I'd like you to stop smoking") when that patient is in the precontemplation stage (e.g., Patient: "Smoking is one of the few pleasures I have in life. I

TABLE 6.1. Stages of motivation for change

Stage	Description
Precontemplation	No plan to change
Contemplation	Plan to change in future (6 months)
Preparation	Plan to change in near future (1 month)
Action	Recent positive change (within 6 months)
Maintenance	Lasting positive change (more than 6 months)

Source: Prochaska J. Prescribing the stages and levels of change, *Psychotherapy* 1991; 28:463–468. Reprinted with permission.

don't want to change that") is a prescription for resistance from the patient and frustration for the clinician. (In this circumstance, the clinician may actually want to contract with the patient *not* to bring up discussion of behavior change for some period of time. This approach acknowledges the power that the patient actually has in his or her own health, and will either result in no change or in the patient moving from precontemplation to contemplation as he or she takes charge of the problem, rather than the clinician.) A collaborative approach allows the clinician to assess the patient's motivation for change and to construct a collaborative and realistic plan for change when patient motivation increases.

Clinicians always consider the influence and resources of the family in family-oriented primary care. Family members can be an important resource and support with behavior change (e.g., when a wife changes the family meals because her husband needs to lower his cholesterol); however, families can also provide disincentives for change (e.g., when a spouse refuses to stop smoking in the face of her partner trying to stop after a diagnosis of chronic obstructive pulmonary disease). For these reasons, any assessment of a patient's motivation for change is incomplete without understanding the impact of family members and significant others (see the Protocol at the end of this chapter for a list of questions corresponding to each stage of change).

Finally, the clinician may experience resistance to treatment when he or she does not fully understand the meaning of the symptom to the patient or the family. The patient's and his or her community's beliefs about the behavior, the meaning they give to it, and the rewards that it offers underlie any resistance or motivation for behavior change. As discussed in Chapter 1, in addition to causing pain or hardship, some symptoms or illnesses may also serve some adaptive function for the patient. In these cases, the patient may fear at some level that giving up the symptom may be more painful than having the illness. This is a frequent problem with patients on disability or children who are school phobic. The clinician needs to assess whether the gain from the illness is greater than the fear of what the treatment might bring. A woman who believes that her workaholic husband pays attention to her when she is ill may similarly be quite ambivalent, consciously or unconsciously, about carefully following medical recommendations for treatment. These cases are certainly not routine; however, when a patient or family's resistance to treatment persists, it is useful to explore the risks of a cure for this patient (e.g., "How would your life change if suddenly, overnight, you were cured of this problem?" "How would your significant relationships change?") It can be helpful in this situation for the patient and family to examine whether the cure is worse than the illness. Treatment then can either proceed, be changed, or be discontinued without ambivalence being expressed indirectly through not complying with the clinician's recommendations.

> Dr: Jane, I just don't understand why your sugars are so high. I am well aware that you understand the regimen you are supposed to be following. And I know you're a bright girl. Perhaps there's something we don't understand about your situation.
>
> Jane: I don't know, Doc. It's a mystery to me.
>
> Dr: I wonder what would happen if suddenly, overnight, you were cured and no longer had to deal with this diabetes.
>
> Jane: It would be heaven, Doc. All my problems would be solved.
>
> Dr: I wonder how it would change your relationship with your parents?
>
> Jane: Well, I guess they would have to interfere in some other part of my life.
>
> Dr: So, treating your diabetes is one area right now that you and your parents struggle over. They try to tell you what to do, and you are determined to do it your way.
>
> Jane: That's right. It's my body.
>
> Dr: You do it your way, even it if it's occasionally bad for you?
>
> Jane: Well, maybe.
>
> Dr: How about if I invite your parents in to discuss your diabetes? Perhaps we could find a way for you to be in charge while still reassuring them you are going to be okay.

In this example, treatment for diabetes in a teenage girl has become intertwined with her struggle for independence from her parents. She feels intruded upon and rebels when they advise or chide her about taking care of herself. Trying to manage the treatment without understanding what function it has come to serve in this family is likely to fail.

Clear recognition of what one does and does not have control over as a clinician is fundamental to establishing collaborative relationships with patients. Even though we can offer advice, prescribe medications, recommend treatment, and be persuasive with our patients, in the end we can only directly change ourselves. Our patients have the right and ability to choose how to participate in what we recommend. In the process of treatment, then, we must focus on our own behavior (e.g., on connecting with our patients and those closest to them, on structuring the interview in the most useful way, on having the strongest treatment plan possible, and on using the patient's and family's strengths and resources to help the patient heal). This will no doubt decrease our frustration and promote our own job satisfaction.

Clinicians' Contributions to Resistance

Clinicians' personal experiences can be humanizing and can result in increased empathy for patients and a wider range of strategies for patient care (15) (see Chap. 26); however, unresolved personal issues can negatively affect our ability to see patients clearly and to function optimally. This interference in clinician functioning is the clinician's contribution to resistance and can come from many sources. Cases may resemble our own current family situations in ways that cloud our judgment. For example, a clinician whose father just died of a sudden myocardial infarction may begin sending many more patients for catheterization and argue strongly with patients who object. Patient situations also may recapitulate our own unresolved family-of-origin issues (16, 17). For example, a clinician whose mother was alcoholic may become unusually angry when dealing with alcoholic patients. Less exotic problems (e.g., fatigue, illness, and general energy level) can affect our ability to think clearly when a patient appears resistant to what we feel is clearly the correct medical course. Interactions with patients seen early in a given afternoon may influence us in ways that affect our treatment of patients seen later that afternoon (18).

A patient's or family member's behavior sometimes so offends a clinician's sense of values that the clinician has difficulty forming or maintaining an alliance, or developing any understanding of that person's offensive behavior. Cases of physical or sexual abuse, or other criminal activity, are common examples of situations many clinicians find challenging in forming good working alliances with the patients involved. Even a mild suspicion of such problems, or some other circumstance that breaches the clinician's own code of ethics, can contribute to difficulties in building therapeutic relationships between the doctor and the patient and family.

> Dr. R. was a Ashkinazi Jewish woman active in the feminist movement who enjoyed her obstetrical practice. She was very supportive and capable of guiding women through the physical and emotional challenges of pregnancy, labor, and delivery.
> Mrs. Hernandez came to see Dr. R. at 18 weeks of pregnancy. She spoke broken English because she just moved to this country from Puerto Rico after meeting her husband, becoming pregnant by him, and then marrying him rather quickly. The pregnancy went along smoothly, though Mrs. Hernandez was clearly stressed by all the changes she had encountered in such a short period of time. Dr. R. saw her frequently and tried to be as supportive as possible.

At 36 weeks, Mrs. Hernandez came in complaining that she was having some light intermittent bleeding that seemed to occur after her husband insisted they have intercourse. Upon questioning, Mrs. Hernandez acknowledged to Dr. R. that she did not want to have sex at this point with her husband, but that he disregarded her feelings. Dr. R. had met Mr. Hernandez only briefly, but felt his behavior was reprehensible and unacceptable. She took out a prescription pad and wrote out a prescription stating Mrs. Hernandez was to engage in no sexual intercourse until after delivery for medical reasons.

Mr. Hernandez had been vocal about his reluctance to attend his child's birth, but he was in the room when Dr. R. walked in to do the delivery. She felt herself bristle as she thought of how Mrs. Hernandez described his earlier behavior. Mr. Hernandez did not change Dr. R.'s impression as he spent the next few hours laughing inappropriately and making wisecracks while his wife endured her labor pains. He made it especially clear that this baby was to be a boy named after him. No girls' names were even considered. Dr. R. was very cool and did not speak to him at all, continuing her supportive relationship with Mrs. Hernandez.

Mr. Hernandez left the room during the last hour of labor. He re-entered just as the baby was delivered: a girl. Dr. R. continued to address only Mrs. Hernandez and the baby, telling the child: "You have such a nice mommy. She's going to take very good care of you." The next morning on rounds, Dr. R. found Mrs. Hernandez somewhat depressed saying her husband had not yet visited, and she knew he wouldn't have left the hospital if the baby had been a boy.

Dr. R. later discussed this experience with a colleague. She wondered how joining could ever occur with someone so obnoxious. The colleague raised several questions that helped her reconsider the situation: What motivated Mr. Hernandez's obnoxious behavior? What role did anxiety, insecurity, and cultural values play in the scenario? In the end, would some alliance between the clinician and the father have been helpful to the patient?

In this situation, Dr. R. struggled with her own sense of values, and her commitment and responsibility to help her patients. Discussing the father with a colleague made her realize that she had an incomplete understanding of him and of his relationship with her patient. Avoiding contact with him probably did not help to protect her patient or to facilitate a healthier bond between him and his wife, or between him and his new daughter. Strong negative feelings about patients or family members signify important information about the patient, the clinician, or both, and they deserve a discussion with a trusted colleague.

Finally, interactions with colleagues can play an important role in how we treat certain patients, and how we take care of ourselves. Some cases brew controversy. If consultants are drawn into a struggle and become divided over the case, clinician difficulty as well as patient resistance can intensify rather than decrease. For example, an oncologist may wish to give a 5-year-old with a malignant brain tumor every possible treatment available, even when the side effects of the treatment are severe and the prognosis is not affected. The child's primary care clinician in this situation may wish to consider stopping invasive treatments when the child appears certain to die. Because of his long-standing relationship with the family, they look to him for advice about treatment. In such intensely emotional situations as this, struggles between consultants and a primary care clinician are common and can mimic the ambivalence the family has over whether to continue treatment.

Family-systems consultations and Balint groups offer some of the best solutions to "clinician resistance." Family-systems consultations can occur when a clinician has a systems-oriented colleague who is willing to trade consultations with difficult families. It is rare that another clinician does not see a patient or family differently, enabling some new approach to treatment (19). Balint groups are also important vehicles for clinicians to examine their own reactions to patients among trusted colleagues (20, 21). Every primary care provider needs to have a system for dealing with the inevitable personal issues stimulated by our work. This process allows for the most creative and useful treatment to occur. It also allows challenging patients to facilitate our own growth, both personally and professionally.

References

1. Kaplan SH, Gandek B, Greenfield S, Rogers W, & Ware JE: Patient and visit characteristics related to physicians' participatory decision-making style, *Medical Care* 1995;**33**:1176–1187.
2. Leopold N, Cooper J, & Clancy C: Sustained partnerships in primary care, *J Fam Prac* 1996;**42**:129–137.
3. Stewart MA: Effective physician–patient communication and health outcomes: a review. *Can Med Assoc J* 1995;**152**:1423–1433.
4. DiMatteo MR: Health behaviors and care decisions: an overview of professional–patient communication. In: DS Gochman (Ed): *Handbook of Health Behavior Research*. New York: Plenum Press, 1997.
5. Minuchin S, Fishman C: *Family Therapy Techniques*. Cambridge, MA: Harvard University Press, 1981.
6. Sullivan HS: *Schizophrenia as a Human Process*. New York: WW Norton, 1962.
7. Marvel K, Epstein R, Beckman HB, & Frankel RF: Soliciting the patient's agenda: have we improved? *JAMA* 1999;**281**:283–287.
8. Levinson W, Roter DL, Mullooly JP, Dull VT, & Frankel RM: Physician–patient communication: the relationship with malpractice claims among primary care physicians and surgeons. *JAMA* 1997;**227**:553–559.
9. Neill J, Kniskern D (Eds): *From Psyche to System: The Evolving Therapy of Carl Whitaker*. New York: Guilford Press, 1982.
10. Campbell T, Patterson J: The effectiveness of family interventions in the treatment of physical illness. *J Marital Fam Ther* 1995;**21**:545–584.

11. Doherty W, Baird M: *Family Therapy and Family Medicine*. New York: Guilford Press, 1983.
12. Watzlawick P, Weakland J, & Fisch R: *Change*. New York, WW Norton, 1974.
13. Prochaska J: Prescribing the stages and levels of change. *Psychotherapy* 1991;**28**:463–468.
14. Botelho R: Beyond Advice: 1. Becoming a Motivational Practitioner & 2. Developing Motivational Skills. 2002, www.MotivateHealthyHabits.com.
15. Candib L, Steinberg G, Bedinghaus J, Martin M, Wheeler R, Pugnaire M, et al.: Doctors having families: the effect of pregnancy and child-bearing on relationships with patients. *Fam Med* 1987;**19**: 114–119.
16. Crouch M: Working with one's own family: another path for professional development. *Fam Med* 1986;**18**:93–98.
17. Mengel M: Physician ineffectiveness due to family-of-origin issues. *Fam Syst Med* 1987;**5**:176–190.
18. Seaburn D, Harp J: Sequencing: the patient caseload as an interactive system. *Fam Syst Med* 1988;**6**:107–111.
19. McDaniel SH, Campbell T, Wynne L, & Weber T: Family systems consultation: opportunities for teaching in family medicine. *Fam Sys Med* 1988;**6**: 391–403.
20. Balint M: *The Doctor, His Patients and the Illness*. New York: Internatonal Universities Press, 1957.
21. McDaniel S, Bank J, Campbell T, Mancini J, & Shore B: (1986) Using a group as a consultant. In: Wynne L, McDaniel S, & Weber T (Eds) *Systems Consultation: A New Perspective for Family Therapy*. New York: Guilford Press, 1986.

Protocol: How to Help Patients Change Risky Health Behaviors**

Principles

1. Discover the meaning of the behavior to the patient and family (e.g., "What does smoking mean to you right now?" "To you partner?").
2. Support the patient's autonomy (e.g., "It's your decision").
3. Find out what the patient is considering or doing currently (e.g., "Have you considered stopping smoking recently?").
4. Solicit family support for the change, wherever possible (e.g., "Why not bring your partner in next time to talk about how she might support you in this?").
5. Offer professional support or help in moving to the next stage of change (e.g., "How can I help you with this?").
6. Encourage the patient to set specific goals (e.g., "What specific behaviors would you like to change in the next month?").
7. Schedule regular follow-up.

Assessing Motivation for Change

- Have you considered making a change in this risky health behavior?
- What kind of change?
- When?

Questions for Each Stage of Change

Precontemplation

- What are the benefits to you of not changing? Benefits for your family?
- Are there any warning signs that indicate you should change this behavior? Do family members worry you about it?
- What would be some advantages if you decided to change?

Contemplation/Preparation

- How did you decide to do something about this problem?
- Would you like some help?
- What specifically are you going to do to make the change?
- What might make it hard to change? How will you handle these difficulties?
- Who can help you with the change?
- How does your family feel about your plan? Is their involvement helpful or problematic? Would you like to meet with them and me to discuss the planned change?

** *Source*: Prochaska J, 1991. Adapted with permission.

Action/Maintenance

- I'm very impressed by what you've accomplished. How did you make this change?
- What have been the benefits to you of changing your behavior? To your family?
- What might make it hard to maintain the change? How can you deal with these challenges?

7
Family Interviewing Skills in Primary Care: From Routine Contact to the Comprehensive Family Conference

Confering with the family is a fundamental part of family-oriented primary care. Contact with a patient's family often provides new and valuable clinical information for assessment and treatment, and it usually serves to build a stronger relationship between the patient and the clinician. For those without guidance or training, however, walking into an exam or hospital room containing more people than just the patient can make one's heart sink. Their presence immediately introduces complexity into the time-pressured practice of primary care. For that reason, it is essential to develop good family interviewing skills (i.e., skills that allow the clinician to facilitate and direct a discussion so that the most amount of information can be shared clearly in the least amount of time).

Chapter 4 described techniques that allow the clinician to gather relevant family information from an individual during the routine visit. This chapter will focus on the multiple-person interview. These interviews can occur informally (e.g., when a family member visits a hospitalized patient and wishes to understand his or her medical condition or when a spouse accompanies a patient to an office visit to report on concerning symptoms. The more extensive family interview can occur when the clinician decides to call a family conference or family meeting. A family conference may involve family assessment (see Chap. 3) to understand the family's contribution to the problem and its solution, information garnered from family members about symptoms, information shared with family members to arrive at a mutually agreeable treatment plan, and so on (see Chap. 5 for a complete description of when a clinician may want to convene the family). Several studies have determined the usefulness of the family conference to the physician (1) and to the patient and family (2). Patients report that they are most interested in family meetings with their doctor when they have a hospitalization, a new diagnosis for serious illness, or depression (3).

Much has been recommended and written about seeing the family together in a medical setting (4–6); however, the pragmatics of family interviewing are rarely specified. That is the purpose of this chapter. We will begin with some principles for family interviewing in common, day-to-day practice. These are principles to be used when a family member accompanies a patient to a routine visit. They are important when families are known to the clinician, as well as when the clinician meets them for the first time. They also provide the foundation for a more extensive family assessment or family conference. After describing these basic principles, we then offer a concrete, step-by-step guide to the family conference in a healthcare setting. When necessary, these more extensive interviews can provide important family assessment information that impacts directly on the health of the patient, breaks a deadlock in treatment, or provide essential information to the family about the care of a complex patient. Sections of the comprehensive family conference can be used in brief, frequent routine visits to the office or informal contacts with family members in the hospital.

This guide to family interviewing integrates techniques from a variety of approaches. We draw from both the family therapy literature (7, 8) and the family medicine literature (9–11) to produce a format that addresses the issues involved in interviewing a family in a primary care setting. This guide is not intended as family therapy, or even family counseling. The interview format is generic. It can be used for the diversity of reasons a family meeting is called (e.g., facilitating lifestyle changes, grief work, improvement with compliance, referral, or as a precursor to primary care counseling). It is a blueprint for helping family members communicate about issues of concern to them and to you as their clinician. It draws on the family's resources to establish a collaborative plan between them and the healthcare system.

General Principles for Interviewing Families

General *goals* for interviewing patients and family members, whether in a routine visit or a more extensive family conference, include:

1. Socialize and *develop rapport* with the family; get to know each member; accommodate the interpersonal style of family members; create an environment in which each family member feels safe and supported.
2. Organize the group so that communication is clear; *establish goals* for the interview that are concrete, mutual, and attainable.
3. Gather information and *facilitate discussion* from each person present about the issue of concern; *transmit information* about the medical issues involved, as is appropriate.
4. *Identify strengths, resources, and supports* that are available to the family.
5. Establish a *plan* that allows the family to collaborate with you in addressing the issue(s) of concern.

Once goals are established, the clinician works to create a supportive environment in which the family interview results in increased information for the clinician and the family and a shared plan that increases the likelihood of compliance. It is the clinician's responsibility to ensure that all members are respected and heard. The following Dos and Don'ts allow the clinician to create a context for clear communication among clinician, patient, and family members.

Dos

- Greet and shake hands with each family member.
- Seat the family member(s) beside the patient to allow for easy communication (no one should be sitting on the exam table).
- Affirm the importance of each person's contribution.
- Recognize and acknowledge any emotions expressed.
- Encourage family members to be specific; ask for examples.
- Help family members to clarify their thoughts.
- Maintain an empathic and noncritical stance with each person.
- Emphasize individual and family strengths.
- Block interruptions from others if persistent.
- Note disagreements among family members. If the following simple conflict resolution skills are not successful, consider referring to a family therapist.
    — Clarify in a supportive manner the concerns that underlie each person's position (e.g., "Mrs. Gonzalez, you are opposed to your son taking Ritalin. Can you tell us more about your thoughts on this?").
    — Recognize the feelings underlying strong disagreements (e.g., "Mr Smith, you seem frustrated by how long it is taking to find your father a nursing home bed").
    — Emphasize areas of common interest or concern (e.g., "It is clear that you all have Joey's best interest at heart. You just disagree about what should be done to help him right now").

Don'ts

- Do not let any one person monopolize the conversation. If necessary, interrupt and ask for another person's opinion on the topic.
- Do not allow family members to speak for each other. Encourage each person to offer his or her own point of view on the problem.
- Do not offer advice or interpretations early in an interview, even if asked.
- Do not breach the patient's confidentiality. Allow the individual patient to take the lead on how much of his or her concerns are revealed.
- Avoid taking sides whenever possible. Even when one member has a good point, taking sides will draw you into a family conflict and may render you unable to resolve the conflict.

A Blueprint for the Family Conference

Our guide for a family conference is a compendium of specific tasks designed to accomplish these five goals. It is oriented toward a family interview or a network session of family, friends, and involved professionals, although it can easily be adapted for a couple or a family-oriented individual session. We assume that the major issues around convening the family (i.e., who to ask and how) have already been resolved (see Chap. 5).

We include sections on both preconference preparation and postconference tasks. A successful session depends on attention to information already known about the patient and family that can lead to the development of appropriate goals and strategies for the conference. After the conference, it is likewise important to evaluate whether the goals of the conference were met, and record the information and the treatment plan efficiently in the chart so that treatment can proceed effectively.

See Table 7.1 for an outline of the stages involved in a family conference. Although the phases are clearly demarcated, and may even be assigned approximate time frames for efficient pacing, the actual process of conducting a family conference demands a good measure of sensitivity to the natural flow from one phase to another. Phases can overlap or take place concurrently in an actual session. The sensitivity and flexibility required to adjust to the various tasks develops as clinicians gain more experience in working with families.

Steps for Conducting a Family Conference

Preconference Tasks

Set the Stage

The goal of this first phase of preconference preparation is to make contact with the patient and family and to plan for the family conference. This planning may occur as the result of a concern expressed during a regular patient visit or may be initiated during a phone conversation.

1. Choose your contact person.

It is important to choose the appropriate contact person because this person will set up the conference successfully or unsuccessfully. The contact person typically should be the patient if he or she is a capable adult. If not, the contact person may be a patient's son or daughter (i.e., if the patient is elderly and mentally incompetent) or some other responsible party.

TABLE 7.1. Stages of the family conference

Preconference Tasks
1. Set the stage
2. Review the genogram
3. Develop hypotheses

Conference Tasks
Phase 1. Greeting
Phase 2. Clarify and further develop goals
Phase 3. Discuss the problem or issue(s)
Phase 4. Identify resources
Phase 5. Establish a plan

Postconference Tasks
1. Revise the genogram
2. Revise the hypotheses
3. Document the meeting in the patient's chart

2. Establish a rationale.

The conference can be for the purpose of discussing the prognosis for an illness, gathering information, providing support to a family coping with a difficult illness, answering questions, or any reason why a clinician might want to communicate with a family or a family with a clinician.

The stated rationale should be clear, purposeful, and nonthreatening to the contact person and the family (e.g., "I'd like to meet with the rest of the family, the people most important to you, to discuss the dietary changes necessary with your type of diabetes").

3. Establish who in the patient's network will attend.

Help the patient identify family, friends, and other involved professionals who are relevant to the issue of concern. Make it clear that people other than family members are welcome.

4. Clarify with the patient what may be discussed in the conference.

It is important to reach agreement with the patient prior to the family meeting about what will and will not be discussed so that no breaches of confidentiality occur. For example, a man who had just had a myocardial infarction agreed to a family meeting to discuss his health and necessary lifestyle changes with his wife and adult children. He told his physician and his wife, however, that he did not want the couple's marital struggles discussed during the meeting.

5. Set the appointment.

Ask your secretary to mail a reminder or call the relevant parties (see Chap. 5 for suggestions regarding convening the family).

Review the Genogram

The goal of this second phase of preconference preparation is to review what is currently known about the patient and his or her family with regard to the issue of concern.

1. Prepare or revise the genogram.

Based on information in the chart and your contact with the patient, prepare or revise to genogram. The genogram should represent the most up-to-date picture of the patient and the family. Information depicted should include names, ages, marital status, children, households, significant illnesses, dates of such traumatic events as deaths, and occupations. It can include emotional closeness, distance, or conflict between members, significant relationships with other professionals, and any other information you deem important to the case. Putting together a genogram may reveal repeating dysfunctional emotional patterns, common medical problems, and other important considerations in the process of evaluation and treatment planning (see Appendix 3.1 for a summary of standard genogram symbols). McGoldrick, Gerson, and Shellenberger (12) give a complete review of standard symbols, as well as helpful hints in creating and revising genograms.

2. Note the patient and family's life cycle stage.

The family life cycle stages give a framework for predicting individual and family developmental issues that may influence the symptom or issue of concern (13) (see Table 3.1 for a description of the family life cycle stages).

It is important to identify at least three generations and note their developmental issues. For example, the family of a man recovering from a myocardial infarction may be facing the following life cycle issues:

patient—contemplating retirement
wife—going through menopause
teenage son—leaving home for college
couple—"empty nest" syndrome
patient's   mother—failing   health,   nursing   home   placement   being
   considered.

Develop Hypotheses

The goal of this third phase of preconference preparation is to develop initial hypotheses about the issue of concern and how the family is functioning to deal with the concerns. These hypotheses will help guide the exploration of issues in the family conference.

1. Set your own goals for the interview.

For example, in a family conference held just after the death of a family patriarch, goals might be to answer remaining medical questions, to facilitate the grieving process for the survivors, and to support the new leaders in the family. In a family conference held to assess the treatment of a non-compliant juvenile diabetic, goals might be to assess the functioning of the parents with regard to the medical regime, assess the relative independence of the adolescent from his parents, review other stressors in the household, and complete any necessary patient or family education about diabetes.

2. Develop tentative hypotheses.

These hypotheses which are to be tested in the meeting, will be expanded and revised as new information is gathered throughout treatment.

   a. Begin with the life cycle stage of the family, relevant and current medical problems, and the issue of concern.
   b. Build hypotheses using such other data as the emotional tone con-veyed by the contact person (e.g., flat affect after a death) or your knowledge of how a family has dealt with similar issues in the past (e.g., excellent coping early in a crisis followed by a deterioration in functioning). An example might be hypothesizing an acute grief reac-tion in a middle-aged man with chest pain and no biomedical findings when the symptoms occurred soon after the funeral of his best friend.
   c. Hypotheses are typically generated after setting the appointment with the contact person. With a particularly difficult patient or family, you may wish to sit down, review the chart, and develop hypotheses before inviting the family in.

3. Develop a strategy for conducting the conference.
   a. Include specific questions, observations, or tasks that will facilitate data-gathering and help test the hypotheses. The strategy will help prevent muddled thinking and drifting about in the session.
   b. Once you have developed initial hypotheses and a working strategy, be careful to remain open to information that supports alternative hypotheses and to the unique needs of this particular family.
   c. With a particularly difficult family, consider asking a family therapist or other mental health professional to join you in conducting the meeting.

Five Phases of a Family Conference

Phase 1. Greeting (approximately 5 minutes). The goal of this first phase of the family conference itself is to welcome the family, get to know them better, build rapport, and help them become comfortable in the setting of the conference.

1. Greet the family.
   a. Introduce yourself. Shake hands and greet each person attending the meeting. Use formal names for adults unknown to you; be sure

to greet and make contact with all children attending, regardless of age.

b. Invite family members and others to sit where they wish. This information may be used to hypothesize about who is close to whom, and so on.

2. Orient the family to the room.

a. Inform them of any colleagues behind an observation mirror or students sitting in on the conference.

b. Show children where toys or blackboards are located.

c. If you are audio or videotaping, show the equipment to the family and obtain permission from adult members.

3. Talk with each family member.

a. Begin by briefly introducing the agenda for the meeting. This is a restatement of the rationale used in convening the family (e.g., "We are here today to discuss your father's death".)

b. For family members who are not yet known to you, follow this with the comment: "It would help me if I first got some more information about each of you. Please tell me a little about yourself, how you are related to the patient and involved with the illness." It is very important *not* to delve into problem identification, problem-solving, or expression of important feelings prior to the completion of this first phase.

c. Request demographic information from each of them such as their age, work/school activity, education, length of marriage, and so on. Try to find something in each person that is interesting. Attend to and reflect individual and family strengths. Take the opportunity to be human and generally less intimidating to the family. This section of the interview can be brief, if there are a number of people in the room, or more extended, if the family member is obviously reluctant or nervous about the meeting.

d. While talking to the family, remember to give special attention and respect to the adult leaders or spokesperson for the family. Make special efforts to engage those in the family who are unknown to you, distant, or uncomfortable.

e. Note each family member's language and nonverbal behavior. Attempt generally to match this style and language in as natural a way as possible to facilitate communication (without being patronizing).

f. For some families who are especially large or especially uncomfortable, this phase may need to be expanded to 10 minutes, perhaps spending less time on the problems or the plan (e.g., when you have not met a family before, when you suspect family members may worry you will side with the patient against them, or when someone feels blamed).

g. This phase may be shortened, but not overlooked; if all members of the family are already well known to you, brief follow-up questions to previous conversations help demonstrate a commitment to the relationship over time.

h. Thank the group for coming to discuss the issue at end. Recognize the commitment and strength shown by the family in being willing to come and help the patient or solve the problem at hand.

Phase 2. Clarify and further develop the goals (approximately 5 minutes). The purpose of this second phase of the family conference is to clarify the reason for the meeting and establish the group's agenda for the session.

1. Ask the group, "What would you like to make sure we accomplish today?" Solicit ideas from each person who wishes to speak.

2. Translate each goal so it is clear, concise, and realistic. (e.g., "Today we'll focus on Donna's recent depression and how we can all help her," or, "Today we've agreed to focus on your upcoming move and how to handle your son's diabetes, given the new situation.")

3. It is sometimes useful to write the goals up on an easel or blackboard so everyone can see and participate.

4. Propose any goals you feel are important that the family has not mentioned. Be careful not to propose goals the family is not yet ready to deal with. Take your cue from the family's goals and their reactions to your suggestions.

5. Set priorities among the goals. If there are more than two or three, suggest the other goals be addressed at a later time.

6. Note any conflict among the goals mentioned. When peoples' goals converge, the group can move on to a problem-solving phase. When they are widely divergent, time must be spent to resolve these differences or to agree to disagree. If the latter, it is usually best to focus a first conference on the biomedical condition of the patient and on less-conflictual goals in order to build the trust necessary to manage the more conflictual topic at a later meeting. For example, a family met to discuss their mother's refusal to be hospitalized after a myocardial infarction. The first conference focused on her medical condition, and developing an understanding of the mother's view of her illness. By the end of the meeting, a plan was devised balancing the mother's need for independence with her and her children's desire for her to live a longer life. A second meeting was held, from which the mother excused herself, for the adult children to work on the many arguments they had amongst themselves as a result of conflict over their mother's behavior and her healthcare.

Phase 3. Discuss the problem or issue(s) (approximately 15 minutes). The goal of this third phase of the conference is to exchange information with the family.

1. Solicit each participant's view of the issue or the problem.

a. Allow the family to discuss their shared concerns or differences with each other (e.g., "Family members often have different views about what the problem is. Today I would like to hear from each of you about how you see the problem").

b. Address each member of the family, usually beginning with the adult who appears most distant to the issue at hand (e.g., with a child behavior problem, you might address the father first because you have not had contact with him to date about this and because the mother has complained he is uninvolved with the child).

c. Help family members to be more concrete and specific by asking such questions as, "How is this a problem for you?" or "When did this first become an issue?"

d. Explore the involvement of others in this issue: "Who has given you advice about this problem?" or "What is it, and what do you think of their advice?" Include questions about previous treatments and other professionals involved.

e. Ask about other recent changes in the family that could impact on the issue of concern (e.g., moves, illness, death, occupational shifts, marriages, divorces, or births). While keeping focused on the issue at hand, be aware of changes in the family system that influence and are influenced by the presenting concern.

f. Observe repetitive family interactional patterns: Who talks first? Who contradicts whom? Who provides leadership? Final treatment plans should not go against these patterns, unless specifically planned for and negotiated.

2. Encourage the family and the patient to ask any questions they might have of you.

Use this time to share any other information the family needs to have.

3. Ask how the family dealt with similar problems or issues in the past, drawing from the successes and noting past problems to be avoided.

Phase 4. Identify resources (approximately 10 minutes). The goal of this fourth phase of the conference is to recognize the available resources to bring to bear on the issue(s) of concern.

1. Identify family resources and strengths.
   a. List family members and friends that are available to the patient.
   b. Ask participants to volunteer strengths they perceive in the patient and the family. "It is clear to me that, even though you are stressed right now, this is a family with strengths and talents. What do you feel this family (and/or this patient) does really well?"
   c. Record the strengths on an easel or a blackboard. The family often resists this exercise out of embarrassment, but it is powerful both because it is supportive and because it can diminish unnecessary or less effective services outside the family.

2. Identify medical resources.
   a. Identify specialists, nursing services, mental health services, and other allied health professionals that might be helpful to the patients or family.
   b. Help the family members to specify clearly their expectations of physicians, medical staff, and other healthcare providers.
   c. Answer any questions and clarify any misconceptions about what can and cannot be provided.
3. Identify community resources (including nutritional services, visiting nurse, homemaker services, community support groups, etc.).

Phase 5. Establish a plan (approximately 10 minutes). The purpose of this last phase of the conference is to develop a mutually agreed upon treatment plan, and to clarify each person's role in carrying out the treatment plan.

1. At the end of the conference, ask the family about what they believe should happen next.
2. Contribute any necessary medical information and advice.
3. Emphasize those issues that represent common ground.

Negotiate compromises where necessary. If contentious issues remain, either schedule another meeting for further discussion or refer the family for a series of counseling sessions to resolve the issues.

4. Negotiate a formal or an informal contract with the family regarding their concerns.

Check for each person's understanding of and involvement with the suggested plan. Have each person repeat back what they will contribute.

   a. Establish what each family member will do.
   b. Clarify what you will do.
   c. Discuss primary care counseling or referral at this point, if relevant.
   d. Make an appointment for follow up, if appropriate. For example, "Today we agreed that Mrs. W. will monitor her own diet with regard to her hypertension. Mr. W. will ask her once a week how she is doing and take her out to a special dinner if she feels she has had a good week on the diet. Joe and Johnny agreed to leave these issues in their parents' hands. Is this correct?"
5. Ask if family members have any questions.
6. Thank everyone for participating and conclude the conference.

Postconference Tasks

Revise the Genogram

Record on the genogram any new information or correct previous misconceptions that emerged in the family conference.

Revise the Hypotheses

Use the information gathered in the family conference to revise and refine the preconference hypotheses and plan for future treatment.

Document the Conference in the Chart

Several family assessment formats suggested for use in primary care can be adapted as outlines for such conference write-ups as the *PRACTICE* form (14) or the Resident Consultation Evaluation Form (10).

Whatever format is chosen, documentation of the family meeting may include:

1. Attendance.
   a. Who attended the session?
   b. Who was important but did not attend, and why?
2. Problem list.
   a. Issues of concern to the family.
   b. Other issues of concern to you.
3. Global assessment of family functioning, including:
   a. Family structure—note family roles, alliances, and coalitions.
   b. The life cycle stage for the patient and the family, and the relevant developmental challenges of those stages.
   c. Family process—note affect and common interactional patterns (see Chap. 3 for an in-depth discussion of concepts involved in assessing family structure, family process, and repetitive behavioral patterns)
4. Family strengths and resources.
5. Treatment plan.
   a. Medical regimen.
   b. The roles to be played by the patient, family members, and professionals.

References

1. Meyer D, Schneid J, & Craigie FC: Family conferences: reasons, levels of involvement and perceived usefulness, *J Fam Pract* 1989;**29**:401–405.
2. Kushner K, Meyer D, Hansen M, Bobula J, Hansen J, & Pridham K: The family conference: What do patients want? *J Fam Pract* 1986;**23**:463–467.
3. Kushner K, Meyer D, & Hansen JP: Patients' attitudes toward physician involvement in family conferences, *J Fam Pract* 1989;**28**:73–78.
4. Doherty W, Baird M: *Family Therapy and Family Medicine.* New York: Guilford Press, 1983.
5. Christie-Seely J: *Working with the Family in Primary Care.* New York, Praeger, 1984.
6. Crouch M, Roberts L (Eds): *The Family in Medical Practice.* New York: Springer Verlag, 1987.

7. Haley J: Conducting the first interview. *Problem-Solving Therapy*. San Francisco: Jossey-Bass, 1987.

8. Weber T, McKeever J, & McDaniel S: A beginner's guide to the problem-oriented first family interview. *Fam Proc* 1985;**24**:357–364.

9. Talbot Y: Families—the "how." The family in family medicine: graduate curriculum and teaching strategies. Kansas City, MO, Society of Teachers of Family Medicine, 1981.

10. McDaniel, S, Campbell T, Wynne L, & Weber T: Family systems consultation: Opportunities for teaching in Family medicine, *Fam Syst Med* 1987;**6**:391–403.

11. Marvel K: Family interviewing: core and advanced skills, Society of Teachers of Family Medicine Annual Conference. Seattle, April 30, 1999.

12. McGoldrick M, Gerson R, & Shellenberger S: *Genograms in Family Assessment*. New York: W. W. Norton, 1999.

13. Carter E, McGoldrick M (Eds): *The Expanded Family Life Cycle: Individual, Family & Social Perspectives* (3rd Edition). New York: Allyn and Bacon, 1999.

14. Christie-Seely J: PRACTICE—a family assessment tool for family medicine. In: *Working with the Family in Primary Care*. New York: Praeger, 1984.

Protocol: Conducting a Family Conference

General Principles for Family Interviewing

Dos

- Greet and shake hands with each family member.
- Seat the family member(s) beside the patient to allow for easy communication (i.e., no one should be sitting on the exam table).
- Affirm the importance of each person's contribution.
- Recognize and acknowledge any emotions expressed.
- Encourage family members to be specific; ask for examples.
- Help family members to clarify their thoughts.
- Maintain an empathic and noncritical stance with each person.
- Emphasize individual and family strengths.
- Block interruptions from others if persistent.
- Note disagreements among family members (e.g., if these simple conflict resolution skills are not successful, consider referring to a family therapist).
  - Clarify in a supportive manner the concerns that underlie each person's position.
  - Recognize the feelings underlying strong disagreements.
  - Emphasize areas of common interest or concern.

Don'ts

- Do not let any one person monopolize the conversation. If necessary, interrupt and ask for another person's opinion on the topic.
- Do not allow family members to speak for each other. Encourage each person to offer his or her own point of view on the problem.
- Do not offer advice or interpretations early in an interview, even if asked.
- Do not breach the patient's confidentiality. Allow the individual patient to take the lead on how much of his or her concerns are revealed.
- Avoid taking sides whenever possible. Even when one member has a good point, taking sides will draw you into a family conflict and may render you unable to resolve the conflict.

Preconference Tasks

1. Set the stage.
    a. Choose your contact person.
    b. Establish a rationale.
    c. Establish who will attend.
    d. Set the appointment.
    e. Clarify with the patient what may be discussed in the conference.
2. Review the genogram.
    a. Prepare the genogram.
    b. Note the family's life cycle stage.

3. Develop hypotheses.
   a. Set your own goals for the interview.
   b. Develop tentative hypotheses about the family and their concerns.
   c. Develop a strategy for conducting the interview.

Five Phases of a Family Conference

Phase 1. Greeting (approximately 5 minutes).
   1. Greet the family.
   2. Orient the family to the room.
   3. Speak with each family member.
Phase 2. Clarify and further develop the goals (approximately 5 minutes).
   1. Solicit goals for the session from each person who wishes to speak.
   2. Make each goal clear, concise, and realistic.
   3. Add any goals you feel are necessary.
   4. Prioritize the goals.
   5. Note any conflict among the goals mentioned.
Phase 3. Discuss the problem or issue(s) (approximately 15 minutes).
   1. Solicit each person's point of view.
   2. Encourage the family to ask questions of you.
   3. Ask how the family dealt with similar past problems.
Phase 4. Identify resources (approximately 10 minutes).
   1. Identify family strengths.
   2. Identify medical resources.
   3. Identify community resources.
Phase 5. Establish a plan (approximately 10 minutes).
   1. Solicit the family's plan.
   2. Contribute any necessary medical information or advice.
   3. Emphasize issues that represent common ground.
   4. Contract with the family regarding their concerns, including referral or reappointment if necessary.
   5. Ask for any remaining questions about the plan.
   6. Thank everyone for participating and conclude the family conference.

Postconference Tasks

1. Revise the genogram.
2. Revise the preconference hypotheses.
3. Document the meeting in the patient's chart, including:
   a. Attendance.
   b. Problem list.
   c. Assessment of family functioning.
   d. Family strengths and resources.
   e. Treatment plan.

8
When Interactions Are Difficult

Why is it that hospital doctors' rounds are scheduled in early morning and family visiting hours occur in the afternoon and evening? Why do tired residents sheepishly note that they sometimes avoid the rooms of a patient with concerned family members?

Families who seem to question our decisions, repeatedly ask questions, or seem angry with us, may be described as "difficult," "high-maintenance," or even "dysfunctional." This labeling may be therapeutic for the clinician in private discussions, but it can interfere with the often taxing but critical work of including families as integral members of the healthcare team. Although we all recognize that families need additional support during illness crises, we sometimes forget that even a routine visit can be stressful. Some people cope with these stresses in ways that seem combative, argumentative, hysterical, or just counterproductive and inefficient. In today's time-pressured environment, we may be tempted to avoid dealing with the people in these situations and prefer to spend time with people who appreciate our efforts. Ultimately, skillful intervention with these difficult interactions may be the most important thing a clinician does to facilitate the health of the identified patient as well as the family.

> Brianna Kervin, a 16-year-old trombone player, came for a well-adolescent visit, accompanied by her father. Dr. Parks wanted to insure that she had sufficient time with Brianna to discuss personal health decisions, so she briefly introduced herself to Brianna's father, and then suggested that he go to the waiting room. About 10 minutes later, a nurse interrupted Brianna's exam and spoke with Dr. Parks in the hall. Mr. Kervin was making a scene in the waiting room, complaining to the receptionist that he was a very busy man, that he did not appreciate how long he had to wait for the exam, and demanded to know how much longer he would have to wait. The receptionist explained that they had a very busy office, that they tried to see patients promptly, but that Dr. Parks wanted to give all patients enough time. Mr. Kervin told the receptionist that her explanation was not adequate, and he did not appreciate having to wait.

Dr. Parks asked the nurse to convey that she would talk with him after his daughter's visit. When the nurse spoke with Mr. Kervin, he seemed to become more angry, and said he had never seen a health office run in such an unprofessional manner. He told her that he did not see why he had been "kicked out" of the visit, but he was now going to leave the office, and return for his daughter in 20 minutes. The nurse returned to the exam room and, outside of Brianna's view, shook her head so that Dr. Parks could see her disgust.

How could this interaction have turned sour? Does it reflect a father with a personality disorder, or a father who was threatened by the private conversation between the doctor and his daughter? Could the father have just been tired, late for a meeting, or angry with Brianna for something else? Did it reflect some insensitivity by Dr. Parks, who may not have given Mr. Kervin enough time during the visit, or was it a misunderstanding of the routine of an adolescent visit? Did Mr. Kervin's frustration reflect an actual extended wait time, or a disrespectful response from Dr. Parks' staff? Any of these hypotheses, or more likely a combination of them, could have led to this outcome. What, if anything, should Dr. Parks do at this point?

As in this example, clinicians are usually surprised by difficult family interactions. They would rather just go about their business, ignore these interactions, and hope they go away. Clinicians tend to focus on the satisfaction of the patient in the room, and do not feel they have time to worry about the discontent of family members; however, if Dr. Parks did not respond in some way when Mr. Kervin returned, the communication between parent, physician, and Brianna would have been compromised. It is likely that Mr. Kervin would not have let Brianna return to the office, or the staff could feel abused and unsupported. It is even possible that a very angry parent could file formal complaints about Dr. Parks. *As clinicians, we ignore difficult family interactions at our own and our patient's peril.*

Poor communication skills not only result in poor relationships but in inadequate healthcare (1). Good communication and clinician–patient relationships may mediate negative patient responses to poor outcomes, and even a willingness to litigate. Levinson and colleagues (2) identified communication styles during routine visits that distinguished primary care physicians who had malpractice claims from those with no claims logged against them. Those without claims educated patients more, used more humor, and checked patient's understanding and opinions more frequently. Beckman et al. (3) studied depositions from settled malpractice suits. They suggested that the decision to litigate was often associated with patient's perceptions that the physicians did not care about the outcome or did not collaborate with them. Even in the majority of cases that do not proceed to litigation, clinician caring and collaboration with patients makes a significant difference in patient satisfaction and willingness to participate in effective healthcare teams.

Dr. Parks fortunately recognized that this situation could not be ignored, and had the receptionist ask Mr. Kervin to meet with her when he returned for his daughter. She brought him into an exam room, where they both sat down. Dr. Parks noted how there seemed to be some misunderstanding about today's visit, which she hoped they could discuss and resolve. She then asked Mr. Kervin to tell her what happened.

He initially complained about how rude the receptionist was, and how it was not clear how long the visit would take. Dr. Parks apologized for the length of his wait. She then asked if there was something she did that contributed. He told her that he felt "dismissed" from Brianna's exam, and embarrassed in front of his daughter. He spoke about how hard it was to get respect as a single parent, especially since Brianna's mother had abandoned the family.

Dr. Parks told him that it was very helpful to hear this, that she could understand how he could have felt that way, and she was sorry for how it happened. She spoke briefly about how important it was for adolescents to take some responsibility for their own healthcare, and her interest in getting to talk with Brianna.

In retrospect she realized that she and Mr. Kervin had not had much time together. Mr. Kervin said he understood, but he was having a hard time with Brianna ignoring and disrespecting him. Dr. Parks normalized this experience in teens, said she was impressed with his daughter and her maturity, and how Brianna seemed respectful of others. She also stated that it was hard when teenagers acted this way to the ones they loved most.

Within only a couple of minutes, the interaction between Dr. Parks and Mr. Kervin became more relaxed as they each realized how the miscommunication had occurred. Dr. Parks asked if she could do something to assist now. Mr. Kervin thought it would be helpful for them to talk in front of Brianna. Dr. Parks explained that she would have normally done that but felt that she should talk with him first. He also said he was sorry he had been so impatient with the receptionist. Dr. Parks acknowledged that the receptionists have a hard job, but understand that patients sometimes get frustrated. Together they returned to the exam room with Brianna and discussed her health. On his way out, Mr. Kervin briefly apologized to the receptionist, who very much appreciated his comments.

Recent literature addresses difficult doctor–patient relationships (4, 5). There is also specific literature dealing with "hateful patients" (6) and acknowledging mistakes (7). Continuing medical education opportunities through the American Academy of Physicians and Patients (www. physicianpatient.org) and the Bayer Institute for Healthcare Communication (www.bayerinstitute.com) enable clinicians to observe themselves and others and attend to medical interviewing skills. Difficult interactions with families are less frequently addressed, even though families are present in many difficult encounters (8), and individual difficulties often reflect family involvement (9). This chapter includes strategies useful when conflict, communication problems, or intense affect threaten an effective clinician–

patient–family relationship or management plan. (see Chap. 16 for discussion of delivering bad news and coping with grief).

General Strategies When Difficult Interactions Occur

In the previous example, Dr. Parks effectively intervened during what could have been a very disruptive clinical encounter. She demonstrated specific responses useful when family members show extreme affect, or disagree with the treatment plan. She also demonstrated some general strategies useful whenever interactions feel difficult.

Recognize Difficulty Early in the Interaction and Actively Plan How to Address It

In any conflict, there is a natural human tendency to try to be right. Clinicians must ask themselves whether it is more important to maintain a therapeutic connection or to prove themselves right. Dr. Parks and her staff worked collaboratively to head off a crisis. The nurse felt comfortable interrupting a visit to describe the interaction between the receptionist and Mr. Kervin. In turn, Dr. Parks felt comfortable that the nurse could respond to Mr. Kervin and arrange a later time to discuss the difficulty. By waiting to meet with Mr. Kervin, Dr. Parks had some time to think about her response.

An interactional approach recognizes that people try to get others to take their sides during conflict. Patients, perhaps inadvertently, may attempt to create an alliance with a healthcare clinician that may compensate for conflict or deficiencies in the patient's family (9). Hahn and colleagues note that these "compensatory alliances" may not be recognized by the physician, but should be considered whenever a difficult interaction occurs. Brianna may have turned her attention to Dr. Parks in ways that mimicked a maternal relationship, and therefore threatened Mr. Kervin's sense of respect as the sole parent. The response to a compensatory alliance is to have direct communication with other family members as early as possible.

Distinguish How Much of the Difficulty Arises from Miscommunication, Disagreements, or Emotional Affect

In a review of malpractice cases, Beckman et al. (3) identified four themes of problem relationships: deserting patients, devaluing patient or family views, delivering information poorly, or not understanding the patient or family perspective. Legitimate mistakes have sometimes occurred, and clinicians need risk management consultations (see Chap. 23). These themes of problem relationships can more frequently guide the clinician's assessment of difficult interactions.

The first of these themes, desertion, may occur if a difficult interaction is not addressed, and the clinician avoids the patient. The remaining three themes reflect poor communication styles, particularly a lack of recognition of the patient and family's perspective. Thus, clinicians need to ask themselves whether they have heard the patient's concerns and ideas, or whether the patient needs more information. In addition, the clinician should consider whether the poor interaction reflects some frustration, anger, or sadness that comes from the experience of the health crisis, or from other family or life experiences. With the Kervin family, the difficult interaction seemed to reflect a lack of information in that Mr. Kervin did not understand why he was "dismissed" from his daughter's exam. As in many clinical situations, however, his frustration was more acute because it mirrored other occasions with his daughter when he felt dismissed and disrespected (see especially Chap. 13 regarding adolescents).

Monitor One's Response as a Clinician and as a Person

It is clear that "taking one's own pulse" is required to defuse difficult interactions. Farber and colleagues (10) describe how physicians must maintain clear boundaries and self-awareness to be able to assist families during the emotional crises of illness. It requires extra effort to listen to our patients during stressful interactions, yet listening may be the most advanced clinical skill that we possess (11).

It is difficult not to respond defensively when we feel attacked or criticized. It is also difficult not to be discouraged when we are working hard to assist families who may not act appreciative. Finally, our own personal histories with illness and loss impact our responses to our patient's experiences (12) (see Chap. 26). It is particularly helpful for clinicians to have trusted colleagues to discuss difficult interactions in ways that allow the healers to consider their roles (13).

Recognize Differences Among Family Members

Although it is tempting to assume that family members respond similarly to one another, each family member reacts uniquely. Certain family members may complain or argue more vehemently than others. It may be easier to work with the most "reasonable" family member, but difficulties will probably continue unless some attempt is made to speak directly with the most dissatisfied family member. It might have been tempting for Dr. Parks, for example, to finish seeing Brianna and not speak again with her father. Even though her interaction with Brianna was satisfactory, Dr. Parks knew that she should give attention to the most dissatisfied family member. When negotiating treatment plans, particularly when a patient is not adhering to a medical regimen, it is important to find whether someone in the family has an idea that is in competition with the clinician's suggestions.

Insure Safety for Patient, Family, Clinicians, and Staff

Some people respond to intense affect or disappointment with violence, either directed at themselves or at others. At all times, the clinician should consider his or her personal safety, as well as the safety of staff and patients. If a clinician is feeling threatened, it is important to involve other people.

Intense affect is sometimes defused when patients are given a little time to calm down. A clinician can say, "I want to talk with you more about this, but I want to have enough time. I'll go check about my schedule (or another patient) and return." If a patient or family member seems very distraught in ways that may be dangerous, clinicians should always make sure that nothing blocks their ability to leave the room. Stressed patients should not feel that they are being restrained, so there should be sufficient physical space between the clinician and the patient. If staff become threatened, they or the clinician should be prepared to call security or police officers.

Have a Low Threshold for Involving Collaborative Colleagues

If interactions are repeatedly difficult, or if a clinician feels that attempts to defuse intense anger are unsuccessful, behavioral health colleagues should be consulted (see Chap. 25). Families can be reassured that the stress of health crises unexpectedly precipitates feelings of anger, sadness, and difficulties among family members. Hospital social workers, family therapists, and psychologists, or other mental health clinicians can be valuable resources and should be involved when interactions continue to be difficult (14).

Addressing Communication Problems

Even though Mr. Kervin exhibited anger and frustration, it was useful to see if his behavior could be accounted for by misunderstanding. People in conflict are often more amenable to negotiation if differences can be attributed to misunderstanding rather than to personality characteristics. It is often easiest first to try to address communication misunderstandings before having to tell someone that they appear angry or sad. The following suggestions are helpful when communication problems occur.

State That You Believe There Is a Communication Problem That Should Be Addressed Before Continuing

It is the clinician's responsibility to acknowledge difficulties (15). Because interactions occur in the clinician's physical space, the clinician should be considered the "host," and is therefore responsible for trying to insure the comfort of patients. Dr. Parks had help from her staff, who warned her of the difficulty. A clinician notices more frequently that a patient seems to be bothered or annoyed during a visit. It is possible, for example, that Mr. Kervin could have the same feelings of being discounted, but might show it by becoming very quiet, or even avoidant, during an interaction. Clinicians have to trust their instincts that something is going awry with an interaction, and also be brave enough to comment about it.

Acknowledge That the Situation Is Stressful and May Require More Time

Communication difficulties generally occur when people do not have sufficient time to explain their position, or are so worried that they cannot listen well to others. As Dr. Parks examined her role, she recognized that the office pace and her concern about sufficient time with Brianna may have led her to be too brief with Mr. Kervin. Families understand this reality, and appreciate a clinician's acknowledgment that they may have been focused on the health problem and less attentive to the worries of relatives.

Ask Family Members How They Understand the Discussion and What Specific Questions They May Have

When Dr. Parks met with Mr. Kervin, she noted that there seemed to be a problem, asked Mr. Kervin's view, and responded to his feelings with empathy and without defensiveness. By asking his opinion first, before she explained her position, she indicated that she was open to his point of view, and not blaming him for the communication problem. When more than one family member is in the room, make sure that each person has an opportunity to express his or her view.

It may be helpful to restate the patient or family perspectives to make sure that all understand. After Mr. Kervin described how he felt dismissed, Dr. Parks said, "I think I understand how you could have felt pushed out. I was focused on your daughter, and did not ask you a lot of questions about what you were concerned about today." Mr. Kervin had an opportunity to agree or clarify, and said, "Well, you didn't exactly push me out, but I felt like I had to leave fast."

Describe What You Understand, and What Specific Questions You Still Have

After patient and family members state their understanding, the clinician can state his or hers. Brevity is important, as is choosing only one or two areas for discussion. This is also an opportunity to move away from the conflict, and on to a new negotiation or plan. Dr. Parks described how she always tries to spend adequate time with teenagers, and that she was probably focused on that at the beginning of their session; however, she also knows how important it is to learn parents' concerns, and she would like to hear more about Mr. Kervin's hopes and concerns about his daughter.

Find Ways to Underline a Relationship of Cooperation and Partnership

Discussions about conflict can be uncomfortable for all participants, and it is helpful to find ways to make it more relaxed. Thank family members for their honesty. Using the relationship that is formed with each family, identify ways to acknowledge their hard work, and ways that we all make errors or have some awkward communication.

Address Concerns and Provide Information, Using Language That Reflects the Family's Understanding

Negotiations with separate family members, as with Mr. Kervin, may be helpful when communication problems persist. As soon as some understanding is reached with the individual, it is best to move back to the entire family for further concerns and information. Once Mr. Kervin and Dr. Parks felt more comfortable with one another, they returned to the room with Brianna. Dr. Parks told them both that Brianna was very healthy, and that she was impressed with Brianna's maturity and commitment to her health. Dr. Parks then asked if either of them had any questions. This allowed Mr. Kervin to mention that Brianna sometimes did not tell him where she was going or when she would be coming home. This allowed a brief discussion of the normal, but difficult, balance between adolescent autonomy and parent concern. Mr. Kervin and Brianna were able to agree that they could do a better job communicating about their expectations and schedules.

Encourage Family Members to Identify Further Communication Problems If They Arise

Some communication difficulties do not resolve with one discussion. The clinician and family members may clarify their viewpoints, but differences may remain. It may be helpful near the end of the encounter to remind families that differences are a normal part of relationships, and that the stress of illness may make differences more apparent. State that you are happy to talk with any of them further if they need more information or want to clarify anything. Some clinicians may utilize a follow-up telephone call, checking about further questions or concerns. Although this will not be chosen by all clinicians, it is very welcomed by families. The comfort

that the clinician shows will either open or close the door to future discus
sions about awkward communication.

Addressing Disagreements About Treatment

> Rachel and Paul Merton, both in their late thirties, had been married for
> 7 years. During the last 4 years, they were treated for infertility and had
> completed five unsuccessful cycles of hormonal treatment and in vitro
> fertilization. Though they received their infertility treatment at a large
> university hospital, they maintained a strong relationship with their
> family physician, Dr. Barnes, seeing him more frequently than might be
> expected for healthy people of their age. At a visit for a suspected
> bronchitis, Dr. Barnes asked Rachel how she was doing with the
> treatments. Rachel told Dr. Barnes that it was really hard lately because
> it seemed that Paul was having second thoughts about continuing with
> the infertility treatment. Dr. Barnes asked if they had discussed their
> decisions with the infertility specialist, and Rachel said that he had told
> them that he continued to be hopeful about their prognosis. Rachel said
> that it seemed that Paul did not understand because he had an 11-year-
> old son from his first marriage.
>
> Dr. Barnes suggested Rachel and Paul might benefit from talking with
> someone about their dilemma, and that he would be willing to meet
> with them. Rachel thanked him for his offer, and said that she would
> talk with Paul. She did not seem optimistic that more talking would help,
> but thought that they would just need more time. Later that week,
> Rachel called and said she and Paul would like to talk with Dr. Barnes,
> but she made it clear that she did not want to be pushed into changing
> her mind.

When a meeting is called specifically to deal with disagreements about
treatment, the clinician has time to prepare and consider potential difficulties. The conflict occurs more frequently during a standard appointment
(e.g., when a grandmother feels that a child should be getting an antibiotic,
even though the clinician thinks it is not necessary). Whether the disagreements are among family members, or between some family members
and the clinician, care will be compromised or reluctantly received. The
following suggestions address these conflicts in ways that preserve respect
for all.

State That There Are Differing Opinions About
How to Proceed and that It Would Be Helpful to
Consider Each of Them

Family members influence patient's decisions. If clinicians do not ask how
others view the situation, they will not know what barriers or conflicts exist

for the patients (8). The clinician should introduce the discussion of treatment goals by making explicit the principles of agency and communion, and of patient autonomy and family support. Dr. Barnes could describe how this situation is not a clearcut decision about someone making independent decisions about their own health, but is a dilemma that affects them both. Dr. Barnes can also use his knowledge of the couple to recognize their respect for each other, and remind them that there are no right answers. From that position, it seems like a good idea to discuss what factors influence each person's decision.

Ask Family Members About Their Understanding of the Treatment and Their Preferences

An evidenced-based review of research concludes that obtaining patient's priorities on important decisions has been related to better outcomes and patient satisfaction for general medical status, breast cancer, peptic ulcer disease, and diabetes (5). Families have often not heard how different members view the illness or treatment (14). A brief discussion of what each person thinks and hopes reveals areas of discrepancy, and allows the clinician to tailor any information. Rachel and Paul were both very informed about the treatment options, but still may have understood the implications differently. As they heard what the other thought, the differences in their preferences made more sense. As with all family interventions, it is useful to gain the perspective of all relevant and important people.

Ask About Other Sources of Advice About Treatment

Families obtain advice from friends, other health professionals, and multiple media sources. Families have access to extensive forms of health education from the internet (16), sources that range from reputable to biased. Clinicians need to convey their interest in all treatments that patients are considering, whether conventional or complementary.

A gracious and nondefensive discussion of a consultant's opinion is very reassuring for families. Families sometimes fear that they could insult their primary clinician if they want more or different information. If a clinician initiates the discussion of a second opinion, he or she demonstrates a willingness to negotiate and facilitate patient agency.

Describe Your Understanding of the Problem and Why You Suggest a Particular Approach

Because the decision was between Rachel and Paul, Dr. Barnes had no particular preference toward the outcome; however, he was concerned that

Rachel believed that continued treatments had increasing possibilities of success. He wanted her to understand that continued treatment was no guarantee of a pregnancy. Rachel described how her goal was to have a baby, and she worried that Paul was less focused because he already was a father. Paul described how he loved his son, but very much wanted a baby with Rachel. He was concerned that she was the one that had to go through the physical and emotional ordeal of further cycles, and he did not want to do that if it was more likely to bring them sadness than a baby. Dr. Barnes was able to comment on their caring for one another, their joint goals of parenthood, and their responses to facing such uncertainty. He also noted that they had both been through a difficult time, and that they might differ in how much longer they each should continue with the strain of uncertainty.

With Differences Articulated, Attempt to Negotiate a Compromise Plan

When Dr. Barnes noted the similarities and care among family members, the differences between them became fewer, and able to be discussed. Discussion allowed Rachel to describe how her comfort about trying two more treatment cycles would outweigh her discomfort if they were not successful. Paul agreed that if there was a determined end date, and if Rachel really understood that they might not have a pregnancy at the end of the process, he was willing to go through more uncomfortable time and support her further.

Quill and Brody (17) have articulated an enhanced autonomy model in which collaboration between physician and patient informs patient choices. They suggest that clinicians share medical facts and personal experiences in a process of mutual exchange so that patients can make informed and comfortable decisions. This same process of information and belief exchange should be extended to discussions with family members who are an integral influence on patient's decisions.

Acknowledge That You May Agree to Disagree

Patients facing difficult decisions can be over- or under-influenced by their health clinicians (17). The information accorded health professionals places them in a position of power over less informed patients (18). Clinicians can attend to the power discrepancy by discussing how they and the patients may disagree. Paul maintained some reluctance about continuing with treatment, but agreed to accept the plan and support his wife. Clinicians may overtly have to demonstrate their willingness to accept patient's plans as a response to an eroding of public trust in physicians and health systems (19).

Agree on a Specific Plan for Follow Up

When people disagree about treatment plans, one meeting may not result in a mutual solution. A meeting generally allows people to share information with one another, identify the issues remaining for negotiation, and have some new information to consider. With any large decision such as Rachel and Paul's, the family should be encouraged to go home and consider their decisions. The clinician should ask how the family wishes to proceed, and create an opportunity for a later, brief meeting. If no meeting seems necessary, the clinician can clarify the time for the next patient visit or request a call to learn the family's decision.

Addressing Anger

> Mrs. Blau, a 63-year-old woman, was proud of her good health, and rarely saw a physician. She came to her primary care physician, Dr. Scala, with complaints of stomach cramping and bloating. Tests unfortunately revealed esophogeal cancer of an advanced stage. Following unsuccessful surgery and radiation, Mrs. Blau was told that her disease was terminal, and she died within 6 months of her first presentation. Throughout her illness, Dr. Scala met with Mrs. and Mr. Blau, and their adult children, to keep them informed, and eventually to involve hospice workers. Perhaps because of the speed of her decline, the family was reluctant to involve hospice, and Mrs. Blau met with hospice workers only during the last 2 weeks of her life. Throughout the 6 months, Mr. Blau was an upbeat, attentive husband, who seemed informed and cooperative with all aspects of Mrs. Blau's care.
>
> Two months after Mrs. Blau's death, Mr. Blau saw Dr. Scala, for episodes of shortness of breath. In the visit Mr. Blau kept his head down, and Dr. Scala worried that Mr. Blau was depressed following the loss of his wife. Dr. Scala stated that Mr. Blau appeared a little down, and he carefully asked Mr. Blau if he wanted to talk about anything. Mr. Blau emphatically stated that he was here to check out his heart, and "he did not need you or any doctor bothering about how he was doing." Dr. Scala did not know what to make of Mr. Blau's response, so he said he did not want to pry, but he wondered why Mr. Blau felt so strongly. Mr. Blau angrily recalled that Dr. Scala should have noticed his wife's cancer earlier, and his bad judgment was probably the reason for her quick death. Dr. Scala did not know how to respond to Mr. Blau's anger, but tried to listen without agreeing that he had made an error.

Though Anger Can Be Intimidating, Acknowledge and Initiate the Discussion of Anger

A patient's expression of anger is an opportunity for clinicians to demonstrate that they are not frightened by intense affect. In a review of literature on difficult patient interactions, Kemp-White and Keller (20) state that anger, when not acknowledged, often continues in future interactions. Because clinicians are powerful people during stressful times, it is common that anger from the illness may be displaced onto the clinician. Anger toward other providers may also be directed to the primary care clinician. It is also possible that the clinician may have a role in the anger, which needs to be considered carefully (see Chap. 23 regarding making mistakes.) As expected, Mr. Blau had significant distress over his wife's death, and may have only been able to express support while he was caring for her. Delayed responses, particularly after loss or acute trauma, are not uncommon.

Listen Carefully to Elicit Family Perspectives About Why Members Are Angry

As human beings, our natural response to anger is defense, and perhaps we might respond with anger. As clinicians, we must remember that the patient's anger may not have much to do with us, even when it is directed at us. This perspective helps the clinician remain nondefensive, and learn the details of the other person's perspective. The clinician needs to make an extra effort to hear their point of view clearly, and to be sure that the patient or family member knows they have been understood. This reflective listening slows down the process, and just by itself goes a long way to resolving the negative affect. The clinician can respond with statements like, "Just to be absolutely sure I understand what you are saying," or, "I think I know where you are coming from, but correct me if I am wrong. I heard you say" This slowing down of the process also gives the clinician time to think and compose him or herself.

Avoid Defensive Explanations or Responses

It is important not to be defensive, but it is also important to give information that our patients desire. After Dr. Scala listened carefully to Mr. Blau, he said, "I'm really sorry that it's so hard. I understand that you have a lot of questions about what happened. Would you like to go over some of them now, or should we wait for another time?" Mr. Blau was interested, so Dr. Scala listened and responded to some of Mr. Blau's concerns. Dr. Scala also reaffirmed how Mr. Blau's anger was normal, and that he would probably be asking the same questions if he had experienced the same loss.

Validate the Experiences and the Feelings of Anger

Anger often reflects the patient's sense that he or she has not been heard. When we hear a patient's view of a story, we often understand why they are angry. Mr. Blau was furious that his wife had died, and he was trying to make sense of a situation that makes no sense. Dr. Scala was able to say that he was sorry that Mrs. Blau had died, and that it was reasonable for Mr. Blau to continue to question how it could have happened, particularly because it happened so quickly. It also was reasonable that Mr. Blau could be angry at those who were involved with Mrs. Blau's care.

Recognize That Empathizing Is Not the Same as Agreeing

With this explanation, Dr. Scala recognized Mr. Blau's anger, but did not agree that he had done anything in error. To do this effectively, clinicians must be able to distinguish between their feelings and a patient's emotional response. Dr. Scala noted that families are sometimes not comfortable meeting with the clinician who reminded them of the sadness of their loss. Dr. Scala said he would like to continue to be Mr. Blau's doctor, and work with him throughout this time of grief. He also understood that Mr. Blau had to make his choice based on his own comfort.

Be Wary of Triangulation with Others Not Present

When anger is present, it is tempting to make sure that we are not the targets of that anger. In so doing, it is common for people to agree with the angry person in ways that move the anger from ourselves to place it elsewhere. Clinicians are not immune from this process. Though we may be relieved that we are not the direct recipient of anger, we should watch that we do not participate in adding to the blame of a colleague or a family member. As Mr. Blau talked more, he said, "I'm also mad at Dr. Singh (the oncologist), who could have told us more about what was going on." Dr. Scala could have been tempted to remain quiet, and in so doing, convey his agreement; instead, Dr. Scala said, "I have no way of knowing whether that could have been different. I do know that Dr. Singh also cared a great deal for your wife, and was saddened by how quickly her disease took over."

Ask If There Is a Way You Can Offer Further Help

As clinicians, we should recognize that listening, clarifying, and providing information are ways that we help. Without recognizing this, it is easy to think that we are not doing enough, and we can extend ourselves in inappropriate ways. It is helpful to ask if there are other ways that we can be of assistance, particularly by facilitating patients to have access to other providers or information. This may also be a time when clinicians choose to follow up with a telephone call. We show our care and concern primarily by a willingness to meet our patients again and to continue to care for them, even when their affect makes us uncomfortable.

Responding to Sadness and Grief

Michael accompanied Ellen during her regular visit for diabetes and hypertension. Ellen and Michael, both in their mid-fifties, had been married for 12 years, and each had grown children from previous relationships. Ellen, as usual, had blood sugars that were slightly elevated, and Ms. Taylor, the physician assistant, spoke with her about minor variations in diet and exercise. Ms. Taylor said that she was happy that Michael was here today, and asked if he had any thoughts on what could change, particularly around their cooking and diet. Michael said that actually Ellen had not been very interested in cooking lately, and he was doing it all himself. Ms. Taylor asked if that was a change, and Ellen said it was, that she just was not interested in much lately, and with no other explanation, began to cry.

Ellen seemed almost as surprised as Ms. Taylor at her tears, which continued, even when her husband passed a tissue. Ms. Taylor waited a moment, and then asked Ellen if she wanted to talk about what was bothering her. Ellen said she was sorry, she did not want to be a burden, but she could not help feeling so sad. She found herself always thinking about her 26-year-old son, who had recently been jailed in a nearby state. Ellen began to sob as she talked, but eventually stopped crying as she went on and told her story.

Acknowledge and Initiate Discussion of Sadness

Many of us fear that we will not know how to respond when patients show strong emotion. Like Ellen, most people begin to modulate their tears or anger when they talk about it. The concern of another sometimes allows the sadness to come forward, as with Ellen's sobs; however, a clinician's care generally helps a patient to feel calmer. Ms. Taylor gently initiated the discussion with Ellen by asking if she wanted to talk. This allows patients to remain "in control" when they are feeling so "out of control."

Listen with Empathy as Family Members Describe Their Sad Feelings

Listening without judgment is a sophisticated skill. Clinicians have the opportunity to be present with patients, and to assist other family members to listen also, particularly those who may be uncomfortable with displays of sadness. Nonverbal behavior is very important at this time. Even passing a tissue, as Michael did, may feel like a signal for the patient to stop crying, unless it is done with some acknowledgment that it is fine to continue.

Validate and Normalize the Sad Feelings

Validation is demonstrated with verbal and nonverbal cues. When the patient has time to describe some sadness, it is helpful to acknowledge that this must be a difficult time. Though clinicians are encouraged to avoid apologizing for anything that could be construed as a medical mistake, this is a time when it can be helpful to say, "I'm sorry that has happened."

Avoid Trying to "Fix the Sadness"

It is very difficult to hear someone's sadness, and not try to make them feel better. Longer-term treatment includes helping patients cope with sadness, but initially clinicians may be most helpful when they simply listen and let patients know they are heard (11, 21). Ms. Taylor showed sensitivity as she found out more about Ellen's son, and his circumstances, without negating Ellen's feelings.

Help Family Members Support One Another and Identify Outside Supports

After Ellen had the opportunity to cry and regain composure, Ms. Taylor asked who else she had talked with. Ellen said her husband, and reached for Michael's hand. Ms. Taylor stated how helpful that was, and asked about others. Ellen said she had been trying to continue at work, but did not want anyone there to know about her son. Ms. Taylor learned that other family members knew about the situation, but they did not seem comfortable bringing it up in conversation. Ms. Taylor talked about how important it was to have people we trust and with whom we can share these feelings. Together, Michael and Ellen discussed how they could speak with other family members, and how that might help.

Offer Your Support and a Follow-Up Meeting If Necessary

Ms. Taylor thought that Ellen could use further support, and used an efficient two-step process. She asked Ellen to return the following week, at which time she would assess her mood and consider counseling. The opportunity to talk with a clinician often results in improved mood, and patients return with an enhanced sense of agency and communion. In other situations, the follow-up visit provides the opportunity and time to arrange a referral with a family-oriented mental health colleague (see Chap. 25).

There are no easy responses in all of these difficult encounters. The range of patient response, time available, and relationship between clinician and patient mean that each situation requires quick assessment. Within the assessment, however, clinicians can listen carefully and monitor their own responses. Such attention and focus insures that the difficulty is not escalated, and that the clinician does not take personally that which reflects an external stress.

References

1. Platt FW, McMath JC: Clinical hypocompetence: the interview. *Ann Intern Med* 1979;**91**:898–902.
2. Levinson W, Roter DL, Mullooly JP, Dull VT, & Frankel RM: Physician–patient communication: the relationship with malpractice claims among primary care physicians and surgeons. *JAMA* 1997;**277**:553–559.
3. Beckman HB, Markakis KM, Suchman AL, & Frankel RM: The doctor–patient relationship and malpractice: lessons learned from plaintiff depositions. *Arch Intern Med* 1994;**154**(12):1365–1370.
4. Platt FW, Gordon GW: *Field Guide to the Difficult Patient Interview*. Baltimore, MD: Lippincott, Williams & Wilkins, 1999.
5. Taylor TR: Understanding the choices that patients make. *J Am Board Fam Prac* 2000;**13**:124–133.
6. Groves JE: Taking care of the hateful patient. *N Engl J Med* 1978;**298**:883–887.
7. Hilfiker D: Facing our mistakes. *N Engl J Med* 1984;**310**:118–122.
8. Brown JB, Brent P, Steward M, & Marshall JN: Roles and influence of people who accompany patients on visits to the doctor. *Can Fam Physician* 1998; **44**:1644–1650.
9. Hahn SR, Ferner JS, & Bellin EH: The doctor–patient–family relationship: a compensatroy alliance. *Ann Intern Med* 1988;**109**:884–889.
10. Farber NJ, Novack DH, & O'Brien MK: Love, boundaries and the patient physician relationship. *Arch Intern Med* 1997;**157**:2291–2294.
11. Frank AW: Narrative and deep illness. *Fam Syst Health* 1998;**16**(3):197–212.
12. McDaniel SH, Hepworth J, & Doherty WJ: *The Shared Experience of Illness: Stories of Patients, Families and Their Therapists*. New York: Basic Books, 1997.
13. Balint M: *The Doctor, His Patient, and the Illness*. New York: Pitman, 1964.
14. McDaniel SH, Hepworth J, & Doherty WJ: *Medical Family Therapy: A Biopsychosocial Approach to Families with Health Problems*. New York: Basic Books, 1992.
15. Quill, TE: Recognizing and adjusting to barriers in doctor-patient communication. *Ann Intern Med* 1989;**111**:51–57.
16. Mandl KD, Kohane IS, & Brandt AM: Electronic patient–physician communication: problems and promise. *Ann Intern Med* 1998;**129**:495–500.
17. Quill TE, Brody H: Physician recommendations and patient autonomy: finding a balance between physician power and patient choice. *Ann Intern Med* 1996;**125**:763–769.
18. McDaniel SH, Hepworth J: Family psychology in primary care: managing issues of power and dependency through collaboration. In: Frank R, McDaniel SH, Bray J, & Heldring M (Eds): *Primary Care Psychology*. Washington DC: American Psychological Association Publications, 2003.
19. Johnson GT: Restoring trust between patient and doctor. *N Engl J Med* 1990;**322**:195–197.
20. Kemp-White M, Keller VF: Difficult clinician-patient relationships. *J Clin Outcomes Manage* 1998;**5**:32–36.
21. Hepworth J: Listening, perhaps without hearing. *Fam Med* 2001;32:624.

Protocol: When Interactions with Families Become Difficult

General Strategies When Difficult Interactions Occur

- Recognize difficulty early in the interaction and actively plan how to address it.
- Distinguish how much of the difficulty arises from miscommunication, disagreements, or emotional affect.
- Monitor one's response as a clinician and as a person.
- Recognize differences among family members.
- Insure safety for patient, family, clinicians, and staff.
- Have a low threshold for involving collaborative colleagues.

Addressing Communication Problems

- State that you believe there is a communication problem that should be addressed before continuing.
- Acknowledge that the situation is stressful and may require more time.
- Ask family members how they understand the discussion, and what specific questions they may have.
- Describe what you understand, and what specific questions you still have.
- Find ways to underline a relationship of cooperation and partnership.
- Address concerns and provide information, using language that reflects the family's understanding.
- Encourage family members to identify further communication problems if they arise.

Addressing Disagreements About Treatment

- State that there are differing opinions about how to proceed, and it would be helpful to consider each of them.
- Ask family members about their understanding of the treatment and their preferences.
- Ask about other sources of advice about treatment.
- Describe your understanding of the problem and why you suggest a particular approach.
- With differences articulated, attempt to negotiate a compromise plan.
- Acknowledge that you may agree to disagree.
- Agree on a specific plan for follow up.

Addressing Anger

- Though anger can be intimidating, acknowledge and initiate the discussion of anger.

- Listen carefully to elicit family perspectives about why members are angry.
- Avoid defensive explanations or responses.
- Validate the experiences and the feelings of anger.
- Recognize that empathizing is not the same as agreeing.
- Be wary of triangulation with others not present.
- Ask if there is a way you can offer further help.

Responding to Sadness and Grief

- Acknowledge and initiate discussion of sadness.
- Listen with empathy as family members describe their sad feelings.
- Validate and normalize the sad feelings.
- Avoid trying to "fix the sadness."
- Help family members support one another and identify outside supports.
- Offer your support and a follow-up meeting if necessary.

9
Working with Couples in Primary Care: One Plus One Is More Than Two

Couples provide a fundamental and practical working unit for treating many of the problems that bring individual patients into primary care. What primary care clinician has not seen a woman bring a record of all her husband's, tests and consultations, along with a list of questions, to his medications appointment? Who has not seen a man devastated by grief and depression after the loss of his wife; or seen a battered woman continue in that horrific cycle of battering and forgiveness? What clinician has not been touched by the love, dedication, and commitment of a spouse for his or her partner?

Effective work with couples is a critical skill for the family-oriented clinician. A patient's partner can be a tremendous resource for both understanding the patient and implementing an appropriate care plan. Including the partner both provides better care for the patient and will save considerable time in the long run. At first, working with couples in primary care can seem more complex than working with individuals, but the family-oriented clinician who does it well will be amply rewarded.

For most people, their relationship with their partner has profound direct or indirect influence on their health (see Chap. 2). Research has shown that marriage is the most potent family factor that influences health. As early as 1853, William Farr, the registrar general for England and Wales, commented: "Marriage is a health state. The single individual is more likely to be wrecked on his voyage than the lives joined together in matrimony" (1). Subsequent research has confirmed that married individuals have lower death rates and report better health than do those who are unmarried (2). Among married individuals, those who are unhappy in their marriages report poorer health and more depression than do those who are happily married. Among the unmarried, those who have never married are healthier and live longer than those who are widowed or divorced.

There are several explanations for this potent influence of marriage on health. Married individuals tend to lead healthier lifestyles than those who are not married (3). They exercise more, and drink and smoke less than singles, divorcees, or widowers. They also experience less stress and more social support, which appears to have a beneficial impact on their physiology. Conflict can lead to persistent autonomic arousal in married couples, and divorced men and women have been shown to have poorer immune functioning than married individuals (4). Based upon an extensive review of the research on marriage and health, Burman and Margolin concluded that the treatment of marital problems should be considered a preventive health measure, the spouse should be included as part of all treatment regimens, and the impact of an illness on the spouse's health should be assessed on a regular basis (2).

A Family Life Cycle Perspective for Couples

The developmental milestones of pairing—from dating, to marriage or long-term commitment, parenting, retirement, and finally, death—all have health considerations. Contraception, pregnancy, and the diseases of later life most obviously highlight the need for understanding the couple system. Every individual visit for those in a committed relationship, however, may reflect relevant developmental challenges or current family life cycle issues.

> A middle-aged woman, Mrs. Jones, presented with headaches. In reviewing her symptoms, her physician learned that her husband had been offered early retirement, and that the couple had been having many long discussions about the merits of accepting the package. On one hand, Mrs. Jones looked forward to spending more time with her husband, but on the other hand she was not prepared for the change in lifestyle necessitated by less income. She felt guilty about wanting her husband to continue working and had not been able to discuss this with him.

To assess Mrs. Jones' headaches properly without addressing what was happening for the couple would be to overlook what is probably the most important precipitant. Early retirement, which many would consider a welcome change, presented a complex set of challenges and emotions that the couple needed to negotiate. An imaging scan of the head would be of little value in this process.

To apply a developmental family life cycle perspective to primary care, consider the following questions when seeing a patient:

• Are the individuals in the couple in sync developmentally?

As individuals, are they separating from their nuclear families, forming a couple, starting their own family, or in their midlife or retirement years? Are the individuals in the same stage of the life cycle? Is one ready for marriage while the other is still seperating from his or her family of origin? Are they both ready for children or retirement?

• Where in the life cycle is the couple?

As a couple, are they in the initial stages of pairing, or are they having children, promoting their children's independence, or enjoying their grandchildren? Combrinck-Graham (5) describes centripetal (pulling together) phases (e.g., pairing, child-bearing and, retirement) and centrifugal (pushing apart) phases (e.g., adolescence and midlife, for couples and families) (see Chap. 3). Dym and Glenn (6) also describe these natural push–pull phases for couples, but view the cycles happening more rapidly.

• What developmental challenges predominate for the couple?

Are they forming a new identity for themselves as a couple? Are they struggling with the sleep deprivation of having young children? Are they managing to negotiate the time for self/time for work/time for family boundaries? Are they able to launch their teenager(s)? How are they doing now that it is just the two of them again? Do they share similar goals for retirement?

• Are the life cycle stages in sequence or out of sequence?

A couple who marries to become independent of their parents is committing to a relationship before resolving identity or "leaving home" issues and so is out of phase. The couple who becomes pregnant before making a life-long commitment is similarly out of phase. Out-of-phase families are at higher risk for physical and emotional symptoms because of the many simultaneous developmental challenges they must face.

• How is the couple's place in the life cycle related to the presenting complaint?

Is the stress of an out-of-order life cycle development taking its toll on the patient? Is the stress of an illness superimposed on the developmental challenges of the life cycle? The centripetal pull of an acute illness may not fit with the centrifugal developmental forces in the family. For example, a diabetic teenager seeking independence may resist the interdependence needed to care for his or her illness (7). Some couples are better at the dependent centripetal tasks, whereas others are more adept at the independent centrifugal ones. Recognizing what a couple does well often helps them to strengthen what they do not do as well.

New Couple Visits

There are two kinds of "new" couples: those just becoming a couple and those that are new to the clinician's practice. We will discuss both of these types in this chapter because many of the assessment questions are the same.

The early developmental challenges of a newly committed relationship involve the couple's bonding with each other, creating a new family that takes first priority in their lives, and renegotiating relationships with their families of origin. There are often several opportunities for the clinician to learn about the patient's relationship with his or her new significant other. The subject may come up when one sees an individual for a completely unrelated reason, like a sore throat, or the physician or nurse practitioner may be seeing the patient for a reason directly related to a new relationship. The patient may have anxiety or concerns about the new relationship, or may seek contraceptive advice, or prenatal care. Some states still require blood testing prior to marriage, thereby providing an entry for premarital counseling. On the way to the altar couples rarely wish to discuss or be counseled about the wisdom of their choice of mates (8). These discussions may alienate the couple, unless one member has explicitly requested to talk about it. The clinician can instead explain, "As your primary care physician, I find it useful to find out a bit about both of your backgrounds, including your family histories, pertinent medical problems and your plans for the future. This will assist me in caring for both of you in the future."

This transgenerational approach to a visit allows the clinician in just a few minutes both to "bond" with the couple and to open the door for future discussions. It involves constructing together a simple genogram that symbolically joins the two individuals' families (see Chap. 3). In drawing the genogram, it is easy to get a sense for potential trouble spots. There may be emotional cut offs (e.g., "I don't know much about my father, I have not seen him in years"). There may be a pattern of repeated divorce, or alcoholism or substance abuse. The clinician gets clues both from what is said and from how it is said. A patient's mother may have died 10 years ago, but if talking about it still brings a river of tears, this may be an indication of unresolved grief. The healthcare provider may get the impression that there is a lack of parental support for the union, which means additional stress for a new marriage or partnership (9).

The genogram offers a vehicle to collect and record a good family history—information about the history of disease in the two families. At a glance, the clinician can then get a bird's-eye view of the entire biopsychosocial make-up of a couple. This discussion also provides a convenient link to future plans. For example, the clinician may ask about current use of contraception and expectations about having children.

> Joan and Jim came in to see Joan's physician, Dr. M., to discuss their risk of having a child with spina bifida. Joan's cousin had recently delivered a girl with a meningomyelocele and they worried about that possibility for themselves. Dr. M. sat down and drew their genograms together in the chart. This discussion revealed that Jim had been married before and had one son, Jimmy, age 10. This was the first marriage for Joan. Dr. M. asked Jim what he felt was successful in his first marriage

that he would like to bring into this new marriage, and what he intended to make different. Joan then discussed her concerns about becoming a stepmother and part-time parent, and what she had done to solidify her relationship with Jimmy prior to the marriage. Dr. M. asked about "permission" to marry and found that Jim's parents had supported the union all along, whereas Joan's parents had initially resisted lending their support because of Jim's divorce. Joan reported that as her parents spent more time with Jim, however, their affection for him grew, as did their confidence that the two of them could have a successful relationship. The visit concluded with a discussion of Joan's desire to have a baby soon after the marriage, the risks of spina bifida, the role of folate, and the maternal α-fetoprotein test.

A family life cycle approach to this or any other couple would include a consideration of the effect this developmental milestone might have on other members of the family.

Dr. M. was aware of Joan's parents' early disapproval of their relationship. Joan's mother, Mrs. Webb, had come in to see the nurse practitioner in the practice, Kathy P., approximately 3 months ago. At that time, she complained of an increase in her tension headaches. In the course of the visit, Mrs. Webb began discussing her worries about her youngest daughter marrying a divorced man. No one in her family had ever been divorced and Mrs. Webb worried this relationship was a setup for unhappiness and failure. Mrs. Webb also acknowledged that she was going to miss her daughter when she moved out and wondered who would fill the gap. Kathy P. suggested that Mrs. Webb go home and discuss her concerns with Mr. Webb, perhaps while on a dinner date, and that the two of them spend more time with Jim and Joan to observe this relationship and discover whether her worries were well-founded. Kathy P. later discussed the situation with Dr. M.

The same transgenerational format can be used productively with couples in nontraditional relationships (e.g., gay couples). It is important with these patients to explore the additional issue of how their families and friends view their sexual orientation and their choice of a partner. Social or family disapprobation for any couple results in stress that may have considerable health consequences.

In addition to couples in a new relationship, there are couples with a long and established relationship that transfer their care to a new primary care clinician. We live in a mobile society. Older couples may retire to a new community. Younger couples may move for occupational or other reasons. Some couples change to a new doctor because of a change in their health insurance. Whatever the reason, these couples need the same kind of careful assessment as newly committed couples.

Inquiring about strengths is an often overlooked, but critical, part of good quality healthcare. The focus of a visit is too often exclusively on problems and pathology. Learning what the couple has done well can help direct the clinician toward skills that can be used to overcome the current problems. Talking about successes often invigorates the couple and provides a fresh perspective.

> Mike and Abbey were both busy professionals with two young children. As a couple, they had taken a "divide and conquer" approach to life's challenges. They worked beautifully together as a team, with clear expectations of what each was responsible for. When Abbey was diagnosed with breast cancer at the age of 43, their complex but well-organized life was thrown into a paralyzing chaos. Once their strength regarding teamwork was acknowledged, they went right to work deciding who would be in charge of the different parts of Abbey's care, as well as how to redivide their prior responsibilities.

Making past roles in the couple explicit is often a giant step toward successful transition to new roles, however, changing these roles for some may involve considerable inertia. Many elderly couples have worked closely together for years and have deeply entrenched patterns of coping. One must respect the prior success of these roles, as well as their team nature. For some of these elderly couples, it may be unthinkable for them to be treated as separate individuals. For others, there may be more diversity and flexibility.

Health Roles Within Couples

Partners in a couple usually develop a tendency to play one particular health role or another. These tendencies are often determined before the individuals ever meet. These are only tendencies to play a particular role, and a healthy couple has the flexibility to adapt to new situations. The following are roles that are common for spouses or partners to play in coping together with illness:

• The partner as caregiver.

With the increasing sophistication of medicine, more terminal illnesses are becoming chronic illnesses. With the movement toward outpatient treatment, a greater number of very ill patients are being managed at home. As a result, partners and family members are playing an increasing role in "the healthcare team." In today's world, it is often essential for the clinician to work with the informal caregiver to assess the patient's progress, monitor, and even deliver treatment.

When the partner is the caregiver, it is crucial to have him or her present during the visit. Make the partner comfortable and acknowledge his or her opinion. Recognize this person's value explicitly to the patient and note the importance of their input. At the same time, do not undermine the autonomy of the patient. If the caregiver is overly intrusive, it may be necessary to cut that person off or to explain politely the need to examine the patient alone. If the caregiver is going to be implementing any part of the treatment, be sure to clear it first with both patient and partner.

• The partner as customer.

When a patient in the office is vague or seems to be unconcerned about the purpose of the visit, it is often because someone else sent him or her. With couples, that someone is most often the patient's partner. Some middle-aged men who request a "complete check-up" are sent by their wives who feel they are overworking or not paying enough attention to their health. Other wives may be concerned about underemployment or excessive drinking. The men may look similar and clinicians may make incorrect assumptions when the partners' views are not elicited. The customer for treatment, the person who wants the patient assessed or treated, is sometimes crucial to understanding the presenting complaint.

> Mr. Tinney, a 49-year-old healthy truck driver, was seen for a physical. The next day, the physician assistant who had performed the physical received an angry phone call from Mrs. Tinney wondering why his prostate was not checked. After reading an article in *Newsweek*, she had made this appointment for her husband primarily to have his prostate checked. Mr. Tinney had not been asked about, nor had he mentioned, his wife's concerns.

When the partner as customer is not present, ask the patient about the partner's agenda for the visit. "Was there anything your wife was particularly concerned about or wanted me to check today?" It is sometimes worth getting the partner on the phone while the patient is there. The patient virtually always knows just exactly how to reach his or her partner (10). It can save time and later misunderstandings.

• The partner as informant.

At times a patient is unable to provide reliable information, or any information at all. A connection with the patient's partner is then essential for understanding the nature of the problem, as well as for designing a workable solution.

> Mrs. White, a patient with early and undiagnosed Alzheimer's disease, came in for a physical. When Dr. D. asked about her concerns she said, "I don't know. My husband seems to think something is wrong with me." At Dr. D.'s invitation, Mr. White joined them from the waiting room. He told Dr. D. that his wife had become more and more forgetful in the last several months. Mr. White said he decided to schedule his wife for a physical when she left the stove on after cooking one night several weeks ago.

• The partner as consultant.

The patient's partner is often useful in the assessment of an illness or problem. A partner may be willing to provide information that the patient has avoided mentioning or has not noticed. A partner may give another perspective, a second opinion to that of the patient, when the diagnosis is unclear or mysterious.

> In the case of Mrs. White, the patient had denied any significant problems, so Mr. White's consultation was essential to the assessment process. Mr. White also offered that his wife's mother had Alzheimer's disease and wondered if his wife could have the same thing.

• The partner as participant in treatment.

Some medical issues impact directly on a relationship; therefore, in some sense they require the partner to participate in treatment. Any major lifestyle change (e.g., stopping smoking, drinking, or changing diets) affects the larger family. Research has demonstrated that the family influences these lifestyle changes (see Chap. 2).

> For Mrs. White, involvement of her husband in the treatment plan was essential. For example, Dr. D. was able to manage the problem of Mrs. White waking up in the middle of the night and wandering by suggesting that Mr. White sleep on the outside of their bed. That way, if Mrs. White awoke and tried to get out of bed, her husband would wake up and was able to take care of her.

Contraception is another clear issue that affects both members of a couple. It is most efficient in these cases to involve the partner in the treatment process as early as possible.

• The partner as part of the problem.

Blatant relationship or marital problems clearly fall in this category. There are also occasions when a couple's relationship may interfere with medical treatment in more subtle ways (e.g., when a wife does not change her cooking habits after her husband has been diagnosed with coronary artery disease or diabetes). At these times, involvement of the spouse is especially important to the long-term success of the treatment (see Chap. 14 on working with couples with relationship problems).

> With Mr. and Mrs. White, problems emerged after Mr. White complained that his wife had left the stove on. Mrs. White became very angry and said, "Ever since that day, my husband won't let me do a thing. He treats me like a child that has to be watched every minute. I can't even make my own bed." Mr. White acknowledged his fear and

concern had led him to take on all household chores. "It's just easier for me to do everything," he said. Some tasks were clearly important for Mr. White to manage; however, he felt he had to do virtually everything at this point to be safe. Dr. D. was able to alleviate some of the strain for the couple by helping to negotiate what was safe for Mrs. White to do and what was not.

- Illness as a burden for the partner.

Serious acute or chronic illness or severe trauma are very stressful for a patient's partner, and can lead to significant physical and mental health problems for that person.

> In speaking to Mr. White, Dr. D. noticed that he looked quite fatigued and somewhat sad. Mr. White explained that he felt overwhelmed by the physical demands of caring for his wife and the emotional stress of seeing her deteriorate in response to the question, "How are you doing?" After encouraging him to share these feelings, Dr. D. asked Mr. White to schedule a check-up for himself and referred him to an Alzheimer's family support group and to a social worker to obtain home services.

Providing a spouse like Mr. White with information and support can be an important part of preventive medicine in terms of the marriage, the spouse's own health, and the spouse's role as caregiver and informant for the patient. When illness becomes terminal or a patient dies, the partner is clearly affected and deserves attention.

Common Relational Patterns for Couples Around Illness

Families all have health belief systems that determine their behavior at times of illness. Couples often pattern themselves on what they saw their parents do, or what they wish their parents had done, when they have to cope with illness. Healthy couples are flexible and able to take many different roles with each other. Either member of the couple is able to be in the sick role or in the role of caretaker during an illness. Rigid roles can lead to marital strain or dysfunction and affect the sick person's ability to become healthy again. The following are common relational patterns that may occur when illness strikes a couple:

- Sick–healthy pair.

This adaptation, with one sick member and one healthy member, can be one of the most functional if both members of a couple are allowed to play each role as necessary. If the roles are rigid, the couple will have difficulty when the "healthy" member of the pair becomes ill.

Eduardo was seen as sickly because he had many childhood illnesses and that was his role in his family of origin. His wife, Philomena, was seen as strong because she took care of her younger siblings during her childhood. When Philomena was diagnosed with breast cancer, both members of this couple had difficulty doing what was necessary. Philomena (remaining in her healthy role) denied to herself that the lump in her breast could be anything significant. After her surgery, Eduardo (remaining in his sick role) came down with a cold and felt unable to visit his wife or do the necessary household chores.

- Sick–caregiving pair.

This adaptation also can be functional if it is flexible and not driven by either partner's need to be special (by being sick or by being a caretaker). If the pattern is rigid, the caregiving spouse may encourage the sick spouse to be more dependent than necessary so that each partner derives secondary gains from the illness.

Sara Nicoletti babied her husband, Jake, during the 6 months after his myocardial infarction. She suggested that he retire immediately, stop smoking, and generally take it easy. She was so concerned that he not strain himself that she answered all his phone calls, and his friends and physician had to relay their messages to him through her. Handling her anxiety through overinvolvement resulted in serious marital strain.

- Sick–distant pair.

In this pattern, one partner copes with the stress of the spouse's illness by pulling away and turning to work or other people during the time of the illness. The healthy version of this adaptation occurs when the distancing spouse distracts himself with other people or activities but remains connected to the patient in important ways. When this pattern is dysfunctional, the distancing spouse may deny the partner's illness altogether or refuse to spend time with the partner until he or she recovers.

- Competing spouses.

These couples have symmetrical relationships based on similarity, rather than complementary relationships based on difference. Although they are healthy, each member may push the other in a positive way to be all he or she can be. Some of these couples adapt to illness through competitive or dueling symptoms. They can play a never-ending game of, "If you think you feel bad, you should know how I feel. . ." This is an unfortunate adaptation, even if the symptoms are relatively benign, because both members experience themselves as missing the other's attention and feel unable to nurture the partner.

• Shared illness.

Some couples are extremely dependent on each other. Prior to illness, this pattern may function fine. If an illness threatens their interdependence, a dysfunctional adaptation may occur. Somatic fixation is a problem shared by many couples. Some even focus on the same organ functions in a kind of folie à deux.

> Andy became convinced he had contracted chlamydia after having an affair, though tests were unrevealing. His wife, Julie, soon developed exactly the same symptoms as her husband, who believed he had passed on his "infection" to her. The illness was a common focus that functioned to bring the couple closer after the distance that resulted in the affair.

• Coalitions around illness.

Sometimes illness intensifies already existing relationship patterns in a family (11). Prior to illness, families may function well. The presence of illness can exert pressure on relationships, making family dysfunction more likely.

> In the Hicks family, the couple agreed that Mary would be in charge of raising the children, while Mike worked to support the family financially. When one of the children became sick with severe asthma, Mary became quite concerned and worried about the child night and day. She stayed in the hospital with the child, then doted on him when he returned home for recuperation. This pattern persisted long after the child returned to health. Mary remained overinvolved as a mother and Mike grew more and more distant from both his child and his wife. When arguments occurred, Mary always took the side of the child against her spouse. After working with the family over time, the physician decided that the complexities of the case called for the expertise of a family therapist.

Divorced Couples

In 1994, there were slightly over half as many divorces as there were marriages (i.e., 4.6 divorces/1000 population and 9.1 marriages/1000 population). At that time, the median duration of marriage was 7.2 years. Divorce affected more than 1 million children in that year alone (12). Untold thousands of other couples arranged, planned, and anticipated a life-long commitment that was eventually torn asunder. Many, if not most, of these individuals are still connected in some way to their former partner. They may have ongoing financial responsibilities, or important co-parenting responsibilities. Exchanging children at regular intervals usually involves regular contact with one's "ex." Former partners may have ongoing emotional attachments and may still love (or hate) the other.

After separation or divorce, ask about both emotional and financial relationships. Does the patient pay or receive alimony or child support? What kind of contact occurs with the ex-husband/wife? What is the relationship like? Are there arguments about child rearing? How are these resolved? All of these issues need to be brought out to view their impact on the health of one's patients. Many divorced couples have come to terms with their new situation and are healthier, but for others the stress of a problematic relationship continues (see Chaps. 9 and 14).

Guidelines for Working with Couples in Primary Care

1. Have adequate seating for interviewing couples.

To facilitate working with couples, it is important to have proper space and seating available for partners to be comfortably included in the visit. Every exam room should preferably be furnished with two comfortable chairs in addition to the clinician's own seat.

2. Treat as a couple any relationship the patient defines in that way.

The definition of *couple* for the purposes of primary care should be descriptive rather than legal. Much diversity exists in the way people choose to live their lives. A clinician may miss relevant health information (e.g., HIV status) if he or she avoids asking about the possibilities. The "couple" most relevant to healthcare is sometimes not a romantic couple. For example, in a teenage pregnancy the grandmother may be as or more important than the father of the baby. Other examples of this phenomenon also exist.

> Ms. Wisp, a 28-year-old divorced mother, her current boyfriend, and her two children lived in a house with another family composed of a mother, father, and three children, plus the father's father. Ms. Wisp had little money and said she welcomed this family's generosity. Because of Ms. Wisp's recent depression, her physician, Dr. B. invited all the members of the household to a family conference. It became clear during this meeting that the executive pair for this household was Ms. Wisp and her longtime friend, Ms. Barrel. They were the most important people to each other, having supported each other while men came and went in their lives. This pair made most of the families' decisions. It became obvious that Ms. Barrel was a key person in Ms. Wisp's general healthcare and was central to any attempts to alleviate her depression.

3. Develop the art of maintaining simultaneous strong alliances with two or more related people.

Several basic principles can help to facilitate this process:

- Do not talk at any length about a partner who is absent.

Invite the partner in to the office to participate in the conversation (see Chap. 4 for recommendations on inviting partners to a session). This prevents destructive triangulation (Chap. 3) and other potential problems (e.g., the physician coming to be seen as a better listener, or more caring than the partner).

- Build rapport with each person present.

Be sure to make contact with each member of the pair within the first several minutes of the interview. This is especially important if you have a more in-depth relationship with one person than with the other. Spend a few extra minutes at the beginning getting to know the less well-known partner.

- Validate each person's point of view as real and meaningful to that person.

Couples, especially when under stress, often talk as if only one person's point of view can be valid. When considered carefully, each person's point of view usually makes good sense when viewing the world through his or her eyes. The clinician–patient and clinician–family alliance depends on being able to understand each person's perspective. By staying connected with each person, though not necessarily agreeing with all views, the clinician models these same skills for the family.

- Do not collude or keep important secrets with one against the other.

Such statements as, "Do not ever tell my wife I told you this, but . . . ," are often warning signals for present or future dysfunction in a family. The clinician must distinguish between what is "private" and unrelated to others (e.g., an affair of long ago prior to the current relationship), and what is "secret" and directly affecting others (e.g., a current affair). If a secret is disclosed, it is important to consider whether that secret is contributing to dysfunction in the couple. It is also important to consider whether the patient revealing the secret is, in a sense, requesting help in revealing the secret to other significant people. Such statements as, "Please do not ask me to keep a secret that I may feel is negatively affecting your health," can be important in establishing your neutrality in and your commitment to both individual and family health. This issue can become complicated around such issues as affairs, HIV status, and previous pregnancies or abortions. Successful care includes helping patients distinguish between privacy and secrecy, and providing the patient with the support to inform their partner if the secret is harmful in any way (13).

Michael: Doc, I want you to know my father had Alzheimer's disease, but I've never had the guts to tell my partner, Joseph. I've kept it a secret because I don't want him to worry. I worry enough for the two of us.

Dr. O.: I understand how hard that must be for you to wait and wonder if you will get the same disease as your father. I know you want to protect Joseph from the concern he would feel if he knew of this potential problem. At the same time, I myself worry that because he doesn't know he is unable to support you about this. You are unable to be as close as you could be if you shared this issue together. I also worry that if you should get the disease, Joseph will not have had the opportunity to prepare himself for it.

Michael: Well, I hadn't really thought of it that way. My mother said I should tell him, but I didn't want to think of Joseph having to go through what my mother did. Even if it was a good idea, however, I couldn't bring myself to tell him.

Dr. O.: Why don't you think it over? If you decide it is important to tell him, and I think it is, I would be happy to meet with both of you to answer his questions regarding the disease.

Michael: Would you just tell him, Doc, if I asked him to come in and see you?

Dr. O.: No, I won't tell him myself. That's for you to do. But I would be happy to be there and offer support and information.

4. When working conjointly, use the interview to model and teach good communication skills.

The following four suggestions can make a session with a couple therapeutic, independent of what is discussed, because the couple will gain experience in respectful communication.

- Model respectful listening.

Balancing questions to both members of a couple and patiently listening to each of them communicates respect for both parties. This technique can be very useful for couples who take each other for granted, have dysfunctional communication, or just never learned to listen.

- Allow only one person to speak at a time.

This simple principle creates an environment where it is possible for people to listen to each other. It is amazing how often people routinely speak over each other. In their hurry to be understood, they communicate a lack of interest in what their partner has to say. Time-pressured health professionals run a high risk of contributing to this problem, too.

- Reflect back individuals' statements to communicate empathy, understanding, and allow for correction.

This simple technique promotes understanding between people. For the clinician, it is crucial for ensuring accurate diagnosis and being certain the patient understands the treatment plan. For the couple, it is essential for clear communication and intimacy.

- Balance the interview so each partner is able to present his or her point of view.

Do not allow one partner to dominate the conversation. It is important to create space for each person to speak. Most couples look to the physician to provide this structure in an office visit.

> Dr. O.: I am glad you were each able to come in today, Joseph. I understand Michael told you of his father's disease. I would be happy to answer your questions today about Alzheimer's disease.
>
> Joseph: I am very worried, Doc. When do you think Michael will become sick?
>
> Dr. O.: We are unsure whether Michael will get the disease. He may never become sick. If he does, it is likely to happen in the next 10 or 15 years.
>
> Joseph: Well, he told me that, but I guess I wanted to hear it from you. What is the disease like?
>
> Dr. O.: Michael, you haven't said anything yet today. It took a lot of courage and confidence in Joseph to share this information with him. I'm impressed with how much you each care for each other. Rather than my answering Joseph's question, why don't you tell him what you know, and then I'll add to that when you're done.

5. Assess the way the couple interacts around the illness.

Monitor relational patterns such as sick–healthy, sick–caregiving, sick–distant, competing, shared illness, and coalitions. Watch for any rigidity that develops in the individual or the couple's behavior. Frequently, primary care counseling can provide the support needed to introduce more flexibility in the way the couple is handling an illness. If that is not successful, referral to a family therapist is necessary. (For other suggestions regarding conditions for good communication, see Chapter 7 on conducting a family conference.)

6. Assess what role or roles the partner is playing with regard to the illness.

When it is relevant, utilize the partner in that role to facilitate the treatment plan.

- Support the caregiver.

Involve him or her in the treatment plan, but monitor for and try to prevent overfunctioning or burnout in this person.

- Invite the "partner as customer" to at least part of all interviews.

The partner has the most investment in treatment, is usually a great ally, and is often instrumental in implementing a treatment plan.

- Interview any important informant.

A partner, spouse, or friend can offer a wealth of information about the patient's history, symptoms, and current functioning.

- Utilize the consultant.

Ask for suggestions, diagnoses, and reactions to treatment plans. The partner is an expert on the patient and on what the couple can effectively manage.

- When the spouse or partner plays any kind of major role with regard to the illness, give him or her a role as a participant in the treatment plan.
- When the partner is part of the problem, develop a strategy to block the problematic behavior. If it persists, refer for family therapy.
- Monitor the partner for fatigue, symptoms of depression, and other signs that the patient's illness is becoming an intolerable burden for him or her.

References

1. Wykes S, Ford G: Competing explanation for association between marital status and health. *Soc Sci Med* 1992;**34**:523–532.
2. Burman B, Margolin G: Analysis of the association between marital relationships and health problems: an interactional perspective. *Psychol Bull* 1992;**112**: 39–63.
3. Umberson D: Gender, marital status and social control of health behavior. *Soc Sci Med* 1992;**34**:907—917.
4. Kennedy S, Kiecolt-Glaser JK, & Glaser R: Immunological consequences of acute and chronic stressors: mediating role of interpersonal relationships. *Br J Med Psychol* 1988;**61**:77–85.
5. Combrinck-Graham L: A developmental model for family systems. *Family Proc* 1985;**24**:139 150.
6. Dym B, Glenn ML: *Couples: Exploring and Understanding the Cycles of Intimate Relationships*. New York: HarperCollins, 1993.
7. Rolland J: *Families, Illness, & Disability: An Integrative Treatment Model*. New York: Basic, 1994.
8. Friedman E: The family model in church and synagogue: a systems approach to pre-marital counseling. In: Berger M, Jerkovic J (Eds). *Family Therapy in Context: Practicing Systems Therapy in Community Settings*. New York: Jossey-Bass, 1984.
9. Boszormenyi-Nagy I, Sparks G: *Invisible Loyalties*. New York: Harper and Row, 1973.
10. Fishman T: The 90-second intervention: a patient compliance mediated technique to improve and control hypertension. *Publ Health Rep* 1995;**110**(2): 173–178.
11. Penn P: Coalitions and binding interactions in families with chronic illness. *Fam Syst Med* 1983;**1**(2):16–25.
12. U.S. Bureau of the Census, *Statistical Abstract of the United States: 1996* (116th edition). Washington DC: U.S. Bureau of the Census, 1996.
13. Newman, N: Family secrets: a challenge for family physicians. *J Fam Prac* 1993;**39**(5):494–496.

Protocol: Working with Couples in Primary Care

Family Life Cycle Approach

- Are the individuals in the couple in sync developmentally?
- Where in the life cycle is the couple?
- What developmental challenges predominate for the couple?
- Are the life cycle stages in phase or out of phase?
- How is the couple's place in the life cycle related to the presenting complaint?

New Couple Visits

1. Use a transgenerational approach in the interview with the couple.
   Do not overtly question their choice of mates, unless the patient expresses ambivalence or the relationship is abusive.
   - Construct a genogram with them that joins their two extended families.
   - Attend to both content and process while doing the genogram.
   - Review the family history of disease and dysfunction.
   - Update the genogram at regular intervals and as needed. Do not try to do it all at once.
2. Consider the effect of this relationship on any extended family members in your practice, and vice versa.
3. Use new visits by established couples as an opportunity to get background information.

Guidelines for Working with Couples in Primary Care

1. Have adequate seating for interviewing couples.
2. Treat as a couple any relationship the patient defines that way.
3. Develop the art of maintaining simultaneous strong alliances with two related people.
   - Do not talk at any length about a partner who is absent.
   - Build rapport with each person present.
   - Validate each person's point of view as real and meaningful to that person.
   - Do not collude or keep important secrets with one against the other.
4. Use the interview to model and teach good communication skills.
   - Model respectful listening.
   - Allow only one person to speak at a time.
   - Reflect back individual's statements to communicate empathy, understanding, and allow for correction.
   - Balance the interview so each partner is able to present his or her point of view.

5. Assess the way the couple interacts around the illness.
   - Watch for rigidity in the couple's relational patterns around the illness (e.g., sick–healthy, sick–caregiving, sick–distant, competing, shared illness, and coalitions).
   - Consider primary care counseling or referral for family therapy if patterns become too entrenched and dysfunctional.
6. Assess what role or roles the partner is playing with regard to the illness and, when relevant, utilize that person in that role to facilitate the treatment plan.
   - Support the caregiver.
   - Invite the customer to participate in treatment.
   - Interview any important informant.
   - Utilize the spouse or partner as a consultant.
   - Give the partner a role as a participant in the treatment plan.
   - If the partner is part of the problem, develop a plan to block the problematic behavior or refer for family therapy.
   - Monitor the partner for signs that the burden of the illness is becoming problematic or intolerable.

10
The Birth of a Family:
Family-Oriented Pregnancy Care

The birth of a child forever transforms a family. This quantum change affects everything and everyone; what once was true is now completely different. Families become exquisitely vulnerable at this powerful time, and the clinician's influence is magnified and extended. During pregnancy, the clinician has extensive contact with the family and becomes a trusted consultant (1), with families relying on their clinician for most of their information about the pregnancy (2). Family-oriented pregnancy care builds upon traditional obstetrical care, providing an integrated approach that attends to the psychosocial needs of the woman and the family, along with the biomedical aspects of the pregnancy.

The American Academy of Family Physicians, the American College of Obstetricians and Gynecologists, and the International Childbirth Education Association, endorse the definition of *Family-Centered Maternity Care* developed by McMaster University in 1991:

> The birth of a baby represents, as well, the birth of a family. The woman giving birth and the persons significant and close to her are forming a new relationship, with new responsibilities to each other, to the baby, and to society as a whole. Family-centered reproductive care may be defined as care that recognizes the importance of these new relationships and responsibilities, and which has as its goal the best possible health outcome for all members of the family, both as individuals and as a group (3, 4).

Research has demonstrated that family stress, family supports, and aspects of family interaction can influence the course of pregnancy, including obstetrical and perinatal complications and birth weight. Women who receive emotional support and practical help from their spouse and other family members experience less depression during pregnancy and the postpartum period. Highly stressed women with low family and social supports have higher rates of obstetrical complications (5, 6). High levels of family support can buffer the impact of psychosocial stressors. The family can also be a source of stress and have a negative impact on pregnancy outcome.

Poor family functioning has been associated with more labor complications and lower birthweight (7–9). Women who live apart from their families deliver smaller babies than those who live with their partners or families of origin (10). Those women who are excessively close or enmeshed with their extended families, however, also tend to deliver smaller babies, which suggests that the quality as well as the quantity of family support influences health. Ramsey and colleagues have hypothesized that the extended family's overinvolvement during pregnancy may be detrimental by not allowing enough autonomy or psychological space for a new family member (11). Psychosocial factors also influence the actual labor and delivery. One meta-analysis found that women who receive emotional support have an average 19-minute decrease in labor duration (12). Laboring mothers who receive emotional support also are less likely to need intrathecal analgesia and epidural anesthesia (13). Mercer et al. looked at both prenatal and intrapartum factors and discovered that the most important variable in a woman's perception of her birth experience was having a partner present (14).

This chapter will review the developmental issues that families face during this life cycle stage and offer suggestions for implementing a family-oriented approach throughout pregnancy, childbirth, and the newborn period. Because some families experience disappointment with conception efforts, this chapter will also include sections on infertility and adoption. We recognize that most new families are led by a mother and father who are married; however, there are increasing numbers of nontraditional families. A co-parent can be a same-sex partner, another significant other who is not the biological father of the baby, a grandmother, or a sister. The same principles apply to these "alternative" families.

Developmental Issues in Pregnancy and Childbirth

The Birth of a Triangle

For all families, the birth of the first child is a critical period of transition. The couple must accommodate a new member to become a three-person family. The couple reassesses their commitment and responsibility both to the new child and to each other. The couple must make room in their relationship for the new infant, while maintaining the intimacy and sexuality of their marriage. The dyad becomes a triad, and life becomes a more complex balancing act. It is like the difference between balancing on a regular two-sided see-saw, and balancing on a triangular one. In addition to new parent–child relationships, there are opportunities for alliances (e.g., parents working together to care for the child) and risks of coalitions (one parent and child against the other parent). With the addition of each new child, the family constellation will be changed forever (15).

The birth of a first child affects the extended family as well. Everyone moves up a generation: parents of the couple become grandparents; sisters and brothers become aunts and uncles. Combrinck-Graham (16) describes childbirth as a centripetal phase in which the family comes closer together, and the connectedness or cohesion between family members strengthens, whereas interpersonal boundaries become more permeable. Becoming a parent often encourages members of a couple to reflect on their relationship with their own parents, and offers opportunities for reworking these relationships. Subsequent pregnancies and the delivery of additional children have similar developmental challenges. Many parents report that even though having two children is a joy that adds to the family, it is often experienced as more than twice the work of one, and puts additional stress on the family requiring further role negotiations.

Whereas most families successfully negotiate the transitional challenges of a new child, problems can develop that lead to persistent dysfunctional patterns in the family. One common problem occurs when the mother establishes a close relationship with her infant that excludes the father. Feeling left out, the father becomes more involved outside the family, either in work, outside activities, or another relationship. The mother then feels abandoned by her husband and pulls closer to her infant, away from her spouse, and a vicious cycle develops. Another dysfunctional pattern is the couple that abandons their husband and wife roles to be parents. These couples stop spending time alone together. All activities involve the child with a decrease in marital intimacy. Couples with shaky relationships to begin with, especially those who have not accomplished the developmental tasks of the previous stages of the family life cycle, are at the greatest risk for development of these dysfunctional patterns. For example, the adolescent who becomes pregnant, leaves her parents' home, moves in with her boyfriend, probably has neither separated emotionally from her parents nor established an intimate relationship with her partner. The girl's mother, or grandmother, might help with the childrearing, the partner is excluded from this sphere, and the long-term stability of the couple is threatened.

Even in pregnancies where the mother has no ongoing relationship with the biological father and plans to raise the baby alone, there are usually important family members or friends involved. "It takes a village" is a meaningful slogan; encouraging the active participation of these important people in the care of the pregnancy can help ensure a nurturing environment for the child.

Prepregnancy: Family Planning

As discussed in the previous chapter, it is ideal to meet with a couple during routine healthcare visits to help understand their relationship and their approach to health issues. This is particularly important for family planning that involves both members of the couple. Routine gynecological exams are a perfect opportunity to discuss birth control and plans for children. When a woman or a couple expresses the desire to become pregnant and start a family, the clinician can recommend a preconception visit.

At a routine or prepregnancy visit, several issues should be covered:

1. Encourage the couple to discuss their ideas and plans regarding pregnancy and children.

Do they both want to start a family now? If there is reluctance on the part of either partner, identify the difference and encourage them to discuss this further.

2. Evaluate the extended family and their attitudes about pregnancy.

What are their own families' feelings about their plans? Have they put pressure on them to have children?

3. Briefly assess where the couple is in the family life cycle and how they have negotiated the tasks of previous stages.

Have both members of the couple been able to develop a balance in which both are able to maintain connections with their families while also being able to commit to their partner? Is the pregnancy being used to leave home, to get married, or to improve a marriage? If this is the case, it can be helpful to get the couple to acknowledge this explicitly and discuss how successful this plan will be.

> Jenny, an African-American high school senior, came to see Dr. M. for a pregnancy test. She had forgotten to take her birth control pills for several days during the previous month and was now several days late with her period. She was the youngest of five children and was the only one still living with her parents. Her 20-year-old boyfriend, Jim, brought her to the appointment, so Dr. M. invited him into the exam room to discuss the situation. Jenny expressed the desire to keep the baby if she were pregnant and to move in with Jim; however, Jim doubted his ability to support a family and inquired about abortion.
>
> The couple appeared relieved when the pregnancy test was negative. Together, they decided that it was not a good time to have a baby and agreed to continue using contraception at least until they got married or were living together. Jim offered to help Jenny to remember her birth control pills and to use a condom if she forgot.

4. Review biological and psychological risk factors.

Is there anything in the woman's health history that might present a risk in pregnancy (e.g., family history of genetic disorder, medication, smoking, drug or alcohol use)? If so, counseling the woman to stop medication, drugs, or smoking prior to pregnancy is critical. Women who have previously been unable or unwilling to stop smoking or to reduce their alcohol intake, may do so for the benefit of their planned child. Partners can either help or hinder these behavior changes. Risk factors, especially smoking, are often shared by couples (see Chap. 2), and it is more difficult for a woman to stop smoking if her partner smokes. Furthermore, the partner's support has been shown to have a very positive influence on smoking cessation. Thus, it is crucial to elicit the partner's support for behavioral changes.

5. Support healthy habits.

This is an excellent time to promote healthy behaviors in the family. A good diet, regular exercise, adequate sleep are all healthy behaviors that can be advocated. Starting prenatal vitamins, ensuring adequate folate intake, and education about promoting fertility can be done at this time as well.

First Trimester: Initial Prenatal Visit

For the woman, the first trimester of pregnancy is a time of excitement, anticipation, introspection, and adjustment to bodily changes (17). It is also a time of change in the couple's relationship. Even with very committed couples, in addition to joy, there is generally some ambivalence about the pregnancy. For some, there may be serious questions about continuing the pregnancy.

A comprehensive, biopsychosocial evaluation is ideally done at the first prenatal visit. Pregnancy is more often established (or in this era of accurate home pregnancy tests, confirmed) during a brief visit and an extended "initial" appointment is booked for a later date. If the prepregnancy topics have not been discussed previously with the couple, they should be covered during one of these visits. In addition, the following areas should be addressed:

1. Explore whether the pregnancy was desired or planned, and whether there are any thoughts of terminating pregnancy.

"What are your plans for this pregnancy?" Until you know this information, be careful not to congratulate the woman. If the woman is uncertain about continuing the pregnancy, discuss the options with her.

2. Find out what social supports the mother has (e.g., father of child, parents, siblings, friends), and how these people feel about the pregnancy.

"What does your boyfriend think about your pregnancy?" "What has your mother's reaction been?" Tell the woman that you look forward to meeting these important people during the pregnancy. This is a perfect time to do a genogram, or to add relevant family history, medical history, or genetic information to an existing one.

3. Invite the father of the baby to all prenatal visits.

If the father is not in the exam room, ask whether he is in the waiting room, and ask him to join you. Insist on meeting with the father, or other support person if the father is not involved, at least twice during the pregnancy; early on to deal with pregnancy issues, and again toward the end to discuss labor, delivery, and the postpartum period.

> Jean, a 22-year-old Caucasian woman, came to her first prenatal visit with Dr. C. when she was 16 weeks pregnant. The pregnancy had been anticipated by her (she had stopped taking her oral contraceptives), but she had not yet told her husband, Peter. She explained that Peter did not think they could afford a second child. When Dr. C. asked Jean to invite Peter to the next appointment, she said she did not think that he could get the time off from work, nor would he be interested in coming. "He wasn't involved with my first pregnancy," she explained, "and besides, I'm not sure I want him to come to *my* doctor's appointments."

Getting "Reluctant" Fathers in to the Visit

Fathers are usually eager to participate in prenatal care; however, a woman will occasionally say that her partner is "reluctant" or unable to attend any prenatal sessions. Although rigid work schedules sometimes prevent fathers from coming along, it may signal lack of involvement in parenting or some type of marital distress. In these cases, it is particularly important to get the father in as early as possible, and to assess the marital relationship and its impact on the pregnancy. There are occasionally cultural barriers to paternal involvement, and the clinician needs to be sensitive, practical, and flexible with this cultural diversity.

1. Involve the father early on in the pregnancy.

As the pregnancy proceeds, if a woman comes in alone she develops an exclusive relationship with the clinician, making the father feel more excluded and less likely to come in to the office. *Avoid* listening extensively to any complaints about the partner before you have met him or her. Failure to include the father in the intimate experience of prenatal care runs the risk of establishing a very close relationship between the mother and the often male physician, who may be pulled into the role of a substitute spouse (18).

2. Expect the father to come in to the visit.

Be direct about the need for him to participate in prenatal care: "I need to meet with the father of your baby. Can he come in for your next prenatal visit?" Explain that this is part of routine prenatal care. *Avoid* being ambivalent or giving such mixed messages about the importance of the father coming in as, "Do you think your partner would like (or be able) to come in?" Patients pick up your conviction, or lack thereof, in your recommendations.

3. Emphasize the important role of the father.

Tell the woman that you need her partner's help or opinion. *Avoid* accepting the patient's word that her partner is unwilling to come. This can be a projection of her own reluctance or protectiveness. *Stress the benefits* of the partner's involvement to the patient and the pregnancy. *Avoid* blaming the mother or father in any way. Do not imply there are "marital problems" or that the couple is in need of therapy, even if you think the marriage is in trouble. This can increase the couple's defensiveness or fear of coming.

4. Offer to call the partner yourself.

This may be necessary if the patient insists that he will not come in, regardless of what she says to him. It is best to call the partner while the woman is in the office so she can hear what is being said.

5. Request that the father come in for at least one prenatal visit.

He does not need to say anything; he can just listen. Within a few minutes of such a visit, reluctant fathers will typically want to participate.

> Jean: And besides, I'm not sure I want him to come into my doctor's appointment.
> Dr. C.: I'd like to hear more about that, but you need to know that as a family physician, I routinely meet with fathers during the pregnancy because I think it is important for a father to be involved in the care of his developing child.
> Jean: He never helps with the child he already has, so I don't know why he would consider getting involved before the next one's even born?
> Dr. C.: Would you like him to help out with your daughter more at home?
> Jean: Why of course, what woman wouldn't? But he's too busy with his work.
> Dr. C.: In my experience, fathers who get involved during the pregnancy, feel more committed to the family and help out more after the child is born. What if we invite him in for just one of your prenatal visits, and see how it goes?
> Jean: Maybe for one visit, if you can find a time he can make it.

Meeting with the Couple

In general, women see their primary care clinician more often than men do. As a result of routine gynecological care, women also tend to have a more comfortable relationship with their primary care clinician. The doctor's office is often unfamiliar territory to most men in this age group. When meeting with the couple during the pregnancy, extra time and care must be taken to establish a good relationship with the father, while still maintaining a positive relationship with the mother.

1. Establish rapport with the father at the very beginning of the visit.

Thank him for coming in, acknowledge what an important role he has in the pregnancy, and how you will need his help. Find out about his work and demonstrate interest in some aspect of his life.

2. Acknowledge the father's importance throughout the pregnancy and after delivery.

Refer to *their* pregnancy and *their* child. Use him as a consultant and ask him how he thinks the pregnancy is going. Encourage the couple to attend prenatal classes together.

3. Encourage the father to attend prenatal visits whenever possible, and to listen to the fetal heartbeat.

A doptone stethoscope with two headsets or a speaker allows couples to enjoy listening to the fetal heartbeat together. Both can be taught how to feel the uterus and where the baby is situated.

> Dr. C.: Hello, Peter, I am delighted that you could come it today. Did you have to take some time off from work to come in?
>
> Peter: Yeah, I had to leave my shift early today.
>
> Dr. C.: I see. What kind of work do you do?
>
> Peter: I'm the supervisor at one of the darkrooms at Kodak.
>
> Dr. C.: That must be challenging work. I appreciate the effort it took to get here. As I told your wife, I believe that the father plays a very important role in the care of his developing child, and I'd like to get your thoughts on how the pregnancy is going.
>
> Peter: Well, I'm not really sure. She doesn't tell me much. I am concerned that she hasn't been eating very well recently.
>
> Jean: I'm surprised you even noticed.
>
> Dr. C.: Well, let's talk about it. Jean, I think you should tell Peter how you have been feeling and how the pregnancy has been going for you. Then, we can listen to the baby's heartbeat.

4. Suggest that the father also attend to his health.

Fathers commonly have symptoms that mimic some of the symptoms of pregnancy (e.g., nausea, abdominal bloating, or increased urination, called Couvade Syndrome) (19). An office visit, or even a complete physical, gives the clinician an opportunity to evaluate any physical and psychological symptoms and establish a relationship with the father. It also lets the father know that his physical health is important. A spouse's pregnancy is a good time to suggest routine health screening (e.g., blood pressure, cholesterol) and review health risks (e.g., smoking, substance abuse). Becoming a parent may make some men more attentive to their own health.

5. When there are signs of marital conflict, acknowledge the stress of pregnancy on a marriage.

Focus on strengths and how the couple has coped with challenges in the past. Help the couple problem solve new limitations. For example, the father may need to do more of the shopping, housework, or child care because the pregnant woman is fatigued, or even on bed rest. Avoid blaming partners and focus instead on solutions. Emphasize working together to deliver a healthy baby. Couples will sometimes request help for marital problems, and a referral for marital therapy can be made (see Chap. 12).

Second Trimester: Halfway There

The second trimester (13–27 weeks) is often a period of calm and increased closeness between the couple. Morning sickness has usually resolved, and the woman feels physically and emotionally well. The risk of miscarriage (15% of all pregnancies) is resolved; pregnancy is well-established and very likely to result in live birth. This is the time when the couple can enjoy pregnancy and feel that they really are going to have a child together.

1. Elicit the couple's concerns and fears about the pregnancy, including birth defects.

A natural opportunity for a discussion of birth defects comes early in the second trimester when discussing tests for spina bifida and Down syndrome (e.g., maternal serum α-fetoprotein, triple screen, chorionic villi sampling, and amniocentesis). The couple may not have discussed these worries, concerned perhaps about increasing their partner's anxiety or that their own fears would not be understood. Bringing these out in the open allows the partners to be supportive of each other. Acknowledge and normalize these concerns and discuss any exaggerated or unwarranted fears: "All couples have questions about the baby's development and whether the baby will be normal. What questions or concerns do both of you have?" Some of these fears may be unrealistic. For example, one woman was concerned that her husband, who worked as an X-ray technician, was bringing home radiation that would harm her pregnancy, but was afraid to mention this to him because she thought he might have to quit his job.

2. Have the couple go together for any necessary tests, especially ultrasound.

For many couples, a stronger bond develops with the baby when they can actually see it with ultrasound and receive a picture.

3. Invite important family members and friends to prenatal visits.

Encourage the woman's mother to come for a visit. She is often the most important family health expert, especially regarding pregnancy and childbirth. In many families, beliefs about pregnancy and childbirth are passed on from mother to daughter through the generations. Comments or advice from the extended family may conflict with medical recommendations (e.g., "eat up, you're eating for two now," or "once a c-section, always a c-section") or lead to unnecessary anxiety (e.g., "women usually deliver a couple of hours after they lose the mucous plug"). It is important to establish an alliance with this family expert and to work collaboratively, instead of competitively, with her as much as possible.

> Peter accompanied his wife to several more prenatal visits, during which Dr. C. learned that the first few years of their marriage had been very difficult. Peter returned to school and Jean became pregnant shortly after they were married. For several months after the birth of their first child, Jean's mother lived with them to help care for the baby. When Jean complained to her mother more recently about how busy Peter was with his work, her mother suggested that she might be happier if she had another child.
>
> After learning this, Dr. C. invited Jean's parents to join the couple for a prenatal appointment. At the visit, all four agreed that the arrangement after the first pregnancy had not been satisfactory. Jean had resented her mother's advice and help after the first couple of weeks, and Peter felt excluded from the family. Jean's mother thought she was being taken advantage of and Jean's father felt abandoned by his wife. After discussing plans for the upcoming delivery, Peter decided to take 2 weeks off from work to be home after the child was born. Jean's parents agreed to help care for the 3-year-old and to assist with the new baby only when their daughter asked for help.

4. Discuss sexual issues of pregnancy with the couple.

Include the safety of intercourse throughout pregnancy and the use of different positions. Normalize changes in libido that occur in both men and women during pregnancy. Discuss future birth control options with the couple toward the end of the pregnancy.

5. Begin the discussion about breastfeeding.

Provide information about its benefits to the baby and the family. Find out whether other members of the couple's extended families have nursed their children and what advice they have given. Of all the variables involved with the decision to breastfeed, the support of the father is the most important. It is crucial to enlist his support.

6. Encourage the couple to take a minivacation or "second honeymoon" alone together during the second trimester.

Suggest that the father schedule 1 or 2 weeks of paternity leave for the time of delivery. Have the couple discuss which family members or friends may be available to help during the first few months after birth.

7. Find out what the couple has told or plans to tell the other child(ren) about the pregnancy.

Parents should tell other children by the time that the pregnancy is showing. During the third trimester, invite the other children in to a prenatal visit to discuss the "new baby" and listen to the fetal heartbeat.

8. Discuss with the couple whether and how they want their children involved in the labor and delivery.

Children under 5 or 6 years old generally have difficulty understanding what is occurring and may become quite frightened. This may distract the woman from her own focus on labor. Older children need careful preparation, often provided by hospital educators, if they are going to be present at the delivery. Children at a delivery should always be accompanied by an adult family member or friend who can attend to their needs throughout the labor and delivery (20).

9. Help parents anticipate sibling rivalry and regressions in development by siblings of the new baby (e.g., bedwetting, thumbsucking) and suggest ways the parents can deal with these problems.

These can include giving special attention and privileges to the older child, having the older child give a gift to the newborn, and finding special ways in which the older child can help with the baby's care (e.g., helping with diaper changes).

Third Trimester: Anticipating Labor and Delivery

The third trimester is usually a time of anticipation and some anxiety concerning labor and delivery, and the new baby. Acknowledging and normalizing the impatience and anxiety during this period can be very helpful for couples. At this time, one should review the typical events of labor and delivery, and elicit the couple's desires or birth plan (e.g., use of a birthing center, episiotomy, pain medication, different labor positions, etc.). Have the couple discuss what ways the father can be supportive to his partner during her labor. Options regarding breastfeeding and circumcision should be discussed. The decisions of the couple should be respected and supported. These decisions are often based as much, or more, on family, cultural, or religious tradition than on medical reasons.

The primary goal during labor and delivery is to promote a normal healthy childbirth with only the necessary medical interventions. Encourage families to use a family birthing center, when available. Family birthing centers can offer many of the advantages of home birth with the technology and emergency care available if needed. The homelike atmosphere of these centers helps to demedicalize the birth process and to reduce the anxiety of both mother and father. An office visit or home visit during early labor can allow the woman to remain at home until she has entered the active phase of labor and prevent unnecessary trips to the hospital for false labor. Although controversial, some clinicians provide home birth services, or back up for clinicians who do home births, in order to avoid technological intervention and hospital-based rules.

Labor and Delivery

1. Wisely use such interventions as enemas, fetal monitoring, intravenous fluids, pitocin, prostaglandins, pain medication, and artificial rupture of membranes (21).

Many interventions were performed historically because they were considered "routine," even though they had no grounding in evidence-based medicine. Some interventions cause unnecessary harm or distance the family from the birth process.

2. Recommend continuous support throughout labor.

Encourage the partner to take an active role in assisting during labor. It is often necessary to have the labor nurse and partner negotiate what roles they will have (e.g., who will rub the woman's back, encourage her to push, etc.), or labor nurses may take over, leaving the partner feeling helpless and neglected. Long labors can be extremely exhausting for both members of the couple; the woman cannot take a break, but the partner may need to utilize other family members or support people.

If the partner is not available, or even if he or she is, the use of a doula (i.e., untrained lay person) for continuous emotional support during labor has been shown to have a significant impact on labor. Sosa and colleagues (22, 23) demonstrated that doula supported births had shorter labors, fewer complications (including cesarean sections: 7% vs. 17%), and lower rates of oxytocin augmentation (2% vs. 13%). Kennell (24–26) replicated these studies and also showed lower rates of forceps delivery and use of epidural anesthesia.

3. At the time of delivery, the father's role should depend upon the needs and desires of the woman.

During difficult or long second stages of labor, he may need to support his partner at the head of the bed. If this is not needed, some fathers enjoy helping to deliver the baby or cutting the umbilical cord (27). If the baby is stable, put him or her directly on the mother's chest, skin to skin, shortly after birth. Encourage nursing as soon as desired. Early mother–infant contact has been shown to improve bonding (28), and early breastfeeding reduces the need for oxytoxics.

> Jean ruptured her membranes at home 4 days after her due date, but had no contractions. This was confirmed in the office and she was sent home with Peter. Several hours later she was in active labor and referred to the hospital. Shortly after settling into the birthing center, she

delivered a 9-pound baby boy without an episiotomy or laceration. Peter cut the umbilical cord and helped the nurse with the babys' first bath. An hour later, Jean's parents brought their granddaughter into the birthing center to see her parents and her new baby brother.

4. If complications arise during labor or delivery, it is important to explain clearly to the couple what is happening.

They usually will be very frightened and assume the worst (i.e., that the baby is dying) unless told otherwise. Choose consultants who have good communication skills and will work with the family. If a Ceasarean section is required, many hospitals now allow the father to be present in the operating room. Even if the baby requires resuscitation, the father should be allowed to be present and observe (out of the way). Even when the outcome is bad, fathers are reassured by observing everything done for the infant.

5. At the time of birth, parents are usually anxious to be told that the baby is normal.

This is best done by examining the baby at the bedside and explaining the normal findings to both parents. When birth anomalies are present, parents should be told immediately, but the overall health of the baby should be stressed. "Your baby appears to be very healthy; however, he has a cleft lip that can be corrected surgically." Going into detail about the problem is not useful at the time of delivery, but is best left to later when the parents can attend to and remember what is said.

Postpartum: Adjusting to a New Baby

1. Encourage feeding on demand and rooming-in, and avoid supplementing breastfeeding with formula or glucose water.

First-time mothers are usually anxious about their ability to breastfeed their infants and deserve lots of encouragement. If the mother is having difficulty with breastfeeding, observe a feeding to see what the problems are. Find out whether her mother breastfed her, and if possible use her as a consultant; unfortunately, a generation ago, fewer women breastfed so the grandmother may be just as anxious as the mother. A sister, sister-in-law, or close friend who has successfully nursed, or such a group as La Leche League can provide advice and support.

2. Encourage siblings to visit when the mother and infant are in the hospital.
3. At the time of discharge from the hospital, meet with both the father and mother.

Conduct the newborn's discharge physical at the mother's bedside, detailing normal findings again to the couple. Many first-time parents are reluctant to handle the newborn for fear of injuring the infant. Having the couple participate in the examination, feeling the fontanels, and lifting the unswaddled child in their hands can help them feel more comfortable with infant care.

Provide preprinted postpartum and newborn instructions and review these with the couple. Explore ways in which the father can participate in care of the child. For couples that breastfeed, the mother can pump her breasts for at least one bottle per day, and the father can do one feeding at a convenient time. Keeping the baby adapted to a bottle allows the mother and couple greater independence. Birth control and the resumption of sexual activity should be discussed with the couple.

4. At 1–2 weeks, a home visit is an excellent and enjoyable way to assess how the infant feeding is going and how the new family is coping.

In addition, it avoids exposing the infant to patients at the clinician's office with colds and other infections, and accommodates the belief of some cultures that the mother should not leave the house during the first several weeks after birth. At this time, there are usually very few biomedical issues to deal with and only a limited examination is needed; however, a scale may be needed to ensure the baby is back to its birth weight. During the visit, check on how the siblings are doing.

During this period, the family-oriented clinician should support the couple's own parenting skills and avoid giving too much advice. For example, mothers often ask how much formula the infant should be taking or whether he or she is getting enough breast milk. Rather than calculating the amount of formula based upon the infant's weight or age, encourage the couple to learn to assess whether the infant has had enough and is satisfied. This approach does not require a calculator, and it supports the parents' judgement and reduces their dependence upon health experts. With each success, their confidence will generalize to other areas of parenting (well-child care is discussed in Chap. 11).

> Arriving at the home for the 2-week well-child check, Dr. C. was met by the entire family, and a neighbor who "wanted to meet a doctor who really made home visits." After briefly examining the baby, Dr. C. joined the family for tea while they discussed how they were adapting to the new addition. Peter said he enjoyed staying home for the 2 weeks, but now he was eager to get back to work. Jean's parents liked getting to know their granddaughter better, as well as being consultants to the couple. Jean appreciated the help and support of her family and felt much more confident about her judgments and abilities as a mother.

A family-oriented approach that cares for the social, emotional, and biological needs of the entire family during pregnancy and birth provides a stage for promoting a healthy family throughout the life cycle.

Infertility

Infertility is generally defined as the inability to conceive after 1 year of unprotected intercourse. Given this broad definition, many couples fall into this category whose desire for children can be easily fulfilled. Education and advice often result in pregnancy. For many others, a few simple assessments can reveal the problem, and a solution can be provided.

Despite our culture's preoccupation with sex, many couples do not understand some basic principles of conception. Standard preconceptual advice often results in pregnancy. For example, the clinician might suggest that women start prenatal vitamins immediately, couples avoid lubricants that impair sperm motility or vitality, couples have intercourse every other day around midcycle, couples avoid alcohol and substance abuse, and the couple try a home ovulation kit. Depending on the couple's age (i.e., the clinician may want to move faster in the work-up of an "older" couple), a simple history and physical and laboratory tests may soon follow or be coincident with these recommendations. The single most important screening laboratory test that should be done for the couple, especially before any invasive studies are done, is a semen analysis. Many men are reluctant to do this but it is an absolutely essential part of the work-up. The initial advice, work-up, and treatment can be found in any good medical text.

For many other couples, very sophisticated interventions are required to produce any chance of successful pregnancy. For example, 54,383 babies were conceived via in vitro fertilization (IVF) between 1985 and 1995, according to the American Society for Reproductive Medicine, and another 10,000 were born after the use of other assisted reproductive technologies. Infertility presents psychosocial challenges to every family, and provides multiple opportunities for the astute family-oriented clinician to provide support and information that can make a difference.

Couples respond to the diagnosis and treatment of infertility in a variety of ways. For example, a portion of one or the other's identity may be closely linked to the notion of parenthood, and the diagnosis may result in a significant alteration in self-image and self-worth. One partner may blame the other, and/or one partner may feel particularly guilty (e.g. about a previously contracted sexually transmitted disease). One partner may be ready to proceed with treatment, whereas the other is still processing the change in self-image. Anxiety, stress, and depression are common, especially for women (29).

After appropriate primary care treatment, if the couple still has not conceived, referral to a specialist in infertility is warranted. Ongoing contact with the family-oriented primary care clinician is still indicated. The primary care clinician's knowledge of unique family stories about forming a family and parenthood will help as he or she points out special challenges and suggests ways the couple can apply their strengths to the problem(s).

The new reproductive technologies each add their own specific psychosocial challenges. For example, with donor sperm or eggs, some fathers or mothers are concerned about whether they will be less connected to the child because it is not their biological offspring. The American Society for Reproductive Medicine has published guidelines for psychological evaluation of oocyte donors and recipients (30). Donors need to be evaluated and counseled about how they might feel in the future about having offspring with whom they have no contact, or may not even know about. These are specialized issues that require a sophisticated psychological response. Most infertility centers mandate counseling before IVF and egg donor use, but the family-oriented primary care clinician lays the important groundwork and will provide long-term follow up.

As with all referrals, the primary care clinician provides a familiar face to interpret and translate complicated tests and diagnoses that the specialist has ordered or made. The family-oriented clinician provides essential emotional support through the whole process, and will still be there if all attempts are eventually unsuccessful. In addition, the primary care clinician's office may be called upon to provide special services (e.g. injections) because of their relative proximity to the patient.

Helpful tips (adapted from *Medical Family Therapy*, 31) for the family-oriented clinician counseling the infertile couple:

1. Provide education.

Discuss the prevalence of the problem, treatment, and likelihood of success. It may be necessary to translate some of the technical jargon.

2. Encourage communication.

There is frequently a sense of failure and loss of control that is not openly expressed. One may also want to recommend limiting inquiries from family and friends about "how they are doing."

3. Keep it in perspective.

Separate fertility from a sense of potency and self-worth. Externalize the problem and frame it as something the couple needs to work on together. The problem does not reside within one partner or another; it is the couple's problem.

4. Acknowledge the stress.

The work-up and treatment for infertility can be embarrassing, intrusive, invasive, and disruptive to normal living. Many couples will experience episodes of impotence, decreased libido, and anorgasmia. Advise the couple to put general limits on time devoted to the issue. Encourage a periodic vacation from the pressures of trying to conceive, taking time to pause and reflect. Try to decide in advance when to stop treatment.

5. Acknowledge the grief.

First there is loss of a portion of one's self-image, then there is loss associated with each unsuccessful attempt.

6. Mobilize resources.

Have the couple connect with caring family and friends. Many infertility centers provide support groups. Resolve is an excellent national self-help/advocacy/support organization, and the Center for Disease Control also provides useful information (see appendix).

7. When treatment is successful, have parents develop a loving story for the children about conception.

Stress the importance of being honest, in an age-appropriate way, with how the child(ren) was/were conceived.

Adoption

Like treatment for complicated infertility, the adoption process takes couples on an emotional roller coaster. There are many twists and turns, ups and downs, hopes and fears. Unlike the treatment for infertility, however, with enough perseverance (and money), the couple desiring a child is virtually guaranteed success. It is estimated that between 2% and 4% of American families have adopted. At any given time, there are approximately 500,000 American women actively looking to adopt, while another 2 million have at least investigated the process. One out of every five active adoption seekers will ultimately adopt (32). Though many non-relative adoptive couples have been through treatment for infertility, the clinician must keep in mind that adoption is a solution to the desire for a (more) child(ren), not infertility. Clinicians need to be wary of certain motivations for adoption (i.e., solution to a troubled marriage or the desire to replace a child who has died) and be alert for unresolved grief about treatment for infertility.

Successful adoption represents an extraordinary array of individual, family, and societal forces combined with simple luck. Most primary care clinicians have only cursory contact with the process, but they need to be sensitive to the issues as well as to be capable of offering information and advice. Once the adoption takes place, there is much to which the family-oriented clinician needs to watch and attend.

There are two kinds of adoption: private and agency. The legal system plays a crucial role in both cases, but especially so in the case of private adoption. Each method has unique characteristics, strengths, and weaknesses. The couple needs to find a method that is suited to their personal styles, toleration for ambiguity, time frame, and financial situation. In an agency-mediated adoption, there is often considerable contact between the birth mother and the agency staff, and adoptive parents and the staff. Interaction with agency staff often shapes adoptive parents' beliefs about adoption (33). The process is often longer and adoptive parents have more control. Private adoptions have fewer people involved, they tend to be faster, and be more expensive. In addition, there is tremendous variation in the laws of each country and state.

With adoption, there is significant external scrutiny of the couples potential as parents, and many couples resent this kind of intrusion into their personal lives. With biologically conceived children, the couple simply "gets pregnant." In adoption, parents must go before a court of law and be evaluated with a home study. Many couples are unnecessarily anxious about the home study. It is a preplacement report of prospective adoptive parents compiled by a social worker or case worker; basically, they want to ensure financial wherewithal, stability, and love.

The clinician needs to be realistic about what is involved with adoption. The couple will have justified fears about the health of the baby and his or her genetic background. What was the mother's health during her pregnancy? Did she use drugs? Did she have AIDS? Is there a strong family history of cancer, heart disease, or alcoholism? These are all reasonable questions; many can be answered, and some may not. The couple may be so desperate that they are afraid to ask for fear of jeopardizing the adoption, yet their questions may cause ever-increasing anxiety. These questions need to be brought out into the open and answered to the fullest extent possible. The clinician may need to push them a little with questions like, "Many families in your situation wonder about. . . . How have you thought about this issue?"

The couple may also have unrealistic expectations about the power of their love and nurturance to heal and overcome disabilities. Couples adopting children with inborn disabilities, or older children (over age 3) with acquired psychosocial disabilities from sexual abuse or violence, need to be closely counseled about what they can realistically expect. These are tough things to predict, but many couples overestimate their possible influence in these situations.

After a successful adoption, advise the couple to tell the children the story of their adoption. This is an obvious necessity in an open adoption where the birth mother has ongoing contact with the child, as well as in interracial adoptions. Parents should discuss adoption naturally, spontaneously, and in an age-appropriate way. Years ago, adoptive parents were told to keep the adoption a secret. This insulated children from the stigma of "illegitimacy," offered confidentiality to birth mothers, protected adoptive parents from the shame of infertility, and ensured no further intrusion to either biological or adoptive parents. This secrecy, however, inevitably became a barrier in family relationships, and there never seemed to be the "perfect time" to tell the child. An excellent example for how to tell the child is suggested in that time-honored tome of parent advice, *Dr. Spock's Baby and Child Care:*

> Let's say that a child around 3 hears her mother explaining to a new acquaintance that she is adopted, and asks, "what's 'adopted,' Mommy?" She might answer, "A long time ago I wanted very much to have a little baby girl to love and take care of. So I went to a place where there were a lot of babies, and I told the lady, 'I want a little girl with brown hair and blue eyes.' So she brought me a baby, and it was you. And I said, 'Oh, this is just exactly the baby that I want. I want to adopt her and take her home to keep forever.' And that's how I adopted you." This makes a good beginning because it emphasizes the positive side of the adoption: the fact that the mother received just what she wanted. The story will delight the child, and she'll want to hear it many times. (34)

Many adoptive parents enjoy promoting a child's native culture. These families strive to adopt a dual-culture identity. There are multiple support and information groups available to help with this, especially for couples adopting children of Asian heritage. This can be an exciting opportunity for parents (i.e., they can become educated about their child's original culture).

Ample informational resources are now available to adoptive parents. There are many good books for prospective adoptive parents (e.g., *The Complete Adoption Book*), and national organizations (e.g., Adoptive Families of America, National Adoption Information Clearinghouse, North American Council on Adoptable Children). Adopted children may also have some special needs growing up. For example, adopted children may secretly (or not so secretly) fear abandonment, especially during the teen years. There are many excellent resources to help families cope with these issues (see Appendix).

Conclusion

Family boundaries now transcend biological connection. Because of new reproductive technologies that enable unrelated people to conceive; because of increased interracial and intercultural adoptions; because of decreased shame and stigma associated with both infertility and sexual preference; and because of the new role of genetic testing and even the possibility of cloning, we have been forced to rethink what universally constitutes family. Modern treatments for infertility and adoption have pushed the envelope and redirected our focus to the functional relationship between family members. To paraphrase Dostoevsky in The Brothers Karamazov, "It's not just that they are your children, it's the relationship you develop with them over time" (35).

References

1. Klein M: Contracting for trust in family practice obstetrics. *Can Fam Clinician* 1983;29:2225–2227.
2. Prindham K, Schutz M: Preparation of parents for birthing and infant care. *J Fam Pract* 1981;13:181–188.
3. Young D: ICEA Adopts definition of family-centered maternity care. *Int J Childbirth Ed* February, 1987.
4. Scherger J: Family-centered childbirth: a philosophy well suited to family practice. *Family Practice Recertification* 1989; **11**, (1).
5. Nuckolls KB, Kaplan BH, & Cassel J: Psychosocial assets, life crisis and the prognosis of pregnancy. *Am J Epidemiol* 1972;95:431–441.
6. Norbeck JS & Tilden VP: Life stress, social support, and emotional disequilibrium in complications of pregnancy: A prospective, multivariate study. *J Health Soc Behav* 1983;24(1):30–46.
7. Reeb KG, Graham AV, Zyzanski SJ, & Kitson GC: Predicting low birthweight and complicated labor in urban black women: a biopsychosocial perspective. *Soc Sci Med* 1987;25:1321–1327.
8. Pagel MD, Smilkstein G, Regen H, & Montano D: Psychosocial influences on new born outcomes: a controlled prospective study. *Soc Sci Med* 1990; 30:597–604.
9. Smilkstein G, Helsper-Lucas A, Ashworth C, Montano D, & Pagel M: Prediction of pregnancy complications: an application of the biopsychosocial model. *Soc Sci Med* 1984;18:315–321.
10. Abell TD, Baker LC, Clover RD, & Ramsey CN Jr: The effects of family functioning on infant birthweight. *J Fam Pract* 1991;32:37–44.
11. Ramsey CN Jr, Abell TD, & Baker LC: The relationship between family functioning, life events, family structure, and the outcome of pregnancy. *J Fam Pract* 1986;22:521–527.
12. Larimore WL, Cline MK: keeping normal labor normal. *Prim Care* 2000;27(1):221–236.
13. King VJ: Passion and compassion. The healing arts. *NC Med J* 1992;53(4):177.
14. Mercer R, Hackley K, & Bostrom A: The relationship of psychosocial and perinatal variables to the perception of childbirth. *Nurs Res* 1983;32:202–207.
15. Midmer D, Talbot Y: Assessing post-partum family functioning: the family FIRO model. *Can Fam Clinician* 1988;34:2041–2048.
16. Combrinck-Graham L: A developmental model for family systems. *Fam Proc* 1985;24:139–150.
17. Friederick MA: Psychological changes during pregnancy. *Contemp OB/GYN* 1977;9:27–34.
18. McDaniel SH, Naumburg E: Gender issues: family medicine's family secret. *Fam Med* 1988;20:408–410.
19. Lamb GS, Lipkin M: Somatic symptoms of expectant fathers. *Am J Maternal Child Nursing* 1982;7:110–115.
20. Clark L: When children watch their mothers deliver. *Contemp OB/GYN.* Aug 1986;69–78.
21. Klein M, Lloyd I, Redman L, et al.: A comparison of low risk women booked for delivery in two different systems of care. Part 1: obstetrical procedures, and neonatal outcomes. *Br J Obstet Gynaecol* 1983;90:118–122.

22. Sosa R, Kennell J, Klaus M, et al.: The effect of a supportive companion on peri-natal problems, length of labor, and mother-infant interaction. *N Engl J Med* 1980;303:597–600.
23. Klaus M, Kennell J, Robertson S, Sosa R: Effects of social support during par-turition on maternal and infant morbidity. *Br Med J* 1986;293:585–587.
24. Kennell J, Klaus M, McGrath S, et al.: Medical intervention: the effect of social support during labor. *Pediatr Res* 1988;23(4):211a.
25. Kennell J, McGrath S, Klaus,M, et al.: Labor support: what's good for the mother is good for the baby. *Pediatr Res* 1989;25(4):15a.
26. Kennell J, Klaus M, McGrath S, et al.: Continuous emotional support during labor in a US hospital. *JAMA* 1991;265:2197–2201.
27. Block RA: We've let 1500 fathers deliver their own babies. *Med Econ* Aug. 9, 1982, pp. 181.
28. Klaus MH, Kennel J: *Maternal-Infant Bonding*. St. Louis: CV Mosby Co., 1976.
29. Greil AL: Infertility and psychological distress: a critical review of the litera-ture. *Soc Sci Med* 1997;45(11):1679–1704.
30. The American Society for Reproductive Medicine: Psychological assessment of oocyte donors and recipients. *Fertil Steril* 1998;70:4 (Suppl. 3):9S.
31. McDaniel SH, Hepworth J, & Doherty W: *Medical Family Therapy*. New York: Basic Books, 1992.
32. National Center for Health Statistics: Fertility, family planning, and women's health: new data from the 1995 national survey of family growth. National Center for Health Statistics, Vital Health Statistics 23, no. 19, 1997 (can be accessed at adoption institute web site: www.adoptioninstitute.org).
33. Gross HE: Variants of open adoptions: the early years. In: Gross HE, Sussman MB (Eds): *Families and Adoption*. Binghamton, NY: Haworth Press, 1997.
34. Spock B, Parker SJ: *Dr. Spock's Baby and Child Care*, 7th Edition. New York: Pocket Books, 1998.
35. Dostoevsky F: *The Brothers Karamazov* New York: Random House, 1996.

Protocol: Family-Oriented Pregnancy Care

Prepregnancy

- Encourage the couple to discuss their ideas and plans regarding pregnancy and children.
- Evaluate the extended family and their attitudes about pregnancy.
- Briefly assess where the couple is in the family life cycle and how they have negotiated the tasks of previous stages.
- Review biological and psychological risk factors.
- Support health habits.

First Trimester

- Explore whether pregnancy was desired or planned, and whether there are any thoughts of terminating pregnancy.
- Find out about social supports (e.g., father of child, parents, siblings, friends), and how these people feel about the pregnancy.
- Invite the father of the baby to all prenatal visits.
- Involve the father early on in the pregnancy.
- Be positive and direct about your need for the father to participate in prenatal care.
- Emphasize the importance of the father in the care of the pregnancy; stress the benefits of the partner's involvement to the patient and the pregnancy.
- Offer to call the partner yourself if needed.
- Request that the father come in for one prenatal visit, just to listen, without asking him to participate.
- Meet with the couple.
- Establish rapport with the father at the very beginning of the visit. Ask about his work, hobbies, or other interests.
- Acknowledge the father's importance throughout the pregnancy and after delivery. Use him as a consultant and ask him how he thinks the pregnancy is going.
- Encourage the father to attend prenatal visits whenever possible, and to listen to the fetal heartbeat.
- Suggest that the father also attend to his health.
- When there are signs of marital conflict, acknowledge the stress of pregnancy on a marriage.

Second Trimester

- Elicit the couple's concerns and fears about the pregnancy, especially regarding possible complications of labor or delivery, pain during labor, and birth defects.

- Have the couple go together for any necessary tests, especially ultrasound.
- Invite important family members and friends to prenatal visits. Consider having the woman's mother come for a visit.
- Discuss sexual issues of pregnancy with the couple, including the safety of intercourse throughout pregnancy and the use of different positions.
- Begin the discussion of breastfeeding early on, and provide information about its benefits to the baby and the family.
- Encourage the couple to take a minivacation or "second honeymoon" alone together during the second trimester; suggest that the father schedule one or two weeks of paternity leave for the time of delivery.
- Find out what the couple has told or plans to tell the other child(ren) about the pregnancy.
- Discuss with the couple how they want their children involved in the labor and delivery.
- Help parents anticipate sibling rivalry and regressions in development of siblings of a new baby (e.g., bedwetting, thumbsucking) and offer some suggestions.

Third Trimester

- Provide anticipatory education about mother's and father's roles during labor and delivery.
- Discuss ways for the father to be supportive to the mother during labor and delivery.
- Make preliminary decisions about:
    where to labor and deliver
    pain medication
    breast feeding
    circumcision

Labor and Delivery

- Encourage families to use family birthing centers, when available.
- Avoid interventions such as enemas, fetal monitoring, IVs, and medication, unless clearly indicated. Encourage the father to take an active role in assisting during labor.
- Recommend continuous support throughout labor.
- If the delivery is uncomplicated, encourage the father to assist as much as he likes (e.g., helping to deliver the baby's head or to cut the umbilical cord); encourage nursing as soon as it is desired.
- Clearly explain to the couple what is happening, especially if complications arise. Allow the father to be present for a Cesarian section if it is required.

- Examine the baby at the bedside and explain normal findings to both parents; when birth anomalies are present, inform parents immediately, but stress the overall health of the baby.

Postpartum

- Encourage feeding on demand and rooming-in, and avoid supplementing breastfeeding; if the mother is having difficulty with breastfeeding, observe a feeding to see what the problems are.
- Encourage siblings to visit when the mother and infant are in the hospital.
- Conduct the newborn's discharge physical at the mother's bedside, and have the couple participate in the examination.
- At 2 weeks, make a home visit to assess how the infant feeding is going and the new family is coping.

Infertility

- Provide education.
- Encourage communication.
- Keep it in perspective.
- Acknowledge the stress.
- Acknowledge the grief.
- Mobilize resources.
- Develop a loving story.

Adoption

- Review motivation for adoption and address any unresolved grief over failure of infertility treatment (if applicable).
- Educate about options for adoption and use knowledge of the family to facilitate appropriate referral.
- Be proactive about addressing risks of adoption and making expectations realistic.
- Acknowledge both emotional and financial stresses.
- Encourage parents to tell their adopted child that they are adopted in an age-appropriate way.
- Provide anticipatory guidance and attend to special cross cultural/ethnic issues; encourage parents to adopt a dual-culture identity.

Infertility and Adoption Resource Guide

Adoption Institute at www.adoptioninstitute.org
Beauvais-Godwin L, Godwin R: The Complete Adoption Book: Everything You Need to Know to Adopt the Child You Want in Less Than 1 Year, Adams Media Corporation, 1997.

Doulas of North America: www.dona.org

Gilman L: The Adoption Resource Book. New York: HarperCollins, 1992.

International Childbirth Education Association: www.licea.org International Journal of Childbirth Education, P.O. Box 20048, Minneapolis, Minnesota 55420

La Leche League International: www.lalecheleague.org

Midwife Association of North America: www.mana.org

Peoples D, Ferguson HR: What to Expect when You're Experiencing Infertility: How to Cope with the Emotional Crisis and Survive. New York: W.W. Norton & Co., 1998.

Resolve: www.resolve.com or at 5 Water St., Arlington, MA, 12174

Society of Teachers of Family Medicine Monograph on Family-Oriented Pregnancy Care

Centers for Disease Control: www.cdc.org

Stork Net: www.storknet.org

Treiser S, with Levinson RK: A Woman Doctor's Guide to Infertility. New York: Hyperion, 1994.

11
Supporting Parents: Family-Oriented Child Healthcare

Parents seek help or advice from their children's primary care clinician for a wide variety of problems. They certainly look for help when their children are febrile, injured, or ill. They more commonly have questions or concerns about such issues as development, behavior, sleeping, eating, and immunizations. In fact, the majority of a pediatrician's time (1), estimated by some as high as 85% (2), is spent dealing with psychosocial and developmental issues that arise during both well-child and acute-care visits. Because most of these requests for assistance are not severe enough to warrant referral, primary care clinicians need skills to assess each situation individually and provide a suitable response. We advocate an approach that expands beyond the traditional biomedical, anticipatory guidance model and takes into account the context of the child while simultaneously assessing the need for intervention.

In the traditional anticipatory guidance model, the clinician uses his or her expert knowledge of child development and child developmental milestones to educate and guide parents in raising their child (1–4). The clinician counsels parents about how to deal with everyday health and behavior concerns and anticipate future changes or difficulties. The clinician also uses his or her expertise to intervene when the child's health is at risk. In the traditional model, the clinician is available to parents as both a medical and childrearing authority.

The traditional model can become a routine checklist where parents and children are scored by the expert clinician. This approach does not place the child's development in context, in relation to his or her parents and siblings. It often does not take into account a particular family's strengths and weaknesses—strengths and weaknesses that should determine the level of intervention, if any, that is needed from the clinician. We are also concerned that the traditional approach can place inappropriate expectations on the clinician to be an expert parent, a better parent than any of his or her patients, while disempowering the parents. It encourages the clinician to assume the role of surrogate parent and give advice, whether needed or not, on everything from toilet training and proper selection of toys to childproofing one's house. It can turn the clinician into a list checker, an inflexible automaton who cannot see the forest for the trees. This approach medicalizes childrearing and inadvertently encourages parents to believe they need expert medical advice to do their job.

In a family-oriented approach to child healthcare, the clinician and parents, as well as other important child healthcare givers (e.g., grandparents) work collaboratively (5). Both the family and the medical system have areas of expertise and the clinician needs to honor, respect, and nurture the family's competence. *The clinician's first priority is to support the parents being in charge of their child's overall healthcare.* The clinician may be an expert on medical matters, but only intervenes when needed. Every patient is unique and the clinician uses his or her knowledge and experience to educate, guide, and intervene, based on the parents' strengths and resources, and the child's level of need (6).

Dimensions of Child Healthcare

A clinician's contacts with a family for child healthcare cannot always be neatly divided into well-child and acute care. It is not out of the ordinary for a "normal" well-child visit to be focused on a parent's unexpected concern ("Why isn't my baby gaining weight faster?") or an acute-care visit to reveal only mild symptoms in the child, but important concerns in the parent ("I'm feeling overwhelmed caring for my child"). One study has indicated that the parent seeking care for his or her child came for reasons other than the primary complaint in one third of acute child care cases (7).

It is important in any child healthcare visit to understand both the nature of the child's symptoms and what they mean to the parents, as well as what the parents are requesting of the clinician. For that reason we view these visits as having two dimensions: one pertaining to the child and the other pertaining to the parent. These dimensions interact to form four different configurations (see Fig. 11.1):

- Well Child–Confident Parent. In these visits, the child is healthy and developing well, and the parents are feeling confident in their parenting.

> Ms. Gleason brought Joey, age 10 months, for a well-child visit. Ms. Gleason reported that their daughter, age 4, was adjusting well to having a baby brother and that both parents were feeling good about how things were going. Dr. B. examined Joey who was developing at a normal rate.

- Well Child–Distressed Parent. In these visits, the child is healthy and developing well, but the parent has specific concerns (e.g., feeding, toilet training, or the use of pacifiers).

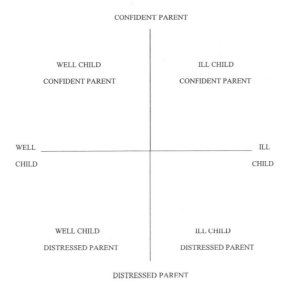

CONFIDENT PARENT

WELL CHILD
CONFIDENT PARENT

ILL CHILD
CONFIDENT PARENT

WELL _____ ILL
CHILD   CHILD

WELL CHILD
DISTRESSED PARENT

ILL CHILD
DISTRESSED PARENT

DISTRESSED PARENT

FIGURE 11.1. Dimensions of child healthcare.

Mr. and Mrs. Tanner, both of northern European descent, had both been previously married, and now had joint custody with their previous spouses of their combined six children. Mrs. Tanner brought her daughter Emily, age 2, for a routine well-child visit. Dr. N. examined Emily and found she was in good health, although she continually opened drawers and tried to play with the medical instruments during the visit. Dr. N. explained to Mrs. Tanner, "We're here to examine your child's health. I know that sometimes in a doctor's office it can be confusing as to who is in charge. If you see your child doing something that you don't feel is appropriate, please feel free to manage her the way you would at home." Dr N. later asked if Mrs. Tanner had any questions or concerns. Mrs. Tanner said they were having a lot of difficulty getting Emily to stop using a bottle, was not sure what to do, and wanted to come up with a plan that would work when Emily was with her father too.

- Ill Child–Confident Parent. In these visits, the child is sick and the parent feels confident to handle the illness, but needs reassurance that he or she is doing a good job as a parent.

  Mr. Conway, a 30-year-old African-American man, brought Mike, age 4, to the doctor's office with a 3-day history of diarrhea. Mr. Conway said Mike's mother had stayed home from work with Mike the day before. They were pushing fluids, treating his fever, staying away from dairy products, and washing their hands frequently. They were not sure if Mike might have been getting dehydrated or if there was anything more they should be doing.

- Ill Child–Distressed Parent. In these visits the child is ill and the parent is distressed both about the child and about his or her own ability to manage the situation as a parent. These visits may also involve a child being brought to the doctor's with mild symptoms by a parent who has his or her own personal concern. (e.g., "Sometimes I don't know what to do next" or "I've been feeling very tired lately"). A more subtle variation of this category is the parent of a very symptomatic child who does not appear to be concerned, but is actually denying his or her distress rather than truly feeling confident. These parents also need extra support from their clinician.

> Mary brought Rachel, age 3, to see Dr. V. because Rachel had symptoms of a cold. Mary, a single parent, reported that her daughter had started day care 2 months prior to the visit and seemed to be "sick all the time." Mary had started a new job and said she felt at her "wit's end" over Rachel's colds. Mary wondered if she was doing something wrong.

Understanding how the child and parent dimensions interact helps the clinician clarify the multiple factors that may be involved in any visit. The clinician is then better able to respond to the concerns related to both dimensions.

> Mrs. Jackson brought David, age 6, to the office with rhinorrhea and a low-grade fever. Nurse practitioner Kathy O. determined that the boy had a cold and the parents had been treating him appropriately with liquids, acetaminophen, and rest. Mrs. Jackson, though, was still distressed about her son's "congestion." Upon further questioning, Kathy O. learned that the Jackson's oldest child had had serious pneumonia at the same age. When Kathy O. said there was nothing to indicate pneumonia, Mrs. Jackson breathed a sigh of relief.

Having taken both the child and parent dimensions into account, Kathy O. recognizes this to be an ill child–distressed parent visit and is better able to address the presenting complaint as well as the concern of the parent. The interplay of child and parent dimensions in an office visit illustrates the importance of considering psychosocial factors in child healthcare. In the next section on psychosocial assessment we will discuss child and family development as well as how child health concerns can be related to other family difficulties.

Psychosocial Assessment in Child Healthcare

Gaining information on child, parent, and family functioning need not be a time-consuming task in the already overburdened schedules of primary care clinicians. Much valuable information can be gained by exploring a few questions with the parent who has brought the child for a visit. In the long run it will save time. Without a clear picture of the multiple factors that contribute to a pediatric visit, the clinician may not be able to respond adequately to the needs of both the parent and child. This may lead to numerous follow-up phone calls and well child–distressed parent visits until the whole agenda of the original visit has been addressed. The clinician will be able to intervene more effectively and efficiently by assessing psychosocial factors early.

There are three valuable questions to explore in child healthcare psychosocial assessment:

1. What are the developmental issues facing the child and his or her parents?

The clinician's frame of reference for assessing child development and behavior is based on cumulative professional knowledge rather than anecdotal or personal experience alone. It is important for the clinician to use such knowledge to both assess the child's growth and functioning, and to identify when parents have inappropriate expectations of their child. In the latter situation, gathering more information before intervening is usually the safest approach.

> Mrs. Rush: Doctor, Jennifer is 15 months old and she shows no interest in the potty at all. I've explained to her that big girls should not be using diapers, but she doesn't understand. My husband thinks I'm on her too much about it.

In this well child–distressed parent visit, the clinician realizes that a concern about toilet training may arise for some parents near their child's eighteenth month (8). He sees that Jennifer has no physiological problem and appears to be a happy child. Mrs. Rush may be premature in her worry about Jennifer. Jennifer does not have the cognitive ability at 15 months to understand her mother's explanation of the importance of toilet training (6, 9). She may not be physically prepared either, as evidenced by her inability to take her pants off. Furthermore, she may not be ready emotionally for the responsibility and reward of using the "potty." The clinician sees that there is an incongruity between Jennifer's level of development and Mrs. Rush's expectations. The clinician explores the situation further rather than giving her advice prematurely.

2. What life cycle tasks are facing the family at this time?

A child's development is part of the larger process of the family development. In the case of the Rush family, Mr. and Mrs. Rush and their new child are moving from one stage in the family life cycle, The Newly Married Couple, to another, The Family with Young Children (see Appendix 3.1 for a description of all the family life cycle stages). The Rushes are working to integrate a new member into what had previously been a dyadic relationship.

The major tasks for families with young children include: (1) adjusting the marital relationship to accommodate new family members; (2) taking on parenting roles; and (3) realigning the parent's relationship to their parents, who now are grandparents. This is a time in the family life cycle when all three generations are drawn closer together, while at the same time trying to redefine their relationships (10). In child healthcare assessment it is important to explore this larger developmental context.

> Dr. S.: This is a time of tremendous change for you and your husband. How has it affected the two of you?
>
> Mrs. Rush: Most of the time I feel overwhelmed. I don't even know how my husband feels. We hardly ever see each other. By the time he's home from work, I'm ready for bed.
>
> Dr. S.: It sounds pretty strenuous for both of you. Are your parents or your husband's parents around?
>
> Mrs. Rush: His parents are out of state. Mine are nearby, but sometimes they help too much. I mean, I feel like no matter what I do I should have done it differently.

Due to the pressing demands of parenthood the Rushes have not had time to renegotiate their relationship as husband and wife. Mrs. Rush's parents are naturally pulled closer to their daughter to help out, but their involvement often feels like criticism. Mrs. Rush feels overwhelmed, inadequate, and alone. Her concern about her daughter's toilet training may reflect the family's difficulty navigating normal changes in the family life cycle. Because it is not clear how Mr. Rush feels, Dr. S. suggests that the Rushes hold off on potty training for now and invites Mr. Rush to the next appointment. This will give Dr. S. an opportunity to further assess as well as support them as a parenting team.

3. Is the child's health or behavior difficulty related to other problems in the family?

A child's illness is sometimes related to worry about a grandparent, school concerns, sibling rivalry, the stress of moving, or a loss. A child's difficulties may play a part in supporting the parents' marriage. For example, a child's health or behavior problems may give a couple with an unstable marriage a common focus of concern. With each new demand the couple may pull together for the sake of their child's health despite problems that may exist in the marriage. In that way the child and his or her difficulties may function as the glue that keeps the parents together. It has also been theorized that one of the ways couples can deal with marital discord is to "project" the conflict onto their children (11–14). The most typical pattern is for the mother to become overinvolved with a child, whereas the father either encourages the overinvolvement by maintaining distance, or challenges it by battling with the mother over parenting questions. In either case, the parents do not have to address the marital problems. Child-related difficulties may receive exclusive attention and become the means by which marital dissatisfaction is also expressed. These patterns can represent quite serious dysfunction, or can be a mild concern, as in the following example:

> Dr. S. (to Mr. Rush): What concerns do you have about Jennifer?
>
> Mr. Rush: None. I don't think there is a problem. No one in my family was toilet trained this young. She's just a baby. It's my mother-in-law who seems to be pushing this.
>
> Dr. S. (to Mrs. Rush): What do you think?
>
> Mrs. Rush: I'm not sure what to think. My mother is concerned.
>
> Mr. Rush: She always seems to be involved in our affairs.
>
> Dr. S.: How do the two of you feel the toilet training should be addressed?
>
> Mr. Rush: I don't think there's a big hurry, do you? (to Mrs. Rush).
>
> Mrs. Rush No, I don't either. I guess I just needed to hear what you thought.
>
> Dr. S.: I think you're both correct. Different generations choose different times to toilet train. The important thing is that the two of you be together on this. It seems that when you have the chance to work together these decisions are easier to deal with.

Dr. S. recognizes that marital stress over the involvement of Mrs. Rush's mother may predate the birth of Jennifer. He also hypothesizes that marital discord may be fueling Mrs. Rush's overconcern about Jennifer's toilet training. It is interesting that the focus on Jennifer has brought the couple together in order to make a decision. Dr. S. supports the parent's capacity to work together and make good parenting decisions. Building an alliance with the couple around this issue will make it easier to address any future marital problems.

In this case example we have illustrated various aspects of assessment and how the clinician can use this assessment process to both involve other family members and support their competence to solve the presenting problem. The family-oriented clinician functions less as the exclusive problem solver and more as a facilitator and consultant in the problem-solving process. In the next section we will discuss specific guidelines for implementing a family-oriented approach to child healthcare.

Guidelines for Family-Oriented Child Healthcare

Child healthcare provides one of the best opportunities for a clinician to implement a family-oriented approach to primary care. The clinician has access to at least one parent on a regular basis for well-child and periodic acute care for many years. This gives the clinician the chance to approach primary care in a way that supports parents and utilizes their strengths in the healthcare of their children. The following are some guidelines for implementing a family-oriented approach.

1. Whenever possible invite both parents to child healthcare visits.

Although both parents do not always need to attend, the clinician's invitation communicates respect for the importance of both parents' roles in their child's healthcare. For physicians who provide pregnancy care, this behavior flows naturally from attitudes established during the pregnancy (see Chap. 10). In more serious or conflictual situations the clinician may communicate the necessity of both parents being involved in order for an effective treatment plan to be developed (see Chap. 12 for a discussion of working with parents on child behavior problems). Even in routine visits, however, it can be valuable either to have both parents come in periodically or to have them alternate bringing their child for visits. This helps the clinician develop a good working relationship with the mother and father so that when and if other critical situations arise, the clinician and parents have already established a foundation for collaboration. For example, if the mother has brought the child, then an invitation to the father can be extended through her:

> Doctor: Mrs. Bailey, your child is doing very well and it sounds like things are going well at home, too. One of the things I do as a normal part of my practice is to involve both parents whenever possible. Sometimes both parents come with their child; sometimes parents alternate accompanying their child. It's very valuable for me to get to know you both because you know your child so well and you each may have a little different perspective. It also gives us a chance to work together for your child's ongoing health. So, I'd like to invite your husband to come in whenever it can be arranged.

2. Discuss the parents' view of how the child is developing.

This gives the clinician a chance to learn the parents' view of how they feel their child is or should be developing. From a family viewpoint, it is also an opportunity to explore the impact of childrearing on parents and significant others. Whether a clinician is seeing one parent, both parents, or a grandparent, valuable questions to pose include:

How do you feel your child is doing?
What do others around you say about how your child is doing?

What is most rewarding in parenting your child (or children)?

What is most challenging in parenting your child (or children)?

What adjustments are you having to make in your marital relationship and daily routine due to the demands of parenting?

How has the birth of this child had an impact on other family members, especially siblings and grandparents?

3. Adjust your level of intervention based on the need.

The strength with which a clinician should intervene will depend partly on the *health risk* involved. When a parent raises the issue of toilet training, the clinician may see the health risks as *absent* or *mild*, and he or she may support the parents in making their own decisions. If the parents are discussing sending their child to bed with a bottle of milk, the clinician may view the health risk as *moderate* and explain the danger to their child's teeth and gums, while supporting the parents in developing a plan to help their child go to sleep without a bottle. If parents report feeding their infant child hot dogs or peanuts, the clinician may perceive the health risk as potentially *severe* and make his or her recommendations actively and strongly.

The level of parental or family anxiety also influences the type of clinician intervention. If the child is well, the parents are confident, and the level of anxiety is low, the clinician can relax and facilitate the parent's decisions. Even if the child is only mildly ill, however, if the parents are very distressed and anxiety is high, the clinician needs to be more directive. The worried parents at 2 A.M. do not really want to be massaged about what a nice job they are doing, they want to know what to do. In situations of high anxiety or crisis, families need a strong, directive response. Once the crisis has passed, a more facillitative stance can be taken to address parental anxiety in the future (see Fig. 11.2).

Individual clinician styles vary, and every clinician finds that at first they tend to be better at one method of intervention than another. Some clinicians are better initially at the kind, nurturing, supportive style of intervention, whereas others are better at the strong, directive, take-charge style. Every clinician eventually needs to be able to incorporate the whole range of styles into their repertoire of relational skills. Different subcultures or training backgrounds may have reinforced a particular style of responding to patient's needs (e.g., the traditional biomedical culture may have so heavily reinforced the level 3 style that clinicians have trouble backing off and letting the parents decide how to resolve an issue). Culturally determined traditional gender roles may also have influenced the clinician's strengths and weaknesses. For example, female clinicians may be better at level 1, whereas male clinicians may be more adept at level 3. In any event, every clinician needs to identify their own strengths, weaknesses, and biases, and be able to diversify their approaches and styles to complement and address the patient and family's needs.

Parental and family anxiety	Medical risk	Level of intervention
Low: Parents just want to double-check something	Low: upper respiratory infections general toilet training question of using a pacifier mild constipation introduction of solid food	1 Support Parental Decision-making
Medium: Parents have concerns and need advice, e.g. about safety of immunizations	Medium: asthma diabetes enuresis/encopresis bottle at bedtime learning disabilities	2 Advise and Collaborate with Patients and Family
High: Family crisis, e.g. divorce.	High: appendicitis lead poisoning infants eating dangerous foods child physical or sexual abuse eating disorders depression with suicidal intent	3 Issue a Strong Directive

FIGURE 11.2. Levels of physician intervention in child healthcare.

Once the health risk and level of distress has been assessed and the decision about how to intervene has been made, remember to use clear, concrete, understandable language in making any suggestions. Boyle and Hoekelman (15) report that interaction with a clinician can be intimidating for parents, and the use of technical language can be a contributing factor. A clinician can help parents feel more comfortable by using layman's language.

4. Support the parents in developing possible solutions.

Parents have primary responsibility for carrying out medical treatment in most child healthcare situations. For that reason it is important to encourage parent involvement in treatment planning, and whenever possible support parents in developing their own solutions to child health-care dilemmas. One study showed that parents were correct 97.1% of the time about whether their child's ear infection cleared up. Letting parents know this bit of research, and leaving a follow-up appointment to their discretion further empowers them as "medical experts" on their children (16).

Even in severe risk situations (e.g., eating lead-based paint) that call for strong clinician interventions it is important to discuss the parents' questions and concerns and, when appropriate, incorporate their ideas into the plan. In many situations the clinician's main intervention may be to engage the parents in discussing and formulating their own solutions. These discussions may range from helping parents decide when to introduce solids into their child's diet to clarifying how their child will receive medication when both parents are working all day.

Before the visit is concluded, if the plan is complex or there is a lot of anxiety, it is valuable to review the plan that the parents and clinician have devised. This may involve having parents restate the plan of action, clarify the areas of responsibility for the parents and the clinician, and specify what follow up will occur. It is sometimes useful to write these things down.

5. When necessary set up a separate appointment to further address any remaining concerns.

Bass and Cohen (7) have shown that in child healthcare visits there is often a difference between the ostensible and actual reason for the appointment. A parent whose son has cold symptoms may also be coming because he or she generally feels overwhelmed with parenting responsibilities. No real dichotomy typically exists between ostensible and actual reasons for a medical visit. It is usually a matter of there being multiple reasons for most visits, the cold may only be the last straw. A parent may both be concerned about his or her child's symptoms and about the anxiety a grandparent may have about the child or the history of a similar illness in the family. It is important for the clinician to explore the possibility of multiple factors in any visit.

If a child's illness provides an opportunity for the parent to ask for help for something else, then it is important to respond to the parent's concern directly. This makes it clear that the child does not have to be ill for the parent to get help in the future. When an agreeable plan for the child has been developed the clinician can suggest an appointment to discuss remaining concerns of the parents. Offering such an appointment shows respect for the parents' concern and provides an opportunity to assess and join with the family further.

In the following case Dr. M. illustrates many of the guidelines for family-oriented child healthcare:

Mrs. Johnson, a 35-year-old professional Jewish woman, brought 8-month-old Judy, the Johnson's first baby, for a well-child visit. During the course of the exam Dr. M asked how Mrs. Johnson felt Judy was doing and learned that Judy had been having some difficulty sleeping in the last month. She had been getting up three times a night and Mrs. Johnson wondered if something was wrong. Dr. M. asked if Mr. Johnson was concerned about Judy. She said her husband was losing sleep as well, and did not know what to think.

Dr. M. completed his exam of Judy and reported to Mrs. Johnson that Judy was developing very well. Dr. M. then asked Mrs. Johnson to describe the impact of Judy's sleep pattern on her and her husband further. Mrs. Johnson said it had been "pretty awful." She and her husband often spent most of the night worrying and feeling they must be doing something wrong. Dr. M. said he was sure there was no physiological problem. He then asked if there had been any other changes recently. Mrs. Johnson said Judy's birth had been the "one big change" in their lives and reported that everything else was going fairly well. Dr. M. said that often a child's sleep, or lack thereof, created concerns for conscientious parents. Dr. M. said he often met with parents who were dealing with these kinds of concerns and offered to meet with Mr. and Mrs. Johnson. Mrs. Johnson felt that would be helpful. They set up an appointment for the following week.

Dr. M. asks about recent life changes in order to learn about losses, job stress, family illnesses, marital difficulties, or other issues that may play a part in the Johnsons' concerns. Dr. M. realizes that there are several factors involved in this visit: Judy's overall health and development, her sleep pattern, the effect of Judy's sleep pattern on her parents, and the Johnson's concern about what to do. Dr. M.'s assessment is that this is a well child–distressed parent case. As the medical expert, Dr. M. assures Mrs. Johnson that there is no physiological cause, except perhaps teething, for Judy's sleep pattern. He then uses this as an opportunity to meet with both parents to support them as a co-parenting team.

During the meeting with Mr. and Mrs. Johnson, Dr. M. learned that both parents got up at night whenever Judy stirred or cried. They picked her up frequently to comfort her and worried that she might not feel well. The Johnsons said they had been trying to have a child for 6 years and just wanted to "do things right." Dr. M. emphasized again that there was no physiological problem, but that infants often enjoyed the comfort their parents offered by picking them up when they cried. Dr. M. said this did not create problems for the baby, but could often be stressful or exhausting for the parents. When that was the case Dr. M. said he suggested letting the child cry longer so that the baby could get used to comforting him or herself. One strategy is to double the time between each visit to comfort the child (i.e. let the child cry for 2 minutes, then go in and comfort the child, then let it cry for 4 minutes, comfort the child, and so on). Although this could make things worse for several nights, it was not dangerous for the child to cry and in a few days he or she tends to sleep better. Dr. M. then asked the Johnsons what they felt they should do. The Johnsons discussed Dr. M.'s suggestion and decided it was worth a try. Mr. and

Mrs. Johnson determined how long they were willing to let Judy cry and how they would alternate checking on her if the need arose. Dr. M. supported their plan and suggested they call to let him know how it was going.

This chapter focused on the clinician's role of supporting parents being in charge of the broad range of child healthcare concerns that may be thought of as "normal." At times, this means the clinician uses his or her authoritative role as medical and child development expert to provide consultation, direction, and even major intervention to distressed parents or seriously ill children; at other times, the clinician is more facillitative and supports the parents establishing directions they deem appropriate. The emphasis is on assessing the need, intervening as appropriate, collaborating with, and empowering parents.

We will discuss child behavior problems that are more extreme in nature in the next chapter. These may involve both high health risk and high parental distress. Parents in these situations feel stuck: They have tried all the solutions they know to try and are unsure what to do or where to turn. Even though parent–clinician collaboration is still the key, the clinician will find it necessary to intervene more actively with these problems while still respecting the parents' authority regarding their child.

References

1. Christopherson ER: Anticipatory guidance on discipline. *Pediatr Clin N Am* 1986;**33**(4):789–798.
2. Brazelton TB: Anticipatory guidance. *Pediatr Clin N Am* 1975;**22**:533–544.
3. Solnit AJ: Psychotherapeutic role of the clinician. In: Green M, Haggerty R (Eds). *Ambulatory Pediatrics*. Philadelphia, W. B. Saunders Co., 1977, pp. 197–207.
4. American Academy of Pediatrics: *Guidelines for Health Supervision*. American Academy of Pediatrics, 1985.
5. Almond, et al. The family is the patient.
6. Parker S, Zuckerman B: *Behavioral and Develpmental Pediatrics: A Handbook of Primary Care*. Boston: Little, Brown & Co., 1995.
7. Bass LW, Cohen RL: Ostensible versus actual reasons for seeking pediatric attention: Another look at the parental ticket of admission. *Pediatrics* 1982;**70**(6):870–874.
8. Talbot Y: Behavior problems in children. In: Christie-Seely J. (Ed). *Working With the Family in Primary Care: A Systems approach to Health and Illness*. New York, Praeger, 1984.
9. Flavell JH: *The Developmental Psychology of Jean Piaget*. New York, Van Nostrand Co., 1963.
10. Combrink-Graham L: A developmental model for family systems. *Fam Proc* 1985;**24**(2):139–150.
11. Bowen M: Theory in the practice of psychotherapy. In Guerin PJ (Ed). *Family Therapy*. New York: Gardner Press, 1976, pp. 42–90.

12. Bowen M: *Family Therapy in Clinical Practice*. New York: Jason Aronson, 1978.
13. Kerr ME: Family systems therapy and therapy. In Gurman AS, Kniskern DP (Eds). *Handbook of Family Therapy*. New York: Brunner/Mazel, 1981, pp. 226–266.
14. Minuchin S: *Families and Family Therapy*. Cambridge, MA: Harvard University Press, 1974.
15. Boyle WE, Hoekelman RH: The pediatric history. In: Hoekelman RH, Blatman S, Friedman S, Nelson N, & Seidel H (Eds). *Primary Care Pediatrics*. St. Louis, MO: Mosbtry, 1987, pp. 52–62.
16. Hathaway TJ, Ksatz Hp, Dershewitz RA, & Marx TJ: Acute otitis media: who needs follow-up? *Pediatrics* 1994:**94**(2 pt. 1):143–147.

Protocol: Supporting Parents in Child Healthcare

Psychosocial Assessment in Child Healthcare

- What are the developmental issues facing the child and his or her parents?
- What life cycle tasks are facing the family at this time?
- Is the child's health or behavior difficulty related to other problems in the family?

Dimensions to Consider in Child Healthcare

- Well child–confident parent visits
- Well child–distressed parent visits
- Ill child–confident parent visits
- Ill child–distressed parent visits

Guidelines for Family-Oriented Child Healthcare

- Whenever possible, invite both parents in for child healthcare visits.
- Discuss the parents' view of how the child is developing.
  - How do you feel your child is doing?
  - What is most rewarding in parenting your child (or children)?
  - What is most challenging in parenting your child (or children)?
  - What adjustments are you having to make in your marital relationship and daily routine due to the demands of parenting?
  - How has the birth of this child had an impact on other family members, especially siblings and grandparents?
- Adjust the level of intervention based on the need.
- Support the parents in developing possible solutions; when necessary, set up a separate appointment to further assess any remaining concerns.

12
When Parents Get Stuck: Helping with Child Behavior Problems

There are no diplomas that insure good parenting, and there are relatively few times that parents hear that they are doing a good job. Disapproving glances exchanged in grocery stores when young children are throwing tantrums are more common. A call from the elementary school teacher can make a parent concerned both about their child's immediate behavior and about whether he or she will have a school career of frustration or ease. Parents often measure the quality of their parenting by the success or happiness of their children. Thus, when children experience behavior difficulties, parents cope both with the annoying or dangerous behavior as well as personal feelings of disappointment and failure.

Parents generally respond to behavior problems first on their own, even though they may consult family members or friends. When they feel stuck in their attempts, parents may turn to a professional, primarily their physician, for help (1). Physicians are resources about common difficulties with daily routine (e.g., refusing to eat, problems with bedtime, toilet training), aggressive or resistant behavior (e.g., fighting, tantrums), overdependent or withdrawing behavior (e.g., separation anxiety, fears), school problems (e.g., hyperactivity or restlessness), and habits that parents do not like (e.g., thumb-sucking, playing with genitals too much) (2). Many of these behaviors diminish with simple strategies, including positive reinforcement, behavioral modification strategies, and consistent expectations among caregivers. Some children, however, perhaps 10–15%, (3), develop behavior problems that interfere with life adjustment.

Most clinicians ask about these concerns at well-child visits, hoping that parents will say that there are no serious problems or concerns. When parents want help with these behavioral problems, clinicians can feel overwhelmed by the perceived time or specialized knowledge necessary to address the concerns. Clinicians can quickly assess whether the problem can be addressed with brief discussion and reassurance, with one or more follow-up visits, or referral to a child specialist or family-oriented therapist. After a brief discussion, a clinician can say something like:

This bed-wetting does seem to be a concern for Tim and for the family. I'd like for us to have enough time to discuss what's been tried, and what strategies we can turn to next. How about if we arrange a visit to discuss this either next week or the one after that?

A referral should generally only occur after follow-up visits with the primary care clinician so that primary care strategies can be attempted, and so the family does not feel dismissed in their concerns. Table 12.1 identifies which childhood behavior problems can generally be addressed in routine or extended visits, or require referral to a specialist.

By the time that parents consult with clinicians, they have tried numerous approaches and feel frustrated. The clinician may be tempted to accept the parents' doubts and try to solve their dilemma for them. Becoming the "model substitute parent" can result in the clinician being pulled into the struggle and feeling as responsible and overwhelmed as the parents. In the case when the clinician is successful, parents can feel like more of a failure.

We believe that one of the clinician's most important jobs is to *help parents recognize and utilize their own strengths in addressing the problem they are having with their child.* This translates into balancing the problem focus by observing and supporting what the parents have done well and how the positive efforts are reflected in their child. For example, the act of requesting help is actually evidence of good parenting and a desire to do the very best for their child.

Working with parents who feel stuck requires that clinicians help parents use their knowledge of their children more effectively. A continuity rela-

TABLE 12.1. Settings for addressing childhood behavior problems

Routine Pediatric Visit
Biting
Night wakening
Primary enuresis
Feeding problems
Temper tantrums
Toilet training

Extended Pediatric Visit
ADHD/hyperactivity
Lying, stealing
School avoidance
Bereavement, witness to violence

Consider Referral
Anxiety
Depression
Eating disorders
Significant family conflict
Behaviors that do not resolve with extended visits

tionship allows clinicians to *catch the parents in acts of good parenting*. These specific examples of good parenting can be useful reminders parents during those times when they feel burdened or overwhelmed. Even during new patient encounters, clinicians can demonstrate respect for parents and help them to harness their expertise. With the recognition that clinicians are not expert parents, but are expert consultants to parents, we offer the mnemmonic, CPR for Parenting:

Consistency. All parents and caretakers must be consistent about expected behavior and consequences. It is much easier when expectations of all adults are consistent, and when children understand that similar behavior is expected in all situations.

Positive Reinforcement. Children generally like to please adults, and are more likely to repeat behaviors that are reinforced. "Accentuate the positive" (and eliminate the negative) is the motto of most child behavior guidebooks.

Realistic Expectations. Clinicians can help parents be realistic about developmentally appropriate behavior and expectations for their children. Anticipatory guidance and normalizing minor behavioral transgressions can help parents select which battles are worth fighting.

Entire sections of popular book stores and developmental pediatric texts are devoted to expanding these principles, including general parenting strategies, and approaches to specific child behavior problems [see especially Parker and Zuckerman (4)]. Our purpose in this chapter is to provide an overall family-focused framework in the context of an efficient office practice. Our goal is to make it easier for clinicians to help parents adopt whatever strategies best suit their values and their family.

Working with Parents on Child Behavior Problems

Getting Started

> Ms. Miner: Doctor, I've tried everything I know to get Mark (age 7) to stop having his temper tantrums, but nothing I do makes any difference. He just ignores me; sometimes he even tries to hit me if he doesn't get his way. I end up yelling at him way more than I want, and half the time I end up in tears. My mother thinks I'm too easy on Mark and is about ready to give up on both of us.

1. Meet with the parent(s), the child or children, and other important child caretakers.

Clinicians should know who are the important caretakers or decision makers for each child. Single parents should be asked about involvement of the other parent and whether grandparents, aunts, or anyone else provides help. In two-parent homes, a grandparent may not provide direct care, but may provide advice. Meeting with all significant caretakers allows for more complete assessment, and any plan has a higher chance of being implemented if all participants are involved. Clinicians, however, should be aware of possible triangulation among parents and grandparents, and strive not to undermine the authority of parents.

Involving both parents in child behavior strategies is particularly important when families are separated or divorced (5). Positive outcomes for children occur when fathers take an active, instrumental role in their children's lives, and when conflict between the parents is diminished. This includes helping with homework, helping set and reinforce rules, and, we would add, being involved with health decisions about their child. Research literature indicates that mere contact with nonresident parents (typically the father) does not impact the emotional adjustment of children after divorce (6).

It may be difficult to have former spouses come to the office together, but it may be important to request that they do so for the sake of their child. Table 12.2 includes suggestions for divorcing or separated parents, including ways that parents can minimize conflict and help children understand that they still have two parents, even though they no longer live together. At a minimum, the physician should talk with both parents separately if a conjoint appointment cannot be made. Contact with both parents helps the physician avoid any unhealthy coalition with either parent and reinforces the significance of both parents' attention to the child and his or her behavior.

> Dr. O.: It sounds like both you and your mother are working very hard to do the best for your son, but you wonder whether what you are doing is working. Your mother seems to disagree with you. How about Mark's father?
>
> Ms. Miner: He mostly leaves it up to me. He sees Mark mostly on weekends, and he asks if he can help me, but he doesn't want to get

TABLE 12.2. Successful co-parenting after divorce or separation

Each parent should:
Make it clear that they love their child and will always be their parent.
Make time with their child a priority.
Be as clear as possible about times when the child is with each parent.
Avoid negative comments about the other parent, either directly or when the child could hear.

The co-parents should try to:
Communicate directly about the child's schedule and expected behavior.
Support the other parent when the child's behavior is difficult.
Encourage the child's contact with all grandparents, and other extended family, and expect them to respect the co-parent.
Support the roles of stepparents, but assume primary responsibility for discipline.
Put aside personal feelings and both attend important events for the child.

into the middle between my mother and me. My mother is with him most days, and we don't really fight about this. She just thinks I should hold my ground more.

Dr. O.: This seems like an important issue—one that deserves more time than we have today. We should have the important people in Mark's life here—what do you think about having his father and your mother come with you?

Ms. Miner: Well my mother always says that she's not the parent, so she wouldn't want to come. I could ask Kevin if he would come.

Dr. O.: OK. That would be great, but I think it would be helpful for your mother to be here too—she sees an awful lot of Mark. Even if she doesn't come, can you ask her what she thinks would help? I'd suggest that you adults each observe Mark's behavior and begin to think about how you would like it to be different (see Fig. 12.1).

2. Clarify what the parents would like to change.

In a meeting with parents, begin by asking the parents what they would like to change. This approach addresses the problem in a way that focuses on constructive change rather than on a litany of failures.

Dr. O.: What would you like to change about your son's behavior?

Ms. Miner: I want him to stop behaving like a baby.

Mr. Miner: He's got to stop these tantrums.

Dr. O.: If he stopped the tantrums, how would you like him to behave?

Mr. Miner: I think he's old enough now to talk respectfully to his mother, instead of yelling and screaming. I tell him that often.

Dr. O. (To Ms. Miner): What did your mother think could be changed?

Ms. Miner: She agrees with Kevin and me. We just can't go on with these outbursts.

Exploring the Problem

The physician needs to assess family patterns that may maintain the problem and investigate other family events that may contribute to the dilemma.

1. Get a detailed understanding of the problem, including onset, duration, and frequency.

Dr. O.: How long have these tantrums been going on?

Ms. Miner: That's the odd thing. When he was little he didn't do this. It only started in the beginning of the school year.

Dr. O.: That would be about 5 months ago? Was there anything else going on at that time?

Ms. Miner: Well, my mother, Mark, and I moved into a new house. I started working more—extra waitressing in the evenings. But that shouldn't account for this.

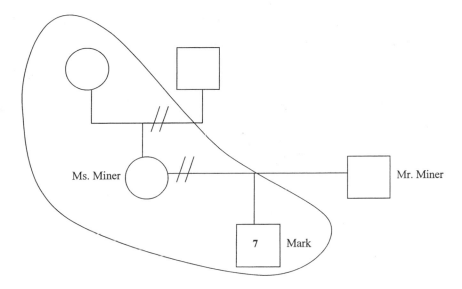

FIGURE 12.1. The Miner family.

Mr. Miner: Nothing changed at my house. Mark still comes on the weekends, and I sometimes see him in the evenings when his mother is
working.

Here Dr. O. learns that the tantrums usually occur after school on days
when Mark's mother has to work. Mark usually asks for something
when his mother is busy getting ready for work. When she cannot
respond immediately he yells at her and throws things. Mother typically ends up in tears, Mark ends up in his room, and grandmother
tries to console both of them.

2. Find out what advice parents have received from significant others.

This helps the physician understand who is important to the family, how
they may be a resource to the parents, and how the parents may be pulled
in different directions by the advice they have received.

Dr. O.: I'm sure you've talked to other people about this. What advice
have you received?

Ms. Miner: My mother says I'm too easy on Mark, but I don't think I
am. She thinks I ought to be more firm with him, and I do try, but
it's so hard when I'm rushing around getting ready.

Mr. Miner: When we went to the parent conference, Mark's teacher suggested that we could structure him more. She talked about behavior charts.

3. Explore the impact of the problem on all family members.

Dr. O. learned that Mark's behavior makes Ms. Miner feel guilty about working, and that she also feels angry that he will not cooperate better. Mr. Miner described how this does not seem to happen when he takes Mark for the evening, but he cannot do that every night. When asked about how Mark and his grandmother are affected, Ms. Miner notes that her mother is left with a frustrated boy at night, which makes her time with him much more difficult. As is common, the parents had a harder time thinking about how this affected Mark, and decided they would ask him.

4. Find out what other stressors may be affecting the family.

It is not unusual for child behavior problems to emerge at times when the family is experiencing other difficulties.

> Dr O.: Earlier you mentioned that some other changes have taken place—a new house, Ms. Miner working more, and more evenings when Mark's grandmother is caring for him.
> Mr. Miner: Some of those nights, I come and get him, but I can't always say when I can be free from work.
> Ms. Miner: Well, what am I supposed to tell him? That maybe his father will come? I never know what to say.
> Mr. Miner: I've got a million things to take care of at work. I can't just change my schedule all the time, especially when you don't know when you're working each week.

5. Do not get distracted by conflict.

Parental conflict does not only occur among divorced couples. Parents often feel embarrassed and frustrated about their perceived lack of control over their child and may blame one another for the failure. When conflict emerges, the clinician may want to avoid getting caught in the middle, and may get derailed from the specific behavior of the child. A common pattern is that parents begin to talk about a problem, reach some conflict, and then get frustrated and never achieve a plan to address their child's behavior. The clinician can recognize how this pattern occurs, and help parents stay focused on the behavior and a mutually agreeable plan.

> Dr. O.: You know, I see this a lot—where parents like yourselves are working hard, trying to do a good job, and then get frustrated. It's tempting to get annoyed with each other about how you each handle your son, but this is exactly the time when it's most important to try to work together. From talking with you, it seems that you're in agreement about what you want from your son. And that is. . . ?
> Ms. Miner: We want him to be able to control his temper, especially when I'm alone with him.
> Mr. Miner: Right—that's the main thing right now.
> Dr. O.: OK—That's great. I think that's something that's doable, and I bet that's something that Mark wants too.

Focusing on Solutions

The clinician should move quickly to help parents develop solutions that are clear and specific. This involves supporting the parents' ideas, and finding ways to use their own resources to solve the problem. A clinician can add to these efforts and provide alternative ideas and suggestions.

1. Discuss what the parents have tried in order to solve the problem.

> Dr. O.: It's clear you've both been trying to change Mark's behavior. (to mother) What have you or your mother tried so far?
>
> Ms. Miner: Well, my mother says she doesn't have this problem when she's alone with Mark. She says if she asks Mark to do something, he might whine, but he doesn't lose it with her.
>
> Mr. Miner: Well, I try to talk to Mark about listening to his mother.
>
> Ms. Miner: I've tried everything. I've told him to go to his room; I've threatened to take the TV away. Everything! He just won't listen.
>
> Mr. Miner: But you never follow through. That's the problem.

Dr. O. learns that the adults in this family all believe that Ms. Miner needs to be stronger with her son. Dr. O. also learns that Mr. Miner takes much less responsibility, but often criticizes his ex-wife for not doing a better job. As clinicians, we need to be wary that we do not overtly or subtly blame one or both parents.

2. Find out if there are times when the problem does not occur.

> Dr. O.: Are there ever times when Mark doesn't act this way—times that are pretty good?
>
> Mrs. Miner: Well it never happens when Mark is going to have dinner with his dad.
>
> Mr. Miner: I guess that's true—but really I can't do that every night that you work.

Dr. O. learns that when Mark gets very frustrated on the nights that he is not sure whether he will see his dad or not. He begins to wonder out loud if there is a way that the parents can work out a better system so that Mark will be clear about whether he will see his dad, be with his mother and grandmother, or have the evening with his grandmother.

3. Ask the parents about their strengths.

By helping parents talk about times that go well, or things they do well, the clinician shifts the focus from deficits to assets. The parents can then use those strengths and their more positive assessment of themselves to make constructive changes.

Dr. O.: You know, I've been impressed with the way you two are able to be such good parents, especially when you no longer live together. It sounds like your mother also is very respectful about you folks being the parents, and her role as helping you raise your son. That's a strength I wish I saw in more families. What other strengths do you see in yourselves and Mark?

Ms. Miner: I don't know if that's a strength or not. Sometimes it might be easier if we didn't have to deal with each other all the time.

Dr. O.: It sounds like being good parents means that you two end up with more contact with each other than you might wish. I can understand how that's both a strength and maybe a burden. What are some other strengths of your parenting and how you see Mark doing?

Mr. Miner: His teacher says he's doing well in school.

Dr. O.: Great. That's an area in which you both recognize that Mark is right on track.

4. Engage the parents in developing a plan of action for solving the problem.

Dr. O.: So let's get back to the hard part about you two communicating more than you might like.

Ms. Miner: I was thinking as we spoke that we could probably communicate more about our schedules if it makes it easier on Mark.

Dr. O.: Well, it sounds like that might allow him to know his schedule better, and as you both have noticed, he seems to get frustrated the most when he's not certain what will happen.

Mr. Miner: Well that's something I could work on—either have regular nights that I see Mark, and not worry about which night you're working, or try to be more flexible with work.

Ms. Miner: And I've been at the restaurant long enough that I could probably ask them to be more regular with my schedule.

Dr. O.: Well it sounds like you folks have a lot of possibilities that might help make Mark's life more predictable.

Ms. Miner: But what about if he doesn't change?

Dr. O.: I'd love to say this will make things all better. I do believe this will help, but he's still a kid, and there will be ongoing issues. All I know is that two parents working together, especially with a grandmother, are stronger than any one child. I think it's going to take both of you to make a difference in Mark's behavior.

With Dr. O.'s support, the Miners decide to talk together more about their schedules and make it clear to Mark who will be with him each evening. Over the next few months Ms. Miner notices that Mark has far fewer temper tantrums, and that she and her ex-husband seem able to talk more comfortably. Both parents continue to have active roles in rewarding and disciplining their son.

When Parents Are Stuck

Parents are often ready to work on more effective discipline but do not know where to begin. Clinicians can help by providing several basic guidelines for parents to consider:

1. It is important for both parents to agree about the plan for discipline.

Parents who cannot work together on creating a parenting plan will have greater difficulty following through. Lack of cooperation between parents also makes it easier for the child to split the parents. Parent cooperation about discipline is equally important in families of separation and divorce.

2. The discipline should be clear and concrete.

Grounding a child for "the rest of his life" is often a parental threat, but never an effective plan. Telling Mark he will have a time out if he yells or throws anything, though, is clear and specific enough for everyone to understand.

3. The discipline should be something the parents can monitor and the child can do.

Mark is much more likely to do his after-school chores if an adult is available to monitor the task. Discipline should be clear, concrete, and behaviorally oriented. For example, it is very difficult for a child to know what to do when a parent says, "Change your attitude." Identifying swearing as a behavior to change, and having the child substitute "I am angry because. . ." instead of swearing, however, helps to change his or her attitude at least in the eyes of his or her parents and teachers.

4. Any punishment should be time-limited.

Open-ended punishment ("You can't watch TV until you've shown us you've changed.") often leads to ongoing additional battles between parents and children over the fairness of the punishment. Knowing when a punishment is going to end adds to the likelihood that a child will be able to comply (e.g., "Remember, if there is a tantrum today, there will be no TV tonight."). For "time-out," the common rule is that children can be expected to sit "out" for the number of minutes that corresponds to their age (i.e. 5 year olds can have time-outs of about 5 minutes long).

5. Once a plan is developed, parents should share it with the child and be sure it is understood.

To ensure this, parents can have the child verbally repeat the plan. Another approach involves making a brief written "contract" that outlines the details of the punishment.

6. Parents should encourage positive parent–child interaction.

For some families with child behavior problems, it may seem like parenting is reduced to constant disciplining. Conflict becomes the rule rather than the exception. Without some opportunity for fun, enjoyment, or just time together, parents and children can find themselves at odds a great deal of the time. Because children can express their need for parent attention by misbehaving, giving attention when a child is not misbehaving can interrupt the pattern and bring parent and child closer together.

For many families, time together does not always happen spontaneously, but needs to be planned. Parents can arrange brief, regular, even daily, time with their child in order to talk, play a game, or do some other activity. This plan should also be communicated so that the child will know that he or she can count on time with both parents on a regular basis. The child then does not need to seek attention from parents in other, more problematic ways. Dr. F. illustrates some of the guidelines for working with parents who feel stuck about disciplining their child.

> Dr. F. met with Ms. O'Brien, a single parent, and her mother regarding Ms. O'Brien's 10-year-old daughter, Melinda. Ms. O'Brien lived with her mother, who helped raise Melinda and Caryn, age 15. Last year, on two occasions, Melinda had stolen money from her mother and grandmother. When the corner grocer reported to Grandma O'Brien that the girl had stolen some candy, Ms. O'Brien became so upset that she almost hit Melinda. At the visit, Ms. O'Brien was angry with her daughter and felt at her "wit's end." Dr. F asked if there was anything else that seemed especially troubling right now, and Ms. O'Brien indicated that her mother had been ill with pneumonia, and they had all been worried about her for more than 1 month (see Fig. 12.2).
>
> Dr. F. helped Ms. O'Brien and her mother explore Melinda's problem about stealing and plan an appropriate punishment. They decided Melinda would apologize, pay the store owner for the candy, and do 3 hours of chores at home to pay back her mother for the money. In addition, Melinda would have no TV in the evening for the remainder of the week.
>
> Dr. F. also noted how everyone seemed to be under a lot of stress lately, and asked how it had been during Grandma O'Brien's illness. Ms. O'Brien said she worried "day and night," and even took time off to care for her mother. Melinda had also been very upset by her grandmother's illness, but did not talk much about it. In retrospect, Melinda's behavior seemed to have worsened during this time.
>
> Dr. F. noted that it seemed to be a very hard time for everyone, and Ms. O'Brien talked further about how scary it was to see her mother become ill at her age. Ms. O'Brien said they all seemed to worry more since Grandpa O'Brien's death 2 years ago. Dr F. described how children do not necessarily want to talk about their worries directly, but may express them through things like stealing or other unacceptable behavior. She suggested that the family could mark that the stress was

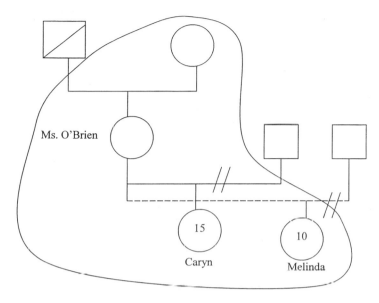

FIGURE 12.2. The O'Brien family.

over, of Grandma's illness and of Melissa's stealing behavior, by returning to some of the usual relaxing, and fun things that they liked to do. Everyone agreed. With relief, Ms. O'Brien said that she would focus on some fun weekend activities with her daughter, and put this sick time behind them. Grandma O'Brien said that she was ready to get back into their after-school routine of special snacks and helping with homework.

Contact with Schools

More than 10% of school children in the United States receive special education and other services because of difficulties with school performance (7). This may be due to learning difficulties, attention deficits, emotional or chronic physical illness, or family dysfunction and social problems. Other children become part of a pattern of school failure and declining self-worth, a type of "failure to thrive" in the school setting (8). Some of these children become identified by the schools, and obtain the assistance of individualized learning plans, which generally include medical as well as psychological and educational assessments. Many more children benefit from physician involvement with the schools for assessment of special needs, attention disorders, or multiple illnesses, and construction of care plans for children with acute or chronic illness. Becoming an effective advocate for students, while maintaining an efficient office practice is a valuable primary care skill. The following guidelines may enhance this process.

1. Stay in the role of consultant.

Healthcare clinicians can offer consultation to school personnel, but are not responsible for solving school behavior problems. Similar to consulting with parents, school consultation is enhanced when all participants can jointly discuss a child's behavior and follow-through on plans, with a focus on consistency of behavior for all settings. It is particularly important to avoid triangulation (i.e., being caught between the parents and the school). Dr. L. demonstrates how to extract oneself from a potentially destructive encounter:

> Mr. Carson: The school wants you to call them about why you won't put Kenny on the ADHD medication.
>
> Dr. L.: Well, I didn't think we had made a final decision on whether the Ritalin might be helpful or not. I could talk with them, but what are you thinking about this?
>
> Mr. Carson: You know that I don't want my son on drugs. I think if the teachers paid more attention to the kids, and didn't expect perfect behavior all the time, Kenny would be doing fine. When he gets out of line at home, we just remind him, and he listens. I'm not saying my son is perfect, but I really think this Mrs. Furman, his fifth grade teacher, has it out for him.
>
> Dr. L.: Well, I'll be happy to talk to her, and see what behaviors she is observing. Would you like me to do that? It sounds like there is a real difference of opinion between you and her. It might be helpful if you make an appointment to talk with her, so you can both feel that you're on the same page, on the side of your son. How about if I let you know how my conversation goes with her, and you can tell me about your talk with her?

2. Stay aware of cultural variability in behavior.

School expectations are generally based on middle class, European-American values (9). Children's activity level, level of participation, and verbal comfort reflect family and ethnic norms. It can be helpful to remind parents that sitting in classrooms for hours may not be an intrinsically natural behavior for many children, and that acceptable behavior is relative to social context. This helps families appreciate the physicality, for example, of their daughter and help her channel her energy into sports, while rewarding the behavior of raising her hand before talking.

3. Structure ways to facilitate communication with schools.

When a practice contains many children from a particular school district, it can be useful to meet once with the special services coordinator to arrange methods for efficient communication (e.g., fax, email, or leaving phone messages). This personal relationship can make future contacts with the school easier because the coordinator could expedite exchanges of information between clinician and teachers. All of these contacts require attention to patient confidentiality.

4. Maintain forms for common school concerns.

The school contact person may provide common behavioral and medical forms that can be distributed from the primary care office. Forms can replace individual letters in many situations, and can be used to provide medical excuses for injury or illness, permission to provide medication, and other special circumstances. The Conners Assessment Form, which is a useful way for parents and teachers to assess a child as the initial work-up for ADHD, should be available in the office (www.widerange.com/conners.html).

5. Unusual situations may call for attendance at a school interdisciplinary meeting.

Physician attendance at meetings is an infrequent event, but it conveys a very powerful statement of support. Having all professionals in one room, with the parents or guardians, allows for negotiation of different perspectives, and a plan that is more likely to be followed. The physician may sometimes be asked to help teachers work with a child with an unusual health condition or disability. A group meeting encourages an exchange of accurate information and questions. When school personnel feel more reassured about their ability to handle a difficult situation, "emergency" phone calls from them or the parents may be diminished.

6. Inform parents of any communication with schools.

Parents should be told when communication with schools occurs, and what will be communicated. This helps to limit triangulation, and underlines the authority of the parents as the experts on their children.

When to Refer

The clinician's most important function is at times to recognize when behavior problems call for a referral to an appropriate mental health professional and then guide the family to this help (see Protocol at the end of this chapter and Chap. 25 for referral suggestions). Referrals may be considered when:

- The parents or parenting figures cannot agree on a plan.
- There is evidence of long-term marital or relationship discord.
- The child's problem has been going on for more than 1 year.
- There is family violence, substance abuse, sexual or physical abuse, suicidal intent, an eating disorder, or evidence of psychosis in the family.
- The clinician does not feel he or she has the time or training to address the matter adequately (10, 11).

Managing Child Behavior Problems During an Office Visit

It is time consuming and difficult to deal with disruptive patient behaviors during an office visit. With a misbehaving child, clinicians may range from taking over the parenting role to ignoring the behavior. In contrast, clinicians can intervene in ways that support and empower parents, and help them effectively manage their child's behavior in other settings. This section will outline ways to work with both passive and aggressive parental responses to child misbehavior.

Child-Friendly Clinical Environments

In all health arenas, the first response is prevention. In an office, prevention of child misbehavior requires attention to the office environment. If children are attended to, they do not need to misbehave to get an adult's attention. Offices should have books, toys, or activities for children in waiting rooms and exam rooms. Nurses can hand out paper and crayons or pages to color. Child-friendly offices post some of these drawings so that families and children see that they are valued. Attention to children includes speaking with all children at a sibling's appointment, and stating that you look forward to their visit. With infant visits in particular, a couple of words with an older brother or sister welcomes a child, and models ways to minimize sibling jealousy.

When a Parent's Response Is Overly Passive

> Mrs. Spencer, a 34-year-old African American woman, brought her son Eddie, age 7, for a routine check-up for school. As Mrs. Spencer and Dr. D. talked, Eddie became louder and louder. Then he opened a drawer of the examining table and began to play with the medical instruments. Mrs. Spencer tried to ignore her son's behavior.

1. Clarify that you are in charge of the office, its contents, and what transpires during the visit.

> Dr D.: I should have mentioned at the beginning that there are some things I do not want children to do in the office. I can't let you play with the instruments or the things in the drawers, to keep those things clean. We also need to talk quietly, so I can talk with you and your mom.

2. Help the parent to be in charge of the child's behavior.

> Dr D.: Would you have Eddie quiet down and also put the tongue blades back in the drawer?

Mrs. Spencer: He doesn't listen to me.

Dr. D.: I think it's important that he listen to you, so why don't you give it a try?

Mrs. Spencer: Come on now, Eddie. (Eddie continues the same behavior.)

Dr. D.: What else could you try?

Mrs. Spencer: I don't know. Maybe you could get him to listen to you.

Dr. D.: I think it's much more important that Eddie listen to you. And I know it can be hard, especially when you have a high-spirited boy like Eddie. Is there anything else you can think of that you could do?

Mrs. Spencer: I can't think of anything.

Dr. D.: Maybe you could tell him what you would like him to do.

Mrs. Spencer: Eddie, stop playing with those things and sit down. (Eddie listens, but continues his behavior.)

Dr. D.: Maybe for today you may need to hold him on your lap. Please do whatever you need to do and if I can help, let me know.

Mrs. Spencer gets up, draws Eddie to her and holds him as he stands beside her. Eddie resists at first but then begins to settle down. Dr. D. acknowledges how difficult this is for Mrs. Spencer and congratulates her for doing an effective job.

3. Plan with the parent how to approach the next visit.

Dr. D.: You handled things well today, Mrs. Spencer. What do you think would make it easier next time?

Mrs. Spencer: I think I'll bring some toys or something to draw with. He likes that.

Dr. D.: Good idea. Sometimes I also encourage parents to bring a family member or friend to help out.

Mrs. Spencer: My husband works and there's really no one else.

Dr. D.: Okay. Maybe your husband could come for a visit in the future. Is there anything else that would help?

Mrs. Spencer: I guess I'll just have to keep him right by my side until he can behave better.

When a Parent's Response Is Overly Aggressive

Ms. Pelham, a Caucasian office manager, brought her daughter Jayne, age 5, for a scheduled immunization. During the visit Jayne walked around the office, made animal noises, and banged the walls with a pencil. Ms. Pelham quickly interrupted her conversation with Dr. L., told her daughter to sit down and stop, and then returned to the conversation. After the second interruption, Ms. Pelham got out of her seat, yelled, "I told you to stop," and struck her daughter twice on the shoulder.

1. **Explore the parent's feelings of frustration.**

> Dr. L.: Boy, it must be hard being a mother at times.
> Ms. Pelham: You see her. Sometimes she just won't listen.

2. **Discuss the frequency of the child's behavior and the parent's response.**

> Dr. L.: Do you have problems with Jayne very often?
> Ms. Pelham: Yeah, a couple times a week; a couple times a day on a bad day.
> Dr. L.: It must be pretty hard on you.
> Ms. Pelham: I take care of it.

3. **Ask how other caretakers respond to similar situations.**

> Dr. L.: How does Jayne's father deal with this?
> Ms. Pelham: Well, he's more patient. He says I shouldn't hit, but he's not there all day, every day.

4. **Find out if the parent was treated in the same way as a child.**

> Dr. L.: How did your parents discipline you?
> Ms. Pelham: What do you mean?
> Dr. L.: Did they hit you at times?
> Ms. Pelham: Sure they did; 10 times more than I hit Jayne.
> Dr. L.: How was that for you?
> Ms. Pelham: I didn't much like it, but I guess they thought that was the best way to make me listen. It worked.

5. **Explore other ways the parent could respond.**

> Ms. Pelham: Don't get me wrong, I love Jayne, but when she gets doing something and won't listen, there's only one way to get her to stop.
> Dr. L.: Nothing else seems to work?
> Ms. Pelham: Uh-uh.
> Dr. L.: And I'll bet you've tried a lot of different things.
> Ms. Pelham: Have I ever! I've tried groundings and time-outs, and they don't last 5 minutes. I threaten her, but she doesn't seem to care. She gets so defiant. That's when the only thing I feel I can do is spank her. I usually don't, but sometimes I have to.
> Dr. L.: You don't like it when she makes you that mad.
> Ms. Pelham: No, I don't. My fuse can get pretty short when she doesn't listen.
> Dr. L.: I'm sure it does. Would it be easier to deal with Jayne if she didn't make you angry so quickly?
> Ms. Pelham: What do you mean?
> Dr. L.: Well, is there any way to make the fuse a little longer?
> Ms. Pelham: If there is, I haven't found it yet.

It took Dr. L. several visits over the next year to help Ms. Pelham find different ways to manage Jayne's behavior. Mr. Pelham was only willing to come to a visit once during this time, but Ms. Pelham reported that he was being more involved with Jayne, and did not criticize her so much. Ms. Pelham succeeded in "lengthening her fuse" and, even though she still got very angry at Jayne, she was able to discipline her without hitting.

Spanking children as a form of discipline is controversial in our society. The American Academy of Pediatrics (12) has taken a stand against spanking:

Because of the negative consequences of spanking and because it has been demonstrated to be no more effective than other approaches for managing undesired behavior in children, the American Academy of Pediatrics recommends that parents be encouraged and assisted in developing methods other than spanking in response to undesired behavior (13).

The consensus panel also noted that more than 90% of American families reported having used spanking as a means of discipline at some time, and that more than 60% of pediatricians support the use of corporal punishment, at least in certain situations (14). This requires that clinicians examine their own beliefs about discipline, and actively work with families to change the cultural climate around discipline and punishment.

Even though it is very difficult, a clinician's task may be easier in the clear situations when a child appears to be at risk for physical injury, and the clinician is mandated to report the family to protective services (see Chap. 19). It is important in families like Jayne's to respond to the parent's signal, to address the behavior, and to provide follow-up contact. Among other suggestions, the American Academy of Pediatric Guidelines (13) reminds clinicians to:

- Be clear about what constitutes acceptable discipline.
- Try to understand parents' justification of their current practices.
- Let the family lead in creating alternative discipline plans.
- Look for examples of parents' effective discipline practices.
- Follow up on discipline discussions with phone calls or follow-up visits.
- Identify parenting programs and individual counselors for referral.
- Participate in public education and advocacy to change cultural attitudes about discipline.

More serious child behavior problems (e.g., any questions of abuse) require that physicians need to intervene in an active, authoritative manner. The physician can highlight the necessity for change, while still supporting the parents to take charge of their child and his or her behavior. Guidelines for a healthy, effective parent–child relationship change when the child becomes an adolescent and the family enters a new stage. The next chapter will discuss how the physician's role changes to accommodate this individual and family transition.

References

1. Clarke-Stewart KA: Popular primers for parents. *Am Psychol* 1987;**33**:359–369.
2. Chamberlain RW: Prevention of behavioral problems in young children. *Pediatr Clin N Am* 1982;**29**(2):239–247.
3. Schmitt BD: Pediatric counseling. In: Levine MD, Carey WB, & Crocker AC (Eds). *Developmental-Behavioral Pediatrics*. Philadelphia: W.B. Saunders Co., 1999.
4. Parker S, Zuckerman B (Eds). *Behavioral and Developmental Pediatrics: A Handbook for Primary Care*. Boston: Little, Brown and Company, 1995.
5. Visher JS, Visher EB: Beyond the nuclear family: resources and implications for pediatricians. In: Coleman WL, Taylor EH (Eds). *Family-Focused Pediatrics: Issues, Challenges and Clinical Methods. The Pediatric Clinics of North America*, Philadelphia: W.B. Saunders Co., 1995.
6. Marsiglio W, Amato P, Day R, & Lamb M. Scholarship on fatherhood in the 1990s and beyond. *J Marriage Fam* 2000;**62**(4):1173–1191.
7. Dworkin PH: School failure. In Parker S, Zuckerman B (Eds). *Behavioral and Developmental Pediatrics: A Handbook for Primary Care*. Boston: Little, Brown and Company, 1995.
8. Ruggiero M: Maladaption to school. In Levine MD, Carey WB, & Crocker AC: *Developmental-Behavioral Pediatrics*. Philadelphia: W.B. Saunders Co., 1999.
9. Harkness S, Keefer C, & Super C: Culture and ethnicicty. In Levine MD, Carey WB, Crocker AC (Eds). *Developmental-Behavioral Pediatrics*. Philadelphia: W.B. Saunders Company, 1999.
10. Frenck N: A time-conserving protocol for pediatric behavioral problems. *Fam Syst Med* 1984;**2**(2):146–149.
11. Doherty WJ, Baird MA: *Family Therapy and Family Medicine*. New York, Guilford Press, 1983.
12. Friedman SB, Schonberg SK (Eds): The short- and long-term consequences of corporal punishment. *Pediatrics* 1996;**98**:803–860.
13. American Academy of Pediatrics, Committee on Psychosocial Aspects of Child and Family Health. Guidance for effective discipline. *Pediatrics* 1998:**101**: 723–728.
14. McCormick KF: Attitudes of primary care physicians toward corporal punishment. *JAMA* 1992;**267**:3161–3165.

Protocol: Working with Parents on Child Behavior Problems

Getting Started

1. Meet with the parents, the child or children, and other primary child caretakers.
2. Clarify what the parents would like to change.

Exploring the Problem

1. Get a detailed understanding of the problem, including onset, duration, and frequency.
2. Find out what advice parents have received from significant others.
3. Explore the impact of the problem on all family members.
4. Find out what other stressors may be affecting the family.
5. Do not get distracted by conflict.

Focusing on Solutions

1. Discuss what the parents have tried in order to solve the problem.
2. Find out if there are times when the problem does not occur.
3. Ask the family about their strengths.
4. Engage the parents in developing a plan of action for solving the problem.

When Parents Are Stuck Regarding Discipline

1. It is important for both parents to agree about the plan.
2. The discipline should be clear and concrete.
3. The discipline should be something the parents can monitor and the child can do.
4. Any punishment should be time-limited.
5. Once a plan is developed, parents should share it with the child and be sure it is understood.
6. Parents should encourage positive parent–child interaction.

Contact with Schools

1. Stay in the role of consultant.
2. Stay aware of cultural variability in behavior.
3. Structure ways to facilitate communication with schools.
4. Maintain forms for common school-related concerns.
5. Unusual situations may call for attendance at interdisciplinary school meetings.
6. Inform parents of any communication with schools.

When a Referral Should Be Made

1. The parents cannot agree on a plan.
2. There is evidence of long term marital discord.
3. The child's problem has been going on for more than a year.
4. There is family violence, substance abuse, sexual or physical abuse, suicidal intent, an eating disorder, or evidence of psychosis in the family.
5. The physician does not feel he or she has the time or training to address the matter adequately.

Managing Behavior Problems During an Office Visit

1. When a parent's response is overly passive:
   - Clarify that you are in charge of the office, its contents, and what transpires during the visit.
   - Help the parent to be charge of the child's behavior.
   - Plan with the parent how to approach the next visit.

2. When a parent's response is overly aggressive
   - Explore the parent's feelings of frustration.
   - Discuss the frequency of the behavior.
   - Ask how other caretakers respond to similar situations.
   - Find out if the parent was treated in the same way as a child.
   - Explore other ways the parent could respond.

13
Family-Oriented Care of Adolescents

The movie, *Grease*, depicts adolescence as we revere and fear it. The high school students engage in alcohol and cigarette abuse, death-defying driving, and unprotected sexual activity, all with no parents in sight. This fictional description of adolescents in the 1950s is not too different from popular images today, and these common behaviors continue to be the greatest health risks for young people (1, 2). Data indicate that more than three of every four deaths in the second decade of life are caused by "social morbidities": unintentional injuries, homicides, and suicides (1). From a public health perspective, adolescent healthcare requires significant attention to prevention and counseling; however, the media-enhanced images of adolescents contribute to the clinician's uncertainty about how to best approach the necessary counseling.

Popular images of adolescence depict the powerful influence of peers on behavior choices in adolescence. Data from the National Longitudinal Study of Adolescent Health, however, indicates that parent–family connectedness, as well as school connectedness, are protective against almost every health risk behavior (1). This research can be used to support parents as they assist their teenagers with their important life choices.

Adolescence begins with the onset of puberty, as early as age 10, and ends in the early twenties. During this large time span, individuals face dramatic physical, emotional, and relational changes, moving from childhood to adult roles and relationships. To help the busy clinician, the American Medical Association has established comprehensive Guidelines for Adolescent Preventive Services (GAPS) (4, www.ama-assn.org/adolhlth/gapspub), an integrated program of health-risk statistics, screening instruments, and counseling objectives. GAPS suggests that primary care be categorized into care of younger, middle, or older adolescents. The distinctions among the groups are many, but in general younger adolescents are aged 11–14 years, attend middle school, and are significantly involved with their families. Issues for middle adolescents, aged 15–18 years, include concerns with high school and negotiating relationships with parents and peers. Older adolescents are concerned with establishing adult identities, whether through college or job preparation activities, or they sometimes adopt adult roles in their late teen years. These categories are not distinct. A 14-year old, for example, may be pregnant and coping simultaneously with middle school tasks, negotiation of responsibility with parents, and preparing for adult parenting roles. In those situations, the clinician must consider issues relevant to all categories of adolescence and help the patient and family understand why the demands seem so many.

Mandated health maintenance visits related to schooling may occur only two or three times throughout the adolescent period, but GAPS suggest yearly visits to address the unique developmental concerns, and preventive and health behavior measures. These visits, which require counseling skills, are made easier when clinicians have knowledge of each patient, their family, and their unique concerns.

Adolescent development does not take place in a vacuum, but is part of a larger transition for the entire family. We noted in Chapter 3 how Combrinck-Graham (5) describes adolescence as a centrifugal period in the family life cycle in which the normal processes of family development pull family members in different directions. Adolescents are trying to establish their identity, whereas other family members are also changing. Parents may be experiencing a "midlife crisis" as they question career choices, directions for the future, and even their marriage. Along with the changes associated with adolescent development, some teenagers may also have to cope with change in their parents' lives, including separation and divorce, decreased supervision, and illness or death of grandparents.

Adolescence is a period in which parents and teens fluctuate between closeness and distance, dependence and independence, as they all experience the transition from child to adult and anticipate the adolescent's maturity. The family-oriented clinician needs to help adolescents take responsibility for their own health, while enhancing parents' vital role in adolescents' overall health and development. This balance between patient and family communication is a challenge in all medical care, but is heightened during adolescence when issues of identity and privacy are paramount (3, 6, 7). Research repeatedly documents adolescents' fears that communication with clinicians will be conveyed to parents or others (7). In a randomized controlled study of 562 adolescents, assurances of confidentiality increased adolescents' willingness to seek further health care (8). If clinicians want adolescents to talk about what truly matters to them, they must convince these young patients that their communications are appropriately confidential. A trusting relationship between the clinician and the adolescent can "accelerate the process of children becoming independent patients" (9).

Even though we agree with the importance of a one-to-one relationship between the adolescent and the clinician, we also recognize the central role of families in their children's development. In a study of community family physicians, a family member, usually a parent, accompanied adolescents at 73% of visits (10). Parents are present, and studies of adolescents indicate that parents have the greatest influence on the development of values. Even while differentiating themselves from their parents, adolescents derive much of their self-esteem from their parents' approval and support (1, 4). This is not to suggest that adolescence is conflict free. Adolescents must at times challenge parents and other adult authorities. Parents sometimes must set limits to insure safety or continuation of family priorities. As much as adolescents want privacy, parents also are concerned about their children's health and want information. Clinicians can feel caught between these conflicting agendas, but they have a unique opportunity to facilitate communication and mutual respect within families.

The arrangement of who is in the exam room will vary with the purpose of the visit. A parent may be in the room with an adolescent for acute care. A parent may be present for part of the interview and leave for private discussions for a lengthy visit or physical. The adolescent may make his or her own appointment and attend with no adult guardian for sports physicals or requests for contraception. In each of these visits, the adolescent may be concerned that the parent and physician have an additional relationship, and their confidentiality and privacy could be breached.

Confidentiality and Adolescent Healthcare

Although legal attempts have tried to mandate parental notification laws, Supreme Court rulings and state statutes have extended teenagers' rights to confidential healthcare in a variety of areas, particularly family planning services, abortion, and substance abuse care. In 1977, the Supreme Court held that adolescents have a right to privacy regarding the purchase and use of contraceptives (11). The federal Title X Family Planning Program has assured confidential services for adolescents since the early 1970s. This has been challenged, but it was reinforced in 1983 when it was found unconstitutional for the U.S. Department of Health and Human Services to require federally funded programs to notify parents regarding teenage contraceptive use (12).

In 1997, the U.S. House of Representatives reiterated the long-standing Title X policy that parental involvement be encouraged, but not required (13). In general medical care, states require that parental consent be obtained before a minor receives medical treatment, with 18 years being the age of majority. Many states, however, have enacted "mature minor" legislation to authorize adolescents to consent to healthcare specifically related to sexual activity, substance abuse, and mental health (11, 13). Nearly all states authorize minors to consent to treatment of sexually transmitted diseases and substance abuse, and approximately half of all states enable a pregnant minor to obtain prenatal care without parental notificiation. A useful list of specific state requirements is available on the Alan Guttmacher Institute web site (13, www.agi-usa.org/pubs/ib21.html).

This is certainly an area in which professionals, adolescents, and parents have strong opinions, resulting in ongoing legislative and public discussion. Both the American Medical Association (14) and the Society for Adolescent Medicine (11) have taken positions that confidential health care should be available for adolescents, but that clinicians should make every effort to involve parents in those decisions whenever possible.

The law has given adolescents the right to consent to treatment, but the responsibility for judging whether or not the adolescent is capable of exercising that right often falls to the physician. This decision is often influenced by finances and insurance status. Because few adolescents have insurance to cover inpatient care, adolescents are generally not admitted to a hospital for non-emergent treatment without family notification and assumption of financial responsibility (11).

How can clinicians balance the need for encouraging adolescents to seek care, while respecting parental concerns for accurate information? Each family-oriented clinician would do well to create a policy for confidentiality to avoid disruptive conflicts with adolescents or their parents. Family-oriented practices can consider the following guidelines to create confidentiality plans.

1. The clinician's primary priority is to provide necessary and adequate healthcare services for the adolescent.

The purpose of confidential treatment is both to protect the adolescent's right to privacy and to provide healthcare to adolescents who might not seek care if parental consent was required. Confidentiality in cases such as sexually transmitted diseases insures the adolescent's privacy, helps protect the public health, and upholds legal statutes.

2. Blanket confidentiality should not be extended to any patient.

There are conditions in which clinicians are mandated to breech confidentiality with any patient to keep the patient and others safe. Adolescent healthcare also requires this caveat, covering situations such as suicidal or homicidal ideation, a communicable disease, or a history of abuse that must be reported to child protection agencies. In those situations others must be involved to insure safety for the patient or those others endangered by the patient. In most cases, with clear discussion of constraints on confidentiality, adolescents will share their concerns.

> Debbie (age 15): Doctor, there is something I want to tell you, but you can't tell anyone else, especially my parents.
> Dr. D: I'm glad to talk about things that are important to you. I also will respect your privacy as much as is legally possible. If you were to tell me that you were going to hurt yourself or other people, I would

have to involve parents or others, and you would know about that. But for most of our discussions, our communication is confidential because I am your doctor and these are your life decisions.

3. Help adolescents involve their parents in treatment decisions whenever possible.

By involving family members in decisions and for care throughout the treatment period, the adolescent and the clinician have more support and information. As an example, national surveys indicate that more than half of the teenagers who obtain abortions have told at least one parent about their pregnancy and planned abortion (15). Parent involvement and support can be invaluable to teens who face such stressful situations.

When adolescents are reluctant to involve parents, discussion can identify whether including parents would put the adolescent at risk, or if the adolescent is afraid that the parents would be disappointed. For most difficult adolescent decisions, parents, even when disappointed, can be valuable resources, and maintaining secrecy can be a very stressful burden for the adolescent. Clinicians can help adolescents sort out what might actually happen if parents were told, or what it would be like if parents learned about the health decisions from someone else. The clinician can help adolescents consider including others, especially with the difficult decisions of pregnancy, abortion, or substance abuse, in ways that facilitate family communication and demonstrate the need for confidentiality. One can encourage teenagers to speak with their parents, offer to create family meetings for disclosure and discussion, or, as a last resort, offer to contact the parents for the adolescent.

4. Assess what role family dynamics may play in the adolescent's request for confidentiality.

As we have indicated, confidential medical care is often required in order to provide necessary treatment for adolescent patients. At times, though, the request for confidentiality may be related less to healthcare issues than it is to family dynamics. The adolescent may be trying to draw the family physician into a coalition against his or her parents:

> Hector, 14, told Dr. J. he was having problems with his Dominican-born parents, especially his father. Hector said his father hassled him "all the time, for no reason," and that he was so angry at his father that he was going to run away. Hector asked Dr. J. not to tell anyone about his plans.
>
> Dr. J. asked Hector if he was running away because his parents were hitting him or abusing him in some way. Hector said *no*, they just were a "pain." Dr. J. then explained how the parents had no way of knowing how Hector felt unless he told them. There was also no way that things would change without the family discussing how they were all getting along. Dr. J. told Hector that of course he also had to tell parents if a

son said he was going to run away, but he was optimistic that the family could reach a better solution. Dr. J. told Hector he needed to call his parents, but would prefer doing it while Hector was there and could hear the conversation. Hector was angry, but reluctantly agreed. During the call, Dr. J. asked the parents to join him with Hector for a family conference the following day so they could talk further about these concerns.

Parents may also give the physician information that appears to put him or her in a confidentiality bind.

Mrs. Demas asked to speak privately with Dr. L. before Wendy's appointment and explained that she and her husband were worried about Wendy. A family friend had seen Wendy at an unsupervised party. Mrs. Demas said that if Wendy found out how they learned about her behavior, she would be furious and might get "violently angry." Mrs. Demas wanted Dr. L. to "subtly" question Wendy without letting on that she knew anything.

Dr. L. said she could understand Mrs. Demas' concern about Wendy, that she could ask general questions about drug use, but she could not act on this secret information. Dr. L. said it would be better if Mrs. Demas could talk directly with Wendy and offered to help Mrs. Demas do that. Mrs. Demas said she could not risk talking with Wendy. Two weeks later Mrs. Demas called Dr. L. to report a huge fight with Wendy. She asked Dr. L. if she could come in to talk. Dr. L. suggested that Mr. and Mrs. Demas and Wendy come in together. At that point, Mrs. Demas agreed.

In both of these cases, concern with confidentiality is mixed up with one person's effort to draw the physician into a family problem, take sides, and keep a secret. This triangulation, whether intentional or not, usually reflects patterns of indirect communication that may be typical for the families. The physician needs to be vigilant about such triangles and make every effort to have adolescents and parents communicate more directly with one another.

Primary Care of Adolescents: Guidelines for Office Visits

1. Maintain a relationship with both the adolescent and his or her parents.

Avoid entering coalitions with either the adolescent or the parents. Siding with the parent against the adolescent or the adolescent against the parent runs the risk of eventually losing the trust of both. The art of being a family-oriented clinician includes forming supportive relationships with multiple members of a family.

As soon as a child reaches age 10 or 11 years, the clinician can explain to the patient and parents that it is important to routinely see teenagers alone to help them become responsible for their own healthcare. At each visit, a time with the teen and her parents can be followed by some time alone with the clinician and the teen. When this is done routinely and begun early, all family members respect the confidential relationship between patient and doctor, and patients may find it easier to discuss concerns with their clinician.

Parents may also want to talk about their concerns privately with the clinician, and be reluctant to discuss their concern with the adolescent present. In these cases, the physicians should support the parents in their concern, but also underscore the value of the parents and adolescents talking together. The physician should not become a go-between the parents and the adolescent, but may offer to meet with the parents once to hear concerns and help plan how the family can discuss the concerns together.

> Devon's father, Michael, called Dr. G. and said he had found marijuana in Devon's room, but had not said anything to Devon. He was very worried that Devon was using drugs, but felt that he could not ask his son without risking a huge argument. Because Dr. G. knew the family, she suggested that Devon and Michael come in for a visit so they could all talk together.
>
> Dr. G. began the visit, stating that Michael had called because he was very worried about Devon. Michael described that he had found the marijuana, and wanted to make sure that his son was safe and making good choices. Devon was angry that his father had been in his room. Dr. G. interrupted and stated that of course his father wanted Devon to have his privacy, but that as a parent he also had to insure that his son was safe and that there was no risk to the rest of the family. Dr. G. asked if they could talk about what this meant and what they could do now. By focusing on what could be done next, Dr. G. helped the family move from blaming each other to discussing their fears and plans.

2. Be aware of one's own emotional reactions.

Many physicians experience a natural pull to either side with parents against teens or with teens against their parents. This side-taking can reflect the physician's own age and parenting experience, as well as remembered issues from his or her own adolescence. A male physician may see his own efforts to work out a relationship with his father in a 16-year-old male patient. The physician who wants to protect her own 15-year-old daughter may strongly identify with the parents of an adolescent female who has come for a confidential pregnancy test. These responses are normal, and should be considered in the negotiation process among clinician, patient, and parents.

> Dr. M. felt angry after Mrs. Mendoza phoned to ask if 15-year-old Melinda could be given contraceptives because she was afraid Melinda was sexually active, but did not want her to know she had asked. It may

have been that Dr. M. was extremely busy that day and the phone call was just one more intrusion, because it was only the next day that Dr. M. realized it was Mrs. Mendoza's "intrusiveness" that bothered her. It reminded Dr. M. of times in her own adolescence when her mother wanted to know everything she was doing. Knowing this, Dr. M. could now monitor her reactions. By doing so, Dr. M. would be less likely to react to the Mendozas in ways that would disrupt the clinician–patient relationship.

3. Adolescent efforts to individuate impact the delivery of adolescent healthcare.

Individuation or achieving independence can influence everything from discussions about who will come into the exam room for athletics or work, to requests for contraception and pregnancy tests. The physician is in an excellent position to help parents and adolescents appropriately address issues of independence and autonomy with each other.

> Dr. M. saw Melinda alone for the physical exam and talked with her about school friends, as well as other close relationships. Dr. M. learned that Melinda had a boyfriend with whom she was sexually active. When Dr. M. asked about contraception, Melinda said she was not using anything, but that her boyfriend usually used condoms. Dr. M. asked Melinda if she wanted to be pregnant, and Melinda laughed and said of course not. Dr. M. said she thought it would be a good idea for Melinda to use contraception, that she could talk with her about choices, and Melinda agreed to think about it. After Dr. M. completed Melinda's physical, she invited Mrs. Mendoza into the exam room.
>
> Dr. M. (to Mrs. Mendoza): As I explained to Melinda, she is in excellent health.
> Mrs. Mendoza: Good.
> Dr. M.: I was wondering if either of you have any other concerns or questions? (Silence). Was there anything else that either of you wanted to talk about?
> Melinda: No. (silence)
> Dr. M.: Mrs. Mendoza, do you have any concerns?
> Mrs. Mendoza: Not really, just that I worry about her.
> Dr. M.: What do you worry about?
> Mrs. Mendoza: She's growing up.
> Melinda: Of course, I'm growing up!
> Dr. M.: What concerns you about that?
> Mrs. Mendoza: I worry about her when she's out with all these boys; what's going to happen?
> Melinda: Mom! I can't believe you're bringing this up! It is none of your business! (Melinda begins to cry.)
> (Dr. M. nonverbally encourages Mrs. Mendoza to comfort her daughter. Mrs. Mendoza hands Melinda a tissue. Melinda rejects it.)

Mrs. Mendoza (to Dr. M): I'm afraid she could get pregnant if she doesn't watch out. I told her she couldn't date until she was 16, which was 5 months ago. Since then she is out all the time.

Melinda: What do you mean, "out all the time?" I've dated just a few boys, mainly Jack.

Mrs. Mendoza: Have you done anything?

Melinda: That's none of your business.

Dr. M.: This is a tough time for both of you. Melinda is growing up and becoming a young woman and you, Mrs. Mendoza, have all the concerns a good mother has for a teenage daughter. (to Mrs. Mendoza) What are you most concerned about?

Mrs. Mendoza: I guess I don't want her to get pregnant.

Melinda: I don't want that either.

Dr. M.: Have you two ever talked about birth control?

Mrs. Mendoza and Melinda: No.

Dr. M.: I think it's wonderful when mothers and daughters begin to talk about hard things like birth control. I would be happy to talk with each of you or both of you further about various methods.

Melinda: There's nothing to talk about. (silence)

Dr. M.: Well that may be the case now. (to mother) Is it OK with you if Melinda comes in to talk about birth control?

Mrs. Mendoza: Yes. I just want her to be safe, and happy, and also finish school.

Dr. M. (to both): Ok. That's great. I'm available, so let me know how I can help. Melinda makes an appointment to start on birth control pills 1 month later.

It is awkward and unnecessary for parents and teens to discuss the details of a teenager's sexual behavior, but it is very helpful to have a parent assent to contraception. In this case it made it easier for Melinda to take that step when she was ready.

Structuring the Interview When a Parent Accompanies the Adolescent

It is important to talk with both the adolescent and the parent when a parent accompanies the adolescent on a visit, but it is rarely appropriate for the parent to be involved in the exam itself. The physician needs to structure parent involvement in a way that respects the parent's role, but makes it clear that the adolescent is the patient.

1. Meet with the parent(s) and adolescent together initially.

Acknowledge the adolescent first, then the parent, and thank both for coming.

2. Ask how you can help them today.

Let the parent and adolescent decide who will respond first. This gives the physician a picture of how the parent and adolescent interact: Does the parent let the adolescent talk? Do the parents and adolescent agree on why they are here? Does either the parent or adolescent have special concerns? This format is also a way for the physician to model that concerns of parents and adolescents should be talked about together.

3. See the adolescent alone for the majority of the visit.

Once the purpose of the visit has been clarified, the clinician can choose whether to have the parent present for the interview. With a young adolescent, the parent may be helpful to clarify the history, and the parent may be reassured that the teen is describing the full nature of the concern. For general physical exams, parents should be asked to move to the waiting room for the physical exam to affirm that the adolescent is increasingly responsible for his or her own health. For minor health problems (e.g., ear infections), it may not be necessary to see the adolescent alone. A clinician's good judgment and flexibility can set a model for flexibility within the family.

4. Clarify with the adolescent what will be shared with the parent(s).

This should be a negotiated process in which the physician specifies what he or she wants to discuss with the parent and the adolescent has the opportunity to agree or disagree. In cases where there is disagreement, unless there is substantial risk to the adolescent's or someone else's life, the adolescent's wishes should be respected.

5. Meet conjointly with the parent(s) and the adolescent at the end of the visit.

Discuss the findings with the adolescent and parent. Negotiate the treatment plan together. In the following case Dr. V. discovers a significant concern in a routine office visit with an adolescent and his mother. Because of his work with both the adolescent and the parent, Dr. V. is able to help the family address the problem.

> In a routine visit for a school physical, Dr. V. asked Mrs. Chase and Howie if there was anything else either of them was concerned about.
> Mrs. Chase: Well, I wasn't going to bring this up, but, well, Howie has been very moody lately and hard to reach.
> Dr. V.: Hard to reach?
> Mrs. Chase: He just doesn't talk to us. (Howie frowns and sighs.)
> Dr. V.: Do you understand what your mother is talking about, Howie?
> Howie: No.
> Dr. V. (to Howie): Is there anything that you are concerned about? (Howie shakes his head *no*.) What do you think is going on, Mrs. Chase?
> Mrs. Chase: I don't really know.
> Dr. V.: Does Mr. Chase have the same concern?

Mrs. Chase: Oh, yes, he especially doesn't like Howie's new friends.

Howie: Big surprise.

Dr. V.: What doesn't he like about them?

Mrs. Chase: We don't know them very well and they're older than Howie.

Howie: Al is not older.

Mrs. Chase: Well, most of them are (silence).

Dr. V.: Well, Mrs. Chase, I'd like to give Howie a chance to change for the exam. You can wait in the waiting room and I'll call you back in after the exam.

Dr. V. steps out. When he returns, Dr. V. tries to follow up on Mrs. Chase's concern.

Dr. V.: Your Mom seems pretty concerned. (Howie does not respond.) What do you think about what she was saying?

Howie: Nothing.

Dr. V.: Has it been hard on you at home?

Howie: No. (Silence. Dr. V. begins the exam.)

Dr. V.: How is school going?

Howie: Lousy.

Dr. V.: Why is that?

Howie: The teachers are all jerks.

Dr. V.: What do you like to do?

Howie: Hang out, you know, spend time with my friends.

Dr. V.: What kind of things do you like to do with your friends?

Howie: We go out on the weekend, cruise around, get some beer, you know.

Dr. V.: You and your friends like to drink.

Howie: When we can, yeah. Not that much, though.

Dr. V.: How much would you say you drink on a weekend?

Howie: I don't know. Not that much. A couple of six packs.

Dr. V.: Do you ever get together during the week to drink?

Howie: Once or twice, maybe.

Dr. V.: Is this with the friends your mother was talking about?

Howie: Yeah, but they are all great guys. I'm not changing my friends.

Dr. V.: Sounds like they are very important to you.

Howie: Yeah.

Dr. V.: How long have you and your friends been drinking together?

Howie: About 5 months or so.

Dr. V.: Do your parents worry about you drinking?

Howie: They asked me about it once.

Dr. V.: What did you say?

Howie: I wasn't gonna tell them anything because they'll never let me see my friends again.

Dr. V.: Do your parents or relatives drink?

Howie: Not much. My Dad ties one on every once in awhile, but it's no big deal.

Dr. V.: What about relatives?

Howie: Well, I've heard my Dad tell some stories about his Dad, but I don't think he drinks much now.

Dr. V.: What do you enjoy about drinking?

Howie: It's just fun.

Dr. V.: What is most fun?

Howie: Just being with my friends and relaxing.

Dr. V.: Is it hard to relax at times?

Howie: No, not really. School is a pain and sometimes my parents get on my nerves.

Dr. V.: Do you talk to your parents?

Howie: No.

Dr. V.: Would you like to?

Howie: Not really, it just leads to an argument.

Dr. V.: It sounds like being with your friends and drinking is one way you have to relax and get away from things. Whenever I talk with any teenager who drinks from time to time, I'm always concerned that the drinking not become a problem. Do you ever think about that?

Howie: Sometimes, but I think I can handle it.

Dr. V.: One thought I had for making sure it's not becoming a problem is to keep a record of when, what, how much, and how often you drink over the next 2 weeks. Then we could get together and see how you're doing.

Howie: I don't think that's necessary.

Dr. V.: It may not be, but it may be a good idea to check things out to make sure.

Howie: Are you going to tell my parents I drink?

Dr. V.: No, but I would encourage you to talk to them.

Howie: Okay, I guess I'll come back.

Dr. V. leaves the room and returns with Mrs. Chase. Dr. V. briefly discusses the physical with Howie and Mrs. Chase.

Dr. V.: I was wondering, Mrs. Chase, if there was anything else you wanted to say about your concern for Howie?

Mrs. Chase: Well, I guess my husband and I both have wondered if Howie was drinking with these boys. He's been coming in pretty late and a few times we heard him getting sick in the bathroom. He says he just had too much to eat.

Dr. V.: But you wonder.

Mrs. Chase: Yes, I suppose, but he has told us he isn't. You aren't drinking are you Howie? (Howie shakes his head, *no*.)

Dr. V.: I can see why you would worry about your son drinking. Has anyone in your family ever had problems with drinking?

Mrs. Chase: Well, my father-in-law did years ago but not now.

Dr. V.: He's recovering.

Mrs. Chase: Yes.

Dr. V.: That's great. So you have some experience with a family member having drinking problems and what difficulties can arise.

Mrs. Chase: Yes, I do.

Dr. V.: I think you and your husband have done a good job taking these changes in Howie's behavior seriously. I'd like to suggest that you both watch these behaviors for the next couple of weeks and then

all of us can get together to see how things are going. Would Mr.
Chase come?

Mrs. Chase: I'm not sure, I think he would.

Six weeks later Mr. Chase called Dr. V. Howie had come home intoxi-
cated the previous night. Mr. Chase did not know what to do. Dr. V.
suggested a counselor at a local alcohol treatment facility where Howie
could go for an evaluation. Dr. V. contacted the counselor to let her
know the Chases would be calling that day. Dr. V. also suggested that
the Chases come for their appointment with him to follow up on the
steps they were taking for Howie.

In this case, Dr. V. maintained an alliance with Howie and with his mother.
He used that alliance to help Howie monitor his drinking and to support
Mr. and Mrs. Chase's vigilance regarding their son's behavior. This helped
bring the issue to a head so that the family, with Dr. V.'s aid, could get Howie
treatment for the problem.

When Adolescents Refuse to Talk

Jordan, a quiet 14-year-old Caucasian male, was sent by his mother to
see Dr. S. for a follow-up visit regarding a skin infection. Jordan was
doing well and Dr. S. asked about some developmental issues of
adolescence. Dr. S. explained that he wanted to get to know Jordan
and asked him to "tell me about yourself." Jordan looked at Dr. S. and
shrugged his shoulders. Dr. S. tried again, "What can you tell me about
school and other things you enjoy doing?" "Nothing much," Jordan
replied. Dr. S. asked a few more open-ended questions, to which Jordan
responded with assorted shrugs, grunts, and nods. Dr. S., feeling frustrated, told Jordan it would help if Jordan would talk so Dr. S. could get
to know him. Jordan just looked at Dr. S.

Dr. S. was clearly becoming angry and frustrated in a way that could have
detoured the entire interview. It is not unusual for adolescents to be less
verbal with adults, especially those in authority. The physician who pushes
an adolescent to talk may endure many silent visits with teenagers. A clinician who responds to silence by trying too hard to "be cool" will also turn
off adolescents. A clinician should remain in control of the interview, avoid
becoming frustrated, and consider the following suggestions:

1. The physician should continue to talk and give the teenager permission
   to be silent.

It is important to avoid power struggles with adolescents over whether or
not they are going to talk. Such battles will usually increase a teenager's
reluctance to speak. By giving the teen permission to be silent, the physician eliminates potential power struggles and helps make the adolescent
more comfortable. For some adolescents, feeling less pressure to speak

makes talking easier. The physician needs to be active even when the adolescent refuses to talk.

> Dr. S. realized he could not force Jordan to talk. At that point Dr. S. said he understood that going to the doctor's could hardly be at the top of Jordan's list of things he'd like to do, and if he did not want to talk that would be fine. Dr. S. explained that there were some things he wanted to talk about and Jordan should feel free just to listen. Dr. S. then began to talk in a general way about some of the changes that all adolescents face.

2. Start with closed questions and move to open ones.

When talking with nonverbal adolescents, it is often more effective to begin with questions that can be answered in monosyllables and then expand to questions that can be answered in phrases and sentences. Factual questions or ones that require *yes* or *no* answers are safest. The adolescent needs to feel comfortable before he or she will open up.

3. Explore areas of possible interest or accomplishment for the adolescent.

This approach facilitates the joining process and gives the adolescent an opportunity to talk about areas of personal importance. The physician can explore school, peers, and outside interests (e.g., music and sports).

> Dr. S. had another appointment with Jordan 10 months later for a sports physical. Remembering the previous visit, Dr. S. decided to approach Jordan differently:
> Dr. S.: Have you had a birthday since I last saw you, Jordan?
> Jordan: Yeah.
> Dr. S.: So that makes you how old?
> Jordan: Fifteen.
> Dr. S.: And what grade?
> Jordan: Sophomore.
> Dr. S.: Is tenth grade better than ninth?
> Jordan: Not much.
> Dr. S.: So it looks like you're here today for a sports physical. Is that right?
> Jordan: Yeah.
> (Jordan gives Dr. S. a form from school)
> Dr. S.: OK—What sport are you trying out for?
> Jordan: Basketball.
> Dr. S.: I used to play basketball in high school. How long have you been playing?
> Jordan: About 6 years.
> Dr. S.: You must be pretty good by now. Is this JV or Varsity?
> Jordan: Varsity.
> Dr. S.: That's great for a sophomore. What position do you play?
> Jordan: Point guard.

Dr. S.: That's like being the coach on the floor, isn't it?

Jordan: Yeah, you have to know a lot.

Dr. S.: I'll bet. You must practice pretty hard.

Jordan: Yeah, we practice every night except on game days. Those are Tuesdays and Fridays. We practice Saturdays, too.

Dr. S.: That's a lot of work.

Jordan: Yeah, coach is pretty tough.

4. Use the physical exam as an opportunity to talk.

The physical exam is probably the most uncomfortable part of the visit for adolescents. The heightened attention given to the body during a physical can be extremely embarrassing for teens. Sitting in silence while a clinician touches their bodies creates an even more uncomfortable situation. During the physical the physician can continue to talk and gather psychosocial information about the adolescent. This approach helps reduce the adolescent's anxiety, and also gives him or her a chance to talk about personal matters without the parent present.

5. After speaking to the adolescent for some period of time, involve the parent(s) in the interview.

If the parent(s) are available the physician can invite the mother and/or father in for the interview. The physician can explain that they need to get some information from the parent and would like the teen to be present. Teenagers often find it uncomfortable to listen to such a conversation without being an active participant. They will frequently talk voluntarily in order to make sure that a balanced view is presented.

6. When appropriate, facilitate discussion of important adolescent issues.

The physician who has developed rapport with the adolescent patient has an opportunity to explore issues related to the adolescent's health and development. These will typically focus on sexuality, peer conflicts, problems with parents, and the use of drugs and alcohol. At the end of the visit, make it clear that the patient can call or ask questions at any time in the future.

Dr. S. saw Jordan two times over the next year for a minor illness and a sports injury. Their conversations revolved around athletics. Dr. S. usually talked more than Jordan, but Jordan slowly began to talk more freely. In particular, he talked about his friends, hinting at some confusion regarding his relationship with them. Dr. S. used the discussion about friendships to talk about sexuality. Jordan listened intently as Dr. S. described the confusion that all adolescents can experience as they try to sort out their feelings toward females and males. When Dr. S. asked if Jordan had thought about these issues much, Jordan said he had, but he did not want to discuss it. Dr. S. said that was fine and that he would be glad to talk with Jordan further if he ever wanted to discuss it. Dr. S. saw Jordan for the flu 8 months later. During the visit Jordan said he was still having some problems with his friends. When Dr. S. invited Jordan to say more, he told the doctor that he had "odd feelings" toward a boy who was his best friend. Dr. S. guessed that Jordan wondered if he was gay. Jordan had not had any sexual relations with his friend or anyone else, but was feeling very confused and upset. Dr. S. asked if Jordan's parents were aware of his concern. Jordan said, no, and that he wanted to keep it that way. After further discussion Dr. S. offered to talk with Jordan on several more occasions to address these concerns. Jordan appreciated the help and accepted Dr. S.'s offer.

Dr. S. saw Jordan six times over the next year. Jordan gradually began to recognize and accept his homosexuality, although he did not want his family to know at this time. As Jordan became sexually active, Dr. S. talked openly with him about AIDS and the need for safety in his sexual relations. He also referred Jordan to an area gay support and advocacy group. Although Dr. S. continued to encourage Jordan to talk with his parents at some point, Jordan refused.

Two years later, while Jordan, now 20, was home from college for the summer, he called Dr. S., thanked him and said he had decided to tell his parents. Dr. S. offered to see Jordan and his parents together, but Jordan wanted to handle it on his own. Dr. S. helped Jordan clarify what he wanted to say to his mother and father. Jordan's disclosure to his parents led to a great deal of conflict. Dr. S. met with Jordan and his parents once, and recommended they see a family therapist to talk further about their concerns. Dr. S. was able to arrange the referral to a local therapist he knew.

In this case, by going slowly with a reluctant adolescent the physician was able to develop a relationship over time that had a significant impact on the adolescent's development. This case also again illustrates the prevalent concern for adolescents of confidentiality and safety. Many adolescents go through these years with little conflict, and little concern for their relationships with healthcare clinicians. They need information and support for taking on the responsibility of caring for their health. For those young people who feel confused about important aspects of their lives, however, their healthcare clinician can be a very pivotal resource. Providing this support, without undermining parental roles, can be a very satisfying dimension of primary care.

References

1. Resnick MD, Bearman PS, Blum RW, Bauman KE, et al.: Protecting adolescents from harm: Findings from the national longitudinal study on adolescent health. *JAMA* 1997;**278**:823–832.
2. Sells CW, Blum R: Morbidity and mortality among US adolescents: an overview of data and trends. *Am J Pub Health* 1996;**86**:513–519.
3. Purcell JS, Hergenroeder MD, Kozinetz C, Smith EO, & Hill RB: Interviewing techniques with adolescents in primary care. *J Adol Health* 1997;**20**:300–305.

4. American Medical Association: Guidelines for Adolescent Preventive Services. Chicago: American Medical Association, 1994 (www.ama-assn.org/adolhlth/gapspub).

5. Combrinck-Graham L: A developmental model for family systems. *Fam Process* 1985;**24**(2):139–150.

6. Cheng TL, Savageau JA, Sattler AL, & DeWitt TG: Confidentiality in health-care: a survey of knowledge, perceptions, and attitudes among high school students. *JAMA* 1993;**269**:1404–1407.

7. Blum R, Beuhring T, Wunderlich MS, & Resnick M: Don't ask, they won't tell: Health screening of youth. *Am J Pub Health* 1996;**86**;1767–1772.

8. Ford CA, Millstein SG, Halpern-Felsher BL, & Irwin CE: Influence of physician confidentiality assurances on adolescents' willingness to disclose information and seek future health care. *JAMA* 1997;**278**(12):1029–1034.

9. Cogswell BE: Cultivating the trust of adolescent patients. *Fam Med* 1985; **27**(6):254–258.

10. Medalie JH, Zyzanski SJ, Langa B, & Stange KC: The family in family practice: is it a reality? *J Fam Prac* 1998;**46**(5):390–396.

11. Society for Adolescent Medicine (Sigman G, Silber TJ, English A, & Gans Epner JE): Confidential health care for adolescents: position paper of the society for adolescent medicine. *J Adol Health* 1997;**21**:408–415.

12. English A: Old confidentiality principles no guarantee against new challenges. *Am Acad Pediatr News* 1999(15):15.

13. Alan Guttmacher Institute (Donovan P): Teenagers' right to consent to reproductive health care. Alan Guttmacher Institute web site. 1998 (www.agi-usa.org/pubs/ib21.html).

14. American Medical Association: Confidential health services for adolescents. In: *AMA Policy Compendium*. 1996:60.

15. American Civil Liberties Union: Parental notice laws: their catastrophic impact on teenagers right to abortion. American Civil Liberties Union, 1986.

Protocol: Family-Oriented Care of Adolescents

A Family-Oriented Approach to Confidentiality

- The physician's main consideration is to provide necessary and adequate healthcare service for the adolescent.
- Blanket confidentiality should not be extended to any patient.
- Involve parents whenever it is possible and appropriate.
- Assess what role family dynamics may play in the adolescent's request for confidentiality.

Guidelines for Office Visits

The family in transition, developmental considerations:

- Maintain a relationship with the adolescent and his or her parents.
- Address counseling and preventive issues pertinent for each stage of adolescent development.
- Be aware of one's own emotional reactions.
- Adolescent efforts to individuate and create autonomy.

Structuring the Interview When a Parent Accompanies the Adolescent

- Meet initially with the parent(s) and adolescent together.
- Ask how you can help them today.
- See the adolescent alone for a majority of the visit.
- Clarify with the adolescent what will be shared with the parent(s).
- Meet conjointly with the parent(s) and the adolescent at the end of the visit.

When Adolescents Refuse to Talk

- The physician should continue to talk and give the adolescent permission to be silent.
- Start with closed questions and move to open ones.
- Explore areas of possible interest and accomplishment for the adolescent.
- Use the physical exam as an opportunity to talk.
- After speaking to the adolescent for some period of time, involve the parent(s) in the interview.
- When appropriate, facilitate discussion of important adolescent issues.
- Reiterate clinician availability for future discussion.

14
Recognizing the Signs of Strain: Counseling Couples in Primary Care

In a busy office practice, why would primary care clinicians consider working with couples in distressed relationships? Why would a clinician not immediately refer to a couples therapist? Referral is the appropriate treatment for some couples. Other couples will resist referral and will need time with their primary care clinician to prepare for formal counseling. Many others, however, benefit from attention and primary care counseling. Treatment for these subthreshold disorders requires that primary care clinicians have skills in primary care couples assessment and counseling.

It is common, for example, for a woman to feel isolated and embarrassed if her husband loses his job, and she finds herself more depressed. Reluctant to tell friends, she may find herself crying or unable to sleep, and may turn to her physician for assistance with sleep or a letter to excuse her from work. The physician can address the sleep or work concerns, and perhaps suggest a therapist. In these acute situations, however, many people are not ready to go to a therapist. They may be far more comfortable talking about their concerns with the person with whom they began speaking—their physician. They may also be more willing to continue the discussion, perhaps by bringing the partner in for one or two visits, with a clinician who offers to see them both.

Counseling couples is not a new role for physicians. In the 1940s, primary care physicians, along with psychiatrists, social workers, and clergy, founded the profession of marriage counseling, now generally termed *couple and family therapy* (1). Clinicians have used their unique knowledge of each family, and their position as a trusted "outsider" to help couples negotiate normal, but distressing, life cycle crises, and differences in their relationships. For the following reasons, the primary care clinician is both the first and perhaps the most effective professional to assist couples with relationship challenges.

TABLE 14.1. Ways in which couple stress presents in primary care

Stress, depression, "worry"
Change in parental responsibilities
Change in work responsibilities
Affairs—concern about STDs, guilt
Sexual complaints or concerns
Domestic abuse
Partner response to a patient's medical condition

1. Problems in intimate relationships, especially marriage, are often factors for patient visits in a primary care setting.

Research supporting the link between relationships and health is increasingly strong (2) and was cited in Chaps. 2 and 9. Family conflict and criticism are among the most important risk factors for a number of health outcomes (3), and marital problems often underlie a patient's presentation of vague physical complaints. Throughout the couple's lifecycle, the physician has the opportunity to respond when patients are most distressed. Table 14.1 notes the common ways in which couple concerns are presented.

2. Patients view their primary care clinician as a resource.

Like clergy, physicians and nurse clinicians are recognized as confidential sources for compassionate and pragmatic help. It has been estimated, for example, that more than 1 in 10 adult visits involves a sexual problem (4). In research in a primary care setting, patients indicated that they would be more likely to consult their family physician about sexual problems than any other professional (5). These patients' willingness to consult depended on whether or not they perceived their physicians as being interested or concerned about sexual matters in general. When physicians initiate questions and indicate their interest to discuss sexual concerns, patients are more likely to raise concerns in later visits.

3. A primary care clinician can recognize when stressful primary relationships may be impacting health.

A primary care clinician can monitor how couples are coping with care plans, or a new or chronic condition. Brief couple counseling may be particularly indicated when one member of the couple has a chronic disease, or when role change occurs with caregiving responsibilities (6).

4. The primary care clinician can normalize relationship crises, and facilitate coping strategies.

Clinicians are viewed as experts in helping people in crisis, and their experience and advice is valued. A clinician is in a powerful position to assure patients that even welcome developmental stages also lead to stress, including the transition to parenthood, the launching of children, or caring for an elderly parent. A confident clinician can reassure couples that these normal stresses and resulting differences are treatable.

From well-child visits and acute illnesses, to the experience of loss, the physician has contact with a couple throughout the life cycle and can be the one to whom a couple turns; yet, only a fraction of these couple problems are either identified by healthcare providers or recognized as an appropriate target for intervention. Realistic concerns exist about time and about how to manage couple distress, Other barriers include assessment difficulties when only one partner is at an office visit, or vague somatic complaints that may reflect a relationship problem. A clinician may be concerned that questions about a patient's relationship may seem intrusive or embarrassing. Finally, working with couples can remind clinicians of their own imperfect relationships and create anxiety about how to control anger or conflict when more than one person is present. Clinicians who are attuned to signs of marital strain and who can comfortably talk with couples can help them take the first steps toward resolving their problems. Recognizing the barriers around couple counseling, this chapter will consider some common relationship patterns, show how to recognize marital difficulties, and offer guidelines for efficient couple counseling in primary care.

Pursuers and Distancers: Recognizing Common Relationship Patterns in Couples

The following example illustrates a common relationship pattern that can become exaggerated and problematic. Helping couples recognize this pattern, particularly when it relates to healthcare, can be a useful aid for clinicians and for couples.

Elna and Burt Washington, an African-American couple in their thirties, had been married for 7 years. They had one child, Ron, age 6 years. From Elna's perspective, their marriage had been fine until the last several months, when there had been considerable conflict. A beautician, Mrs. Washington felt her husband had been preoccupied and never in the mood to talk. He did not have an answer when she asked him about this. When Burt got angry, he often became quiet and left the house. Elna complained that no matter how hard she tried, her husband would not "open up to her." She became increasingly convinced that her husband was rejecting her, and perhaps interested in another woman.

From Burt's perspective, he wished his wife would stop nagging him. No matter what he did, she thought it was never right and it was never enough. Did she not know that he had to answer complaints all day long as an apartment building maintenance supervisor? He did not want to come home and listen to more problems. He often said that he needed time to himself, not more pressure from her.

Fogarty (7) suggests that there are two primary ways people respond to anxiety: to pursue or to distance. When stressed, a pursuer tends to move toward other people for support or attention. The pursuer believes in togetherness and that happiness can be attained through attachments to others. Distancers want relationships, but also see them as difficult. When anxious, distancers withdraw, fall silent, and shoulder their difficulties alone. Distancers try to be rational and objective and are confused by the emotionality of pursuers. Pursuing and distancing styles can characterize roles in couple relationships, as well as in work, doctor–patient, or other important relationships. Everyone uses pursuing and distancing responses, but most people tend toward one primary style much of the time. With some issues (e.g., sex) a person may pursue, while distancing for things like expressing feelings.

It is of interest that pursuers and distancers are typically attracted to each other (8). Their differences can be a resource for a relationship as long as there is flexibility for each to pursue or distance at times. In this way a healthy balance of togetherness and separateness (i.e., of intimacy and privacy) can be maintained. When the relationship pattern is more rigid, one person primarily pursues while the other distances, and the relationship may feel like an endless and exhausting struggle. The more the distancer withdraws to refuel, the more the pursuer feels anxious and unloved and looks to the distancer for acceptance. A cycle continues such that the distancer feels more intruded upon and pulls further away, and the pursuer feels more alone and increases the pursuit. (See Fig. 14.1).

> Mr. and Mrs. Washington were caught in such a cycle. Elna pursued her husband in the hope of getting more closeness. Burt perceived her questions as nagging, and felt that more talking would only make things worse. He then avoided Elna, left for work earlier, and stayed later in the evening. Elna had more trouble sleeping, felt exhausted, and often had headaches. She described these symptoms at her annual physical with her nurse practitioner, Ms. Furman.
>
> Ms. Furman's examination revealed nothing remarkable, and asked what else might be of concern. Elna discussed the pressures about raising her son, working, and keeping up with the house. Ms. Furman listened and was supportive. When Elna asked about "tricks" for reducing stress, Ms. Furman suggested deep-breathing exercises. She also suggested that she return in 3 weeks for follow up. Ms. Furman was glad she had helped, but felt slightly perturbed when she realized she was 15 minutes late for her next appointment.

Pursuers are more likely than distancers to seek help from a professional, including a physician. Distancers may withdraw into their work, as does

Recognizing the Signs of Strain

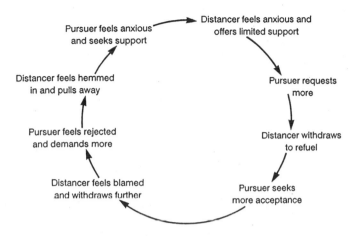

FIGURE 14.1. The pursuing and distancing cycle.

Burt, use substances, or have affairs to decrease the intensity of the primary relationship. If Elna's emotional needs are met by the attention she receives during healthcare, she may pursue her clinician further and become a more frequent visitor at the medical office. One signal that the patient may have underlying relationship problems is the physician's mixed reaction to her visit.

> Elna appreciated her visit with Ms. Furman. She talked to her husband about how "lousy" she had been feeling. Burt was pleased that his wife had no serious illness, but he had always believed that she was overly sensitive to aches and pains. Elna said her nurse believed she was under too much stress. Burt wondered if this comment was a criticism of him, and told his wife he did not want to talk about it; he had "enough on his mind."
>
> Two days later, Mrs. Washington again had a significant headache. Ms. Furman was on call when she called to say she was upset that she was not feeling better. Ms. Furman spoke to her for 10 minutes, and offered an appointment for the following day. When she hung up, Ms. Furman realized she was angry at Mrs. Washington for calling and realized she did not want to see her the next day.

What happened to Ms. Furman and Mrs. Washington is not unusual. Clinicians often find themselves in pursuer–distancer relationships with certain patients. When patients do not adhere to their medication plan, the physician is often the pursuer. He or she tries hard to get the patient to cooperate in treatment (e.g., increasing the frequency of visits), whereas the patient appears to sabotage treatment (e.g., "forgetting" to take medication). With other patients, physicians may feel pursued and find themselves distancing in response (e.g., taking greater time to return the patient's frequent phone calls).

A problem exists when clinicians find themselves consistently pursuing or distancing from a patient. The solution begins with the recognition that the physician can alter his or her behavior, and develop a more balanced approach to the patient. Distancing often encourages the patient to pursue, and pursuing encourages the patient to distance. For example, a physician can request regular meetings with patients who pursue, while setting appropriate limits about contact between visits or on call. Approaches can emphasize patient autonomy with distancing patients. For example, the physician may ask a patient to determine the frequency of their contact, while alerting the patient and the family about risks of not complying with treatment (see Chap. 8 for additional suggestions).

A pursuer–distancer pattern in clinical care may indicate similar patterns in the patient's relationships with significant others. Patients who pursue physicians, for instance, are often not getting their needs met in their closest relationships. Physicians may not see distancers in their office very frequently, and these people may be less revealing with their families as well. Asking about the patient's primary relationships may result in more rewarding patient encounters.

> Ms. Furman recognized that her strong reaction to Mrs. Washington may have been a sign that there were other issues contributing to her request for medical care. She decided to explore Mrs. Washington's psychosocial situation further.
>
> Mrs. Washington (as Ms. Furman enters the room): I thought the exercises would work, but I just feel worse everyday. The headaches are stronger. They go down the back of my neck. . .
>
> Ms. Furman: It sounds like you've been in a lot of discomfort.
>
> Mrs. Washington: . . . I can't get any rest, but I've got to keep working. Sometimes I have to get up at night two or three times.
>
> Ms. Furman: So all of those symptoms have been pretty constant since you were here a few days ago?
>
> Mrs. Washington: Yes, I've felt awful.
>
> Ms. Furman: I'm sure you have. Have you talked with your husband at all about this?
>
> Mrs. Washington: Yes, a little.
>
> Ms. Furman: So, he's aware of how you've felt.
>
> Mrs. Washington: I would think anyone would notice. I really am uncomfortable.
>
> Ms. Furman: This must be very exhausting. What does your husband say about it?
>
> Mrs. Washington: Well, I think he thinks it's all in my head. But he's around so little, how would he know. . . (Mrs. Washington went on to talk about some of the conflict that had occurred in the marriage.)

Ms. Furman: It sounds like this has been a hard time for both of you. Your husband is working a lot of hours. You have been working hard, too, at home and on your job; and both of you are trying to be good parents. At times you haven't felt as close as you'd like. To top it off, you've been feeling pretty sick.

Mrs. Washington: That about sums it up.

Ms. Furman: This is what I would suggest at this point. I would like to invite your husband in to get some of his thoughts about how you are feeling and how he thinks this could be improved.

Mrs. Washington: Well, if you think it's necessary. I don't know if he'd come. He can't get off work very easily.

Ms. Furman: Do you think it would help if I give him a call to invite him?

Mrs. Washington: Maybe. I'll give you his number.

Ms. Furman remained sensitive to Elna's physical problems, while gaining valuable psychosocial information. By inviting the husband to the next appointment, Ms. Furman interrupted the pursuer–distancer cycle that had begun between herself and Mrs. Washington. It also gave her the opportunity to assess the role that marital discord might play in Elna's complaints.

Assessing Couples' Relationship Problems

Burt Washington came with his wife for the next medical appointment. He wondered how sick his wife "really" was and stated that he seldom knew how to help her. In the session, Elna became angry with her husband, stating that he never tried to understand. Ms. Furman quickly stopped the conflict:

Ms. Furman: Elna, I understand you are frustrated, and I can see that this is a difficult situation for both of you. I am willing to speak with you further about how you might be able to understand and help each other a little bit more. Do you think that might be worthwhile?

The Washingtons agreed that things had not been good between them for months. Ms. Furman offered to meet with them for a longer visit to discuss the difficulties they were having and to follow up on Mrs. Washington's symptoms. Elna was willing to return, but Burt was skeptical about the value of "just talking more" and wanted time to think about it. Ms. Furman agreed that this was an important decision that they both should think about. Ms. Furman suggested the Washingtons call in 1 week with their decision. Elna called 2 weeks later. Things had gotten worse and they had decided to talk with Ms. Furman about it.

By reading the signs correctly, Ms. Furman recognized the existence of a problem and succeeded in stimulating the couple's willingness to discuss their marital difficulties. She recognized that Burt was "distancing," and that he would not have cooperated if she pushed him into making an appointment. By having them take responsibility for future interactions, she pulled herself out of a pursuer–distance pattern. Ms. Furman assessed the Washington's relationship in the next visit. An assessment session should: (1) gain additional information about the couple and their problems; (2) help the couple clarify their concerns and wishes for their relationship; and (3) assist the clinician and couple in deciding the next steps. Couples relationships can be assessed according to the nature of the problem and attempted solutions, brief history and family background, strengths of the marriage, sexual intimacy, and the couple's motivation to change.

Problems and Attempted Solutions

Helping couples clarify why they are at the visit, as well as their expectations, helps to decrease anxiety and create expectations for honest discussion. When couples come for counseling, they generally are frustrated with one another, blame one another for the problems, and also feel that they have been blamed. One person is generally more invested in trying to talk together, but there is often not much hope for change.

For a short period, the clinician should help the couple discuss their problems and how they have tried to resolve them. Careful attention should insure that each partner has an equal amount of time to talk and present their view. This includes seating patterns, so that the clinician is in a triangle with the couple and so that all can talk together, but where the clinician is not sided with one partner or another.

This brief discussion can allow observation of couple interaction. How do they communicate verbally and nonverbally? Does one partner intellectualize whereas the other is emotional? Who pursues and who distances? Does one blame whereas the other accepts guilt? The following questions can help assess whether the problem is chronic or situational, severe, or mild:

- How do you each view this problem?
- How long has there been a problem?
- What changes have occurred in your life during this time?
- How do you think these changes have affected your relationship?
- What do you think is the cause of the problem?
- How have you tried to solve the problem in the past? Any previous counseling?
- What has worked? What has not worked?
- What have family and friends said to you about your problems?
- Has anyone else in either of your families had similar problems?
- Ideally, how would you like things to be?

Mr. Washington felt his wife was always upset about something. Nothing he did for her was right. Mrs. Washington was angry that her husband was "never affectionate" and did not listen to her. She said her husband had always been quiet, but that things had been much worse in the last 5 months. Mr. Washington had not noticed a problem until several weeks ago, although he acknowledged that something was up over the last few months.

It was apparent to Ms. Furman how much both parents loved their son. Ron had been very ill with pneumonia 7 months ago and Mrs. Washington had taken time off from work to care for him. Mrs. Washington said it was very stressful for her, especially because her husband had to work a lot of overtime during the illness. Mr. Washington reported that he worried about his son all the time. The couple reported arguing several times during their son's illness and not being able to resolve the tensions between them since that time. They now reported fighting "at the drop of a hat."

As the clinician sums up the discussion, he or she should make it clear that no one is to blame because the difficulties reflect differences rather than right or wrong. The clinicians should also express hope and confidence that change can occur. Ms. Furman used a concrete technique that can be very helpful. She pointed to the floor between the couple.

Ms. Furman: This space between you represents your marriage. So there are really three things for us to pay attention to here each of you and the marriage. If you two acted the same way and wanted exactly the same things from the marriage, there would be no difficulty. It also would be rather boring.
(Mr. and Mrs. Washington laughed, and Ms. Furman continued.)
Neither one of you is right or wrong. There is no correct way to behave— no perfect amount of time that you're supposed to talk about an issue, like your son's illness. You are each different people, and want different things, so of course there's going to be conflict. You also obviously care about each other and your family a great deal, and so it's worth it to think about how you can negotiate your differences and make the marriage something that is better for both of you.

Family Background

As part of the joining process, genograms can be initiated or updated (see Chap. 3). Couple difficulties often reflect unresolved issues related to each partner's family of origin or difficulty blending the different relationship styles of two families. Some possible questions include:

- Do your parents live together, and how much contact do you have with them?

- How about brothers and sisters? Are they in relationships? What kind of contact do you have with them?
- Do any of these family members know about the difficulties you are having?

> Mr. Washington was an only child who grew up in what he described as a strict household where emotions were seldom expressed openly. His parents were loving, but not demonstrative. They lived a few states away and visited each other a couple of times a year. Mrs. Washington was the oldest of five children. She reported that her family showed a lot of emotion, fighting often, but always making up. Her widowed mother lived about 1 hour away, and they were able to see one another quite frequently. The communication styles and preferences clearly reflected differences in their family experiences.

Strengths of the Relationship

It is as valuable to understand the strengths of a committed relationship as it is to understand its problems. Couples usually find it easier to discuss problems than strengths when angry or disappointed. Those couples who are able to identify strengths are usually more flexible and open in how they view a marriage; consequently, they are more hopeful about change. Questions that focus on the couple's strengths include:

- Are there times when there are few problems in your relationship?
- What do you do differently at those times that makes them better?
- What do you feel are the strengths of your marriage?
- When was the best time in your relationship?
- What made it good?

> The Washingtons smiled when Ms. Furman asked them about the good times in their relationship. They talked humorously about their ill-fated honeymoon camping trip during which it rained for 5 days, and the excitement and closeness they felt when their son was born. Those were times in which they talked more and felt they were headed in the same direction.
>
> Mr. Washington felt their greatest strength was their "willingness to keep trying." Mrs. Washington said that their greatest strength was their commitment to each other and to their son, although she worried whether or not these commitments would endure. Ms. Furman said he was impressed that even with the difficulties they were having, their marriage obviously had clear strengths that they could draw on to try and solve their current problems.

Sexual Intimacy

Any discussion about couple counseling should include some questions about the couple's sexual relationship. Sexual behavior is a complicated process that reflects intense feelings, gender relationships and roles, societal norms, and sometimes power and abuse. Sexual behavior and satisfaction is clearly a biopsychosocial process, and includes physiological, relational, and sociocultural factors. Although medical conditions may impact sexual functioning in multiple ways (9), sexual functioning also reflects a couple's emotional and intimate relationship (See Fig. 14.2). The primary care clinician is in a unique role to assess how medical processes or medications, as well as a couple's relationship and attitudes, may impact their sexual relationship. Sexual functioning is generally a combination of these factors, which means that treatment may be possible from a number of perspectives.

Assessment of sexual problems depends in large part on the initiative of the physician. Studies show that doctors and patients each believe that the other is more conservative about sexual matters, and that each is hesitant to initiate conversations that might offend the other (9) A clinician who can comfortably ask about sexual functioning and satisfaction within the context of medical and social history will create safety for patients to talk comfortably as well. Lower back pain, abdominal pain, urinary difficulties, and a host of other somatic complaints may include underlying sexual concerns that patients are hesitant to discuss. It is not unusual for a patient who has experienced a lifetime of physical discomfort also to have sexual problems that may never have been discussed with a physician.

In their pioneering and still relevant work, Masters and Johnson (10) have estimated that 50% of all marriages experience sexual problems at

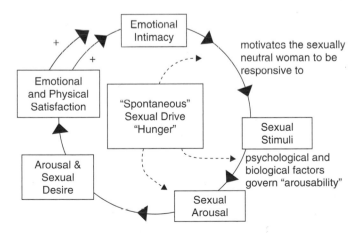

FIGURE 14.2. Intimacy-based cycle (Reprinted with permission from reference 9.)

some time. Studies indicate that physicians who do not inquire about a couple's sexual relationship will only learn about problems 10% of the time, but physicians who routinely inquire will identify sexual problems 50–100% of the time (4). A useful task is to help couples distinguish between normal fluctuations in sexual desire and behavior, and *persistent* difficulties that characterize sexual dysfunction and which require sexual therapy (11).

The most frequent difficulties faced by women include inhibited sexual desire, anorgasmia, vaginismus and dyspareunia, and low sexual desire (12, 13). Among men, with the exception of early ejaculation, most common sexual problems like erectile dysfunction are secondary (13), with the frequency of erectile dysfunction to be more than 50% for men older than 50 years. The introduction of Viagra in 1998 and other medications has created a cultural shift of increasing comfort among couples to discuss sexual difficulties. This medical assistance for erectile problems has also facilitated a corresponding change in attitude that sexual problems reflect primarily physical rather than psychological or relationship issues (13). Thus, it may be even more important now for clinicians to bring in both partners for any discussion of sexual problems, and to stress how sexual problems reflect the full range of biopsychosocial issues, including relationship discord, performance anxiety, lack of sexual knowledge and comfort, and the side effects of medication or disease (14). Ways to initiate these conversations can include the following (9, 12):

- How satisfied are you with the sexual part of your life together?
- How are these issues (that brought you to counseling) affecting your sexual life?
- Has this time of increased conflict made a difference?
- Are there any changes in your sexual interest?
- Are there any changes in your sexual functioning?
- How comfortable are you (two) about talking about these sexual concerns?
- How would you like your sexual relationship to be different?

> Ms. Furman asked the Washingtons if their relationship difficulties affected their sexual relationship. At first they both said everything was "okay," but when Ms. Furman asked if they were satisfied with their sex life, Mrs. Washington said she was not. She felt they should be closer. When asked what she meant by "closer," Mrs. Washington said she wished they could have sex more often. Ms. Furman learned that the Washingtons were having sex approximately once every 6 weeks. Mr. Washington acknowledged that this was less than it had been, but said he often felt too tired at night. He also said that when he was not tired, his wife was angry. Ms. Furman asked if they were able to have intercourse satisfactorily when they had tried. Both said that several times Mr. Washington had not been able to get an erection. Ms. Furman asked more and learned that Mr. Washington had erections at other

times. Mrs. Washington had not had problems until a month go when she reported pain during intercourse, so they stopped. They had not attempted intercourse since.

Motivation to Change

It is a mistake to assume that a couple wants to change their situation without first asking them. It is also important to determine each partner's expectation and motivation. For some, change may involve improving the relationship or considering ending it. Others may not be happy with their marriage, but are not ready to make changes. This reflects a variety of reasons, including anxiety, about giving in to a spouse or fear that discussing problems openly may make things worse. Prospects for effective counseling are diminished if a couple's desire to change is not clarified or if the physician appears more motivated than the couple. Questions that help clarify each partner's motivation to change include:

- Do you want your relationship to continue?
- Do you feel your relationship can change?
- If your relationship does not change, what do you think will happen?
- Do you want to continue to work on the relationship in counseling?

> Ms. Furman asked the Washingtons whether they believed their relationship could change. Mrs. Washington said they could try harder to get along. Mr. Washington did not know what they could do, but felt things had to get better, so that perhaps they could "do things differently." When asked if they wanted to work further on changing their relationship, both said, yes, although Mr. Washington made it clear that he did not want to go off to see some "shrink" for an extended period of time.

Indications for Primary Care Couple Counseling

1. The problem is situational with recent onset.

Such problems include difficulties that have arisen within the previous 6 months related to life cycle changes or specific crises of limited duration. Examples of such stresses include birth of a child, death in the family, recent illness, and job change or loss.

2. The problem is specific rather than general.

Couples seeking to improve their ability to argue productively, for example, are more likely to make changes because they have clearly defined the problem. Couples who have "communication problems" or who want to "make the marriage better" may have multiple or long-standing problems, and may be better treated elsewhere.

3. The couple has a history of a good relationship.

Couples who report a stable, close relationship prior to the onset of the problem have a good foundation to build on in counseling. Couples who have "always fought" or have "never gotten along" should be referred.

4. Neither member of the couple has admitted to an ongoing affair.

Patients may often present to their primary clinician when they learn that their partner is having an affair. The clinician can support the patient, while referring the couple to a couple therapist.

5. Neither member of the couple has a significant individual psychiatric diagnosis.

Partners are impacted when one member has a significant psychiatric diagnosis, as is their relationship. Couple therapy can be effective in these situations (15), but it generally will require referral to an experienced couple therapist.

6. Both members of the couple are motivated to change.

7. The physician has the comfort, skills, and allocated time to work with the couple.

Guidelines for Primary Care Couple Counseling

1. Involve both partners in counseling.

Couple counseling with only one partner may increase the problems that the couple is facing (16). It also encourages the participating partner to depend on the physician inappropriately, which can lead to a pursuer–distancer pattern.

Patients can be coached about how to ask their partner to join them for any counseling session. Clinicians might point out that resistance is very likely if a patient says something like, "The Dr. wants to see you—I don't know why," or, "Ms. Furman thinks that things are stressful at home, and wants to talk with you." It is similar to an adolescent being told that "the principal wants to see you." Patients can say instead that they could use some help managing their stress, and the clinician thinks that their partner could be of some help. A brief conversation about how to approach a partner can make joint attendance more likely.

2. Maintain attention to confidentiality, potential triangles, and alliances.

Primary care couple counseling is usually initiated by one partner, which often results in the concern by the other partner that the clinician is already biased. The clinician should discuss confidentiality, and how any patient confidentiality will not be broken in the couple or later individual sessions. Clinicians should arrange to sit equidistant from each partner in the couple and to insure that each partner has equal opportunity to talk. It can be helpful for the clinician to behave as a "traffic cop" to help couples recognize that both will be heard and both will have a chance to speak.

3. Primary care couple counseling should generally be short term.

This is best accomplished by establishing a clear format for the counseling process that includes:

- number of counseling visits (four to six).
- frequency of visits (weekly, monthly, etc.).
- length of each visit (25–45 minutes).
- clarifying what other contacts between the couple and the physician are acceptable (none, 1 phone call between visits, no phone calls at home, etc.).
- assessing the couple's progress on or before the final contract visit.

4. Primary care counseling is sometimes accomplished in a piecemeal fashion over extended periods of time.

Couples may cope well with a variety of problems, until a stressful event occurs that pushes them "over the edge." At this point, the couple may not need formal referral to a family therapist, but could benefit from a trusted third party. This assistance may take place in combination with medical visits and include either one or both partners.

> Mike and Betsy Smith, a Caucasian couple in their late thirties, had seen Dr. F. for several years, whereas their two children saw a pediatrician in the city. During Mike's physical, Dr. F. learned that about 6 months earlier, their oldest child, Brian, had been diagnosed with brain cancer, had received treatment, and was moving toward hospice status. In that time, Mike had quit his job in a high-tech company to consult from home to have flexibility to care for Brian. Mike complained that Betsy, who had maintained her associate vice-president position, was burying herself in her work, and increasingly unavailable for the family. Dr. F. made a few suggestions and recommended that he meet with Mike and Betsy. Mike doubted whether Betsy would come, but said he would try.
>
> Betsy called and said how difficult it would be for her to take time off from work, but agreed to an end-of-the-day appointment. During the couple session, Betsy and Mike identified their differing coping styles, and Dr. F. supported their differences, as well as their concern for their son and family. As their son had become increasingly ill, they had postponed a family session suggested by the social worker from the

children's hospital. After the couple meeting, they agreed to have the family meeting with Dr. F., who communicated in advance with the social worker. Dr. F. met with all family members about 3 weeks before Brian's death. The family had mobilized many resources, including other family, friends, and the hospice team. They also were able to lean on and support one another.

In the year following Brian's death, Dr. F. saw Mike on several occasions. He monitored his cholesterol, but also provided a place for Mike to talk about Brian and his loss. Dr. F. similarly saw Betsy for a couple of visits for minor tendonitis and routine gynecologic concerns. Betsy had been able to take more time off from work surrounding Brian's death and in the following year, Mike had returned to work at another technology firm. As well as was possible, this couple recovered from this terrible tragedy slowly and with multiple supports. In each of their times with Dr. F., they noted how helpful their brief couple discussions had been. They had been able to stop seeing each other's behavior as a criticism of their own, but as a unique response to an unbearable stress.

5. Negotiating solutions to problems should be the focus of counseling.

The physician should help the couple:

- Clarify which changes they want to make.
- Discuss what each would have to do for the changes to occur.
- Make a clear plan for implementing the desired new behaviors.
- Carry out appropriate tasks between counseling visits.
- Give feedback about progress to each other.

Couples are often so focused on the wrongs in the relationship that they neglect what they can do to find solutions. Counseling should help the couple remember events in which they resolved differences well, or imagine how the relationship would be if they could solve their problem (17, 18). The clinician can help the couple brainstorm ideas and negotiate plans.

The use of "quid pro quo" techniques can be an effective approach to negotiation. In this behavioral process, the couple identifies the behaviors they would like each other to change. Each partner then agrees to try a new behavior in exchange for a new behavior that the other partner will try. In this way the couple builds trust and begins to get their needs met (e.g., Tom agrees to notify his partner Steve when he will be late at work, and Steve agrees to not make social commitments without discussing them with Tom).

6. Couples who are not making progress in primary care counseling should be referred.

By the last contracted visit, the physician and couple should assess whether or not the couple's goals are being met. If change is not occurring, it is unwise to recontract for additional visits with a hope that more sessions would make a difference. It is better to focus on what progress has occurred and how a referral may be the next step in the process of change (see Chap. 25 for a discussion of referrals).

> The Washingtons agreed to meet with Ms. Furman for four times over 2 months and then assess the couple's progress. Ms. Furman asked them during their first session to be more specific about their joint hopes to "get closer." The Washingtons decided they wanted to try to spend more time together and talk more, even with their busy schedules. They decided to plan an evening out together. Elna usually planned these events, so they decided that Burt would arrange for the next evening, with no reminders from Elna.
>
> The Washingtons were very pleased at their second session. They had gone out and enjoyed themselves on two occasions. Ms. Furman encouraged them to share what made it enjoyable to be together. They said they were beginning to talk together for the first time in months. Mrs. Washington felt her husband was more available and Mr. Washington felt less pressured. For the next visit they decided to go out again and also make a list of what they most wanted from each other.
>
> Both Burt and Elna were subdued at the third visit. They had not made their lists although they had gone on another date. Mr. Washington felt things were "not working out," but could not explain why. Mrs. Washington eventually became angry and told Ms. Furman that things had gone well until they had tried to make love. She felt her husband had rejected her, whereas Mr. Washington insisted he was just too tired from a long day at work. Ms. Furman learned that the Washingtons had had sexual problems since the time of their son's birth. In the beginning Mrs. Washington was so involved with a newborn that she seldom felt like making love. When they did she felt her husband was not "tender" with her. Mr. Washington felt his wife criticized him and his interest gradually decreased. He had been unable to maintain an erection several times. The Washingtons eventually stopped talking about sex at all, and made love infrequently.

It is common for couples to have initial success with plans, but then to reach a disappointment or impasse. This sometimes signifies that the work of change will be harder than anticipated. It often allows people to identify a fear or concern that had not been expressed earlier (e.g., the sexual pattern for the Washingtons). These concerns can sometimes be addressed with primary care counseling, but they also may be an indication that the couple is ready to accept a referral for couple therapy.

> Ms. Furman emphasized the progress the Washington's had made on their original goal of increasing their time together and talking more. She suggested that perhaps they were trying to make changes in their sexual relationship prematurely and needed more time to "get to know each other again." Ms. Furman suggested that the Washington's not have sex before the next appointment. She explained that sexual intimacy may be the next step, but for now the Washingtons needed more time

just being together. The Washingtons planned a project to do together and decided to talk together once about their hopes for their sexual relationship.

Ms. Furman learned that the Washington's problem was of longer duration than she had assumed. She saw that the pursuing and distancing process in their marriage may have protected them from the hurt or risks of getting too close and being disappointed. Her ban on sexual intimacy was an attempt to slow the couple down and help to solidify some of the gains they had made.

Restraining the couple from further attempts at sexual intimacy is a common approach in sex therapy (12, 13). The most familiar treatment approach developed by Masters and Johnson involves work on couple communication, the prohibition of sexual intercourse, and the use of sensate focus exercises. Through sensate focus exercises the couple learns to give and receive pleasure by touching and caressing. The couple begins with nongenital touching, moves to genital pleasuring, and is eventually encouraged to have intercourse.

Ms. Furman began this process by encouraging further communication and removing the pressure to perform sexually. In the fourth session Ms. Furman and the Washingtons assessed their progress and decided on future directions. The Washingtons were pleased that they had been successful with their project, which was papering the bedroom. They also noted that they never did discuss sex. Mrs. Washington blamed her husband for being "too busy." Mr. Washington agreed that he was sometimes too angry to talk to his wife.

The Washingtons felt frustrated. They wanted to be more intimate, but they felt stuck. Ms. Furman helped remind them of the progress they had made in a short time and emphasized that couples who are making progress often realize how much more they want from their relationship. The Washingons agreed that there had been some improvement, but that they wanted more time with Ms. Furman to improve their marriage.

Ms. Furman: I'm pleased that you want to continue because you've showed that you can make changes. I also think that with your new commitment, I recommend that you continue counseling with a marriage counselor that I often work with. He is well trained to deal with sexual difficulties that couples are trying to resolve.

The Washingtons agreed to the referral, although Mrs. Washington was concerned that she would no longer be able to see Ms. Furman. Ms. Furman clarified that she would continue to see either of them for her medical concerns and would be in communication with their new therapist.

Recognizing that relationship problems may be a significant factor in a patient's somatic complaints is one of the most important tasks of the physician when working with patients who are in a committed relationship. Early recognition helps the physician avoid developing a relationship with the patient that may only replicate problem patterns in the patient's marriage. The clinician who recognizes the importance of marital dynamics to patient health can either help couples use their strengths to make changes or do the early work that facilitates effective referral to a couple or family therapist.

References

1. Nichols M: *Family Therapy: Concepts and Methods*. New York: Gardner Press, 1984.
2. Kiecolt-Glaser JK, Newton TL: Marriage and health: his and hers. *Psychol Bull* 2001;**127**:472–503.
3. Weiss K, Fisher L, & Baird M: Families, health and behavior. A section of the comissioned report by the Committee on Health and Behavior, Institute of Medicine, National Academy of Sciences. *Fam Syst Health* 2002;**20**(1):7–46.
4. Pauly TB: Human sexuality in medical education and practice. *J Psychiatr* (Australia/New England) 1971;**5**:204–208.
5. Nease DF, Liese BS: Perceptions and treatment of sexual problems. *Fam Med* 1987;**19**(6):468–470.
6. McDaniel SH, Hepworth J, & Doherty WJ: *Medical Family Therapy*. New York: Basic Books, 1992.
7. Fogarty TF: The distancer and the pursuer. *The Family* 1976;**7**(1):11–16.
8. Lerner H: *The Dance of Anger*, New York: Harper & Row, 1985.
9. Basson R: Female sexual response: the role of drugs in the management of sexual dysfunction. *Obstet Gynecol* 2001;**98**(2):350–353.
10. Kolodny RC, Masters WH, & Johnson VE: *Textbook of Sexual Medicine*. Boston: Little, Brown & Co., 1979.
11. Sotile W: *Heart Illness and Intimacy: How Caring Relationships Aid Recovery*. Baltimore, MD: Johns Hopkins Press, 1992.
12. Kaplan HS: *The New Sex Therapy*. New York, Brunner/Mazel, 1974.
13. McCarthy BW: Sexuality, sexual dysfunction, and couple therapy. In Gurman AS, Jacobsen NS (Eds): *Clinical Handbook of Couple Therapy*. New York: Guilford Press, 2002.
14. Steinert Y: Working with couples: sexual problems. In: Christie-Seely J (Ed). *Working with the Family in Primary Care: A Systems Approach to Health and Illness*. New York: Praeger, 1984.
15. Carlson J, Sperry L (Eds): *The Disordered Couple*. Bristol, PA: Bruner, Mazel, 1998.
16. Gurman AS, Jacobsen NS (Eds): *Clinical Handbook of Couple Therapy*. New York: Guilford Press, 2002.
17. Weiner-Davis M: *Divorce-Busting: A Revolutionary and Rapid Program for Staying Together*. New York: Simon & Schuster, 1992.
18. De Shazer S: *Putting Differences to Work*. New York: W.W. Norton, 1991.

Protocol: Counseling Couples in Primary Care

Nature of the Problem and Attempted Solutions

- How do you each view this problem?
- How long has there been a problem?
- What changes have occurred in your life during this time?
- How do you think these changes have affected your relationship?
- What do you think is the cause of the problem?
- How have you tried to solve the problem in the past? Any previous counseling?
- What has worked? What has not worked?
- What have family and friends said to you about your problems?
- Has anyone else in either of your families had similar problems?
- How would you ideally like things to be?

Family Background

- Are your parents together, and how much contact do you have with them?
- How about brothers and sisters? Are they in relationships? What kind of contact do you have with them?
- Do any of these family members know about the difficulties you are having?

Strengths of the Relationship

- Are there times when there are few problems in your relationship?
- What do you do differently at those times that makes them better?
- What do you feel are the strengths of your marriage?
- When was the best time in your relationship?
- What made it good?

Sexual Intimacy

- How satisfied are you with the sexual part of your life together?
- How are these issues (that brought you to counseling) affecting your sexual life?
- Has this time of increased conflict made a difference?
- Are there any changes in your sexual interest?
- Are there any changes in your sexual functioning?
- How comfortable are you (two) about talking about these sexual concerns?
- How would you like your sexual relationship to be different?

Motivation to Change

- Do you want your relationship to continue?
- Do you feel your relationship can change?
- If your relationship does not change, what do you think will happen?
- Do you want to continue to work on the relationship in counseling?

Indications for Primary Care Couple Counseling

1. The problem is situational with recent onset.
2. The problem is specific rather than general.
3. The couple has a history of a good relationship.
4. Neither member of the couple has admitted to an ongoing affair.
5. Neither member of the couple has a significant individual psychiatric diagnosis.
6. Both members of the couple are motivated to change.
7. The physician has the comfort, skills, and allocated time to work with the couple.

Guidelines for Primary Care Couple Counseling

1. Involve both partners in counseling.
2. Maintain attention to confidentiality, potential triangles, and alliances.
3. Primary care couple counseling should generally be short term.
4. Primary care counseling is sometimes accomplished in a piecemeal fashion over extended periods of time.
5. Negotiating solutions to problems should be the focus of counseling.
6. Couples who are not making progress in primary care counseling should be referred.

15
Anticipating Loss: Healthcare for Older Patients and Their Family Caregivers

In Collaboration with Bernard Shore*

> First I am a child to my parent.
> Then I am parent to my child.
> Then I am a parent to my parent.
> Finally, I am a child to my child (1).

Caring for older family members is a normal, but often a stressful, part of the family life cycle. The so-called Geriatric Imperative (i.e., the increasing numbers of elders in all societies) will affect most physicians. By 2030, almost 20% of the U.S. population (70 million persons) will be more than 65 year old. By 2050, one quarter of those elders will be 85 years or more, about 5% of the U.S. population. Those more than 100 years old are now the fasting growing age group in the country and now number more than 50,000 (2, 3)!

Working with people with long and interesting life histories offers the primary care clinician many rewards (4). It also often includes a special poignancy in the course of helping patients and their families resolve important issues before death. As adults live longer and increase in numbers, their reliance upon family members and caregivers grows. The need for a family-oriented approach, therefore, increases with the increasing needs and interdependence of the patient and family as it ages.

Extending the length of an individual's life extends the joys, the pains, and the responsibilities of family life. Three or four generations surviving in one family has become commonplace. Marriages last longer—more than half of the nation's community-dwelling population older than 65 is married. For those older than 75, the large majority of men are married, whereas only 29% of women this age are married, primarily because their spouses have died earlier. Most elderly patients live with or rely on family members. Only 5% of all elders (more than 65 years old) are in a nursing home or other

---

* Bernard Shore, MD, Geriatrician and Medical Director, Jewish Home of Rochester, and Clinical Associate Professor of Medicine, Family Medicine and Psychiatry, University of Rochester School of Medicine and Dentistry, Rochester, NY, USA.

institution, although that increases to 18% for those more than 85 years old (2). The majority live near at least one of their children and visit them often (5). The popular notion of American families abandoning their elderly parents has been shown to be a myth (6, 7). After the relative independence of the empty nest period, family connections and interdependence increase with aging. If physical deterioration occurs along with social and financial changes, there is pressure on elders to rely more on their families. Many come to depend heavily on their offspring and other family members for financial support, transportation, and assistance with activities of daily living. Many, especially women, may face poverty for the first time (2), although social security policy has eased this somewhat since the 1980s (8).

As the physical effects of aging accumulate, the reality of death hangs as a backdrop for elders and their caregivers, making the emotional process between older patients and their families intense and sometimes difficult. The "young old" (ages 65–80) are caring more and more for their "old" (those more than 80) parents. Along with their own advancing age, these caregivers often have significant medical disabilities.

Decision making regarding the medical care or placement of frail elders is often a highly emotional process that highlights family dynamics, unresolved conflicts, loyalties, obligations, and responsibilities. For these reasons the primary care of older patients needs to be consciously family oriented. We will focus on a range of issues relevant to medical care of older persons and their families in this chapter, beginning with a discussion of the clinician's role, then specific adjustments in interview technique, caring for family caregivers, and finally a discussion of issues around nursing home placement.

The Role of the Clinician

The clinician has an influential role for most patients and their families at this phase of the life cycle. He or she is seen as an important supporter, advisor, and healer. For the isolated, a visit to their clinician can provide social contact; for the frail, the clinician can seem to be a lifeline to living; for those confused by the healthcare system, the clinician can act as an advocate and a guide. In addition, many family-oriented clinicians provide care for the patient's extended family, including family caregivers. Clinicians also have an obligation to assess the health and functioning of family caregivers, even when they are not the clinician's patients. Their physical and psychological health can have a major impact on the health, well-being, and living situation of the elder (9). Table 15.1 lists several of the roles that clinicians may assume when caring for patients and families at this stage of the life cycle.

The biopsychosocial model provides a template for integrating the complex issues involved in delivering comprehensive care for older patients. Providers must have a sound practical base in primary care geri-

TABLE 15.1. Roles of clinicians caring for older patients and their families

Guiding patients and families through the intricacies of the healthcare delivery system, and educating them about the appropriateness of various technological procedures.

Coordinating the patient's care with multidisciplinary teams, professional consultants, community agencies, family, and support networks.

Advocating for the patient and family members, especially in preserving autonomy and choice regarding medical care, sometimes to other healthcare workers, sometimes to other family members.

Consulting with the patient and family in their decision-making processes, whether about diagnostic testing or treatment, resuscitation status, or changes in living arrangements.

Collaborating with family caregivers, gathering information, educating them about the care of their loved one, learning from them, and assessing caregivers' capacities.

Supporting the patient and family caregivers, especially in situations where the caregiving is labor-intensive and demanding.

atrics with the aim of distinguishing disease from normal aging. An essential element of good elder care is to remain aware of the person's abilities as well as their disabilities, supporting growth, function, and opportunities despite illness that may occur. Elders show increasing interest in "aging well," and many good references are currently available to share (10–12). Clinicians must relate problems to the level of the older person's functioning, then weigh the benefits of any diagnostic or treatment procedures against the effect these procedures would have on the person. Clinicians should be able to link the older person with other needed healthcare and social services effectively, while coordinating the work of these various professionals to the patient's benefit (13).

To work constructively with elderly patients, clinicians should be aware of their own attitudes and biases toward the aged, the chronically ill, and the disabled. These attitudes are influenced by society's myths about aging, the clinician's experience with his or her own aging family members and patients, and the clinician's personal reaction to becoming older. Prejudices toward the elderly (i.e., ageism) can be subtle, but there is ample evidence that negative stereotypes appear early in life, affect clinicians of many disciplines and experience levels, and powerfully influence the medical care provided (14–17). When reinforced, such stereotypes have even been shown to influence small aspects of an elder's physical function (e.g., the quality of his or her gait) (18). Such attitudes may include discounting the importance of elders' problems or concerns, equating aging with senility, assuming that older patients have (or should have) no sexual life, or thinking that the aged cannot or should not care for themselves. Because older adults have longer and more varied life experiences than most clinicians, they are likely to have different beliefs and attitudes toward health- and medical care. For example, some older persons will be more concerned about maintaining their level of functioning and quality of life, than in prolonging their life.

Interviewing Older Patients and Their Family Members

Interviewing older patients can be challenging. They often have complex medical problems and a number of functional barriers to communication. Family members often accompany older patients to office visits and can be a helpful resource during the visit. In the Direct Observation of Primary Care study, Medalie et al. found that 30% of elderly patients were accompanied by a family member (18). In these visits, the clinician must address and balance the needs of the patient and the family member.

Given this, the clinician should:

1. Be prepared to spend more time with older patients and to pace the interview more slowly.

Although not universally true for all patients, elders' communication style, character, and pace may differ from the more focused, "efficient" model of medical data-gathering. The clinician should be prepared for this. Sensory deficits may necessitate that more time be taken with them. A clinician should evaluate and explicitly ask about communication problems (e.g., hearing, speech, vision, memory, and other aspects of mental status). The issues can be raised in a normative way (e.g., "Many older patients tell me they have some difficulty with hearing, vision, or recalling things. Have you noticed that?"). Direct communication about these issues has a modeling effect and allows patients and family members to explore present or future dysfunction. Any deficits and other physical limitations may put the patient at higher risk for physical and mental health problems and require special accommodations (see Refs. 20 and 21 for specific suggestions). Some patients may require or benefit from a home visit (see Chap. 23 for a discussion of home visits). Working with older patients requires careful attention to effective communication.

2. Always address the patient first.

It can be tempting to find the person in the family who is easiest to communicate with and speak primarily to that person, inadvertently excluding the patient. Communicating with one person may be efficient in the short term, but it can result in hard feelings and even noncompliance from the patient in the long term. Some older people already feel their family is ganging up on them to take away their autonomy, yet it can be difficult to balance the issues of safety and autonomy, as in the following case. It may be helpful to interview the patient alone, then invite the family member in to find out how both patient and caregiver are doing. It is important for the clinician to be supportive to both the patient and the caregivers and to provide each the opportunity to express their opinions.

> Mrs. Feister (daughter): Doctor, you have to help us. My mother, as you
> know, is not capable of driving safely. We have not allowed her to

renew her driver's license and we have sold her car. But she has twice called car dealerships and had them send out new models to her house so she would have a car. We've talked to her about our worries until we're blue in the face.

Dr. M.: I can see you're concerned and frustrated. Mrs. Toms, can you tell me what your concerns are?

Mrs. Toms: I just need to be able to get around, Doctor . . . I'm not in my grave yet, in spite of what my children think. How do they expect me to go to the store, or visit my friends? Am I supposed to just wait until it's convenient for them to cart me around? I know I can't see so well, but my children are busy people with families of their own to take care of. Besides, I just drive during the day.

Dr. M.: Mobility seems very important to your mother, Mrs. Feister. Do you have any ideas?

Mrs. Feister: Well, my brother and I would gladly pay for her to take a cab when she wants to go, if she'd stop calling the car dealerships and trying to buy cars.

Dr. M.: That seems like a solution that really might work. It would allow you to leave home at your discretion, Mrs. Toms. You wouldn't have to rely on your children or friends to drive you. Would this be an acceptable compromise to you?

Mrs. Toms: I don't know. Taxis are awfully expensive, and they never arrive on time.

Mrs. Feister: Mom, we'll pay for the taxis. Why don't you give it a try?

Dr. T.: You know Mrs. Toms, you're right: taxis are expensive. But so is a new car. With taxes, gas, insurance, and upkeep taxis may not be as expensive as they seem at first. Perhaps it's something you could try for a set period of time, then review it together in 3 months.

Mrs. Toms: Okay. I'll try it for a while (see Ref. 21 for a review of driving issue in elders).

3. Involve caregivers and family members early in the patient's care.

In the end, this is a time-saver. Family members can provide important information the patient may not be able to provide.

Dr. T. enters the office to greet a smiling elderly woman, a new patient, still in her coat.

Dr. T.: Hello, how are you?

Mrs. Parrish: (smiles and nods briefly)

Dr. T.: What brings you to the office today?

Mrs. Parrish: (pauses for a moment, then notices the doctor is waiting) Oh, I'm not feeling too badly. It's just these legs. I live with my daughter and she's been on me to see somebody about these legs. They don't hurt at all, mind you, they just swell up a bit at night. I don't think it's very serious.

Dr. T.: Hmm, and how long have you. . . (The door opens and a younger woman peers in, sees her mother and says:)

Mrs. Parrish's adult daughter: Oh, Ma. Sorry to interrupt. I just wanted to bring you your pad and marker. Excuse me, Doctor, it's just that she's deaf and her vision has been blurred a bit lately so we use this big magic marker to write our notes to her. I thought this might help you both.

Dr. T.: Thank you. That will be very helpful. Mrs. Parrish, would you like your daughter to join us for your visit?

Early involvement of family or other knowledgeable people allows the clinician to know about any problems or deficits that are relevant to medical care, deficits about which the patient may be sensitive and trying to compensate. This kind of problem can be particularly important with a demented patient.

When a family member accompanies an elderly patient to a visit, it is important to join with the family member and to find out their relationship with the patient and what role they may have in caring for the patient (see Chap. 6). The clinician should obtain the family member's perspective on how the patient is doing and what concerns the family member may have. This must be done carefully to avoid slipping into talking *about* the elder rather than *to* her or him. It is important to hear from both the older patient and family member and to avoid taking sides in any disagreements. When an older patient comes to a visit alone, it is helpful to inquire how they came to the office (a functional assessment) and whether anyone came with them. The patient's spouse or other family member frequently may be in the waiting room. If asked, the patient may appreciate having the family member participate in the visit.

Over time, many older couples become increasingly dependent upon each other, both physically and emotionally. They may have disabilities that can compensate for each other. A woman with arthritis and congestive heart failure may do the driving and bill paying, whereas the husband with mild dementia does the physical work around the house with his wife's guidance. For many of these couples, it is helpful to see them together for joint visits that address both of their health needs.

It is also important to see the patient periodically by him or herself. During these visits without accompanying family members, the clinician can inquire about the patient's relationship with family caregivers and whether the patient is comfortable having a family member at the other visits. It is also a time when such sensitive issues as sexual concerns or dysfunctions can be discussed. The risk of elder abuse can be assessed (see Chap. 22).

4. Recognize the emotional concerns underlying any explicit requests.

Many patients and caregivers are fearful about the possibility of the patient's functional deterioration, or death, but may not make these concerns explicit to the clinician. Making explicit the emotional concerns underlying the stated requests can allow these concerns to be aired, addressed, and sometimes resolved. For example, in the preceding example

Mrs. Parrish did not draw the physician's attention to her visual and hearing deficits, and she minimized the meaning of her newest symptoms, swelling in her legs. Mrs. Toms, in the earlier example, obviously did not want to accept the lack of autonomy that went with not driving a car (especially with her children wanting to control this part of her life). It should be noted, however, that the elderly patient sometimes accepts the reality of disability better than his or her spouse or children. For example, some elderly patients recognize their need to move into assisted living arrangements before their children have recognized or acknowledged their declining function.

5. Do not make significant changes in a treatment plan based solely on the family's report without evaluating the elderly patient directly.

Even though family members provide invaluable information about an elderly person, they should not be relied upon exclusively. Family concerns can reflect changes in the patient's condition, an increase in other family distress, or intensified fears and anxieties of family members projected onto the elder. When receiving a call regarding a change, assess the level of distress in the caregiver as well as any changes in the patient. In this way, the actual problem can be addressed by the treatment plan, whether it is a change in the patient's medication, placement for the patient, or respite care to prevent caregiver burnout.

> Dr. V. received a call saying his patient, Mrs. Brown, an 88-year-old Russian-American woman, was deteriorating at home and needed to be hospitalized. Mrs. Brown's daughter spoke urgently, saying she had flown in from out of town, had not seen her mother in 5 months, and was worried that her mother was "at death's door." Dr. V. asked to speak to Mrs. Brown, and the patient repeated the complaints she had had since her stroke 3 months ago. Dr. V. told Mrs. Brown and her daughter that he would make a home visit to try and evaluate Mrs. Brown's condition. When he arrived, he found Mrs. Brown to be in stable condition, much as she had been in recent months. He discussed her condition with the patient and her daughter and reassured both that the current treatment plan was appropriate. The daughter spoke about how much the stroke had affected her mother, how difficult it was to see her deteriorate, and her own determination to visit her mother more frequently. Dr. V. invited Mrs. Brown's daughter to call him with any concerns she might have about her mother.

Caring for Family Caregivers

The roles, stresses, and critical importance of family caregivers warrant specific comment. An increasing literature describes the personal, social, economic and healthcare concerns of this previously invisible part of the healthcare system. A poignant anecdote illustrates many of these issues.

In his book, *Patients and Doctors: Life-Changing Stories from Primary Care* (22), Jack Medalie, M.D., describes an event that shaped his career and subsequently the field of family medicine. As a young physician practicing on a kibbutz in Israel, Medalie was caring for an elderly patient recovering at home from a myocardial infarction. Although there were no complications, the man's convalescence was taking much longer than expected. Dr. Medalie made many visits to his patient's home and observed the wife's attentive care. In the middle of one night, he received an emergency request to go to the patient's home. He was surprised to find that his patient had improved significantly, but his wife had committed suicide by jumping off a nearby cliff. Medalie described the wife in this story as "the hidden patient":

> After much thought, the "hidden patient" concept crystallized: in any family in which there is an individual with an acute and life-threatening or chronic and long-term illness or diseases, the caregiver (usually the spouse, the oldest daughter, or sometimes the whole family unit) is under considerable stress. Unless this caregiver receives sufficient support from the family and/or others, coping mechanisms will fail and the caregiver will develop overt or covert signs of illness. (Ref. 22; p. 174)

Medalie went on to devote his career to studying the role of the family in healthcare and to promoting the importance of caring for family caregivers, the "hidden patients."

The stress of caring for elderly family members may be manifest through illness in the caregivers. Research has demonstrated that caregiving exerts a heavy toll on family members. Caregivers have much higher morbidity and mortality than age-matched noncaregivers. One study (24) found that caregivers older than 65 who were experiencing emotional strain were 63% more likely to die than were age-matched noncaregivers over a 4-year-period. Caregivers suffer higher rates of multiple physical illnesses, depression, and anxiety. They often restrict their social activities and reduce their time at work. The financial impact of caregiving on families can be enormous, both in terms of decreased wages of caregivers and the cost of providing equipment and services in the home for the patient.

Nevertheless, for most family members, there are many benefits of caregiving. Caregivers view their work as fulfilling and a way to give back to their parents or spouse. In many studies, there is only a weak association between the subjective and objective measures of caregiver burden. The stress of family caregiving depends as much upon the meaning and satisfaction derived by the family member as the actual work involved. A number of authors have addressed the spiritual and existential dimensions of aging and caregiving, providing a context for weathering challenging times (25, 26).

A number of interventions for the caregivers of patients with chronic illnesses have been developed and tested. An effective, family psychoeducational intervention has been developed and tested by Mittelman. She tested a comprehensive intervention for family caregivers of Alzheimer's disease (AD) patients in a randomized controlled trial (26). These families attended individual and group instructional and problem-solving sessions where they learned how to manage many of the troublesome behaviors of patients with AD. They also attended an ongoing family support group and could access a crisis intervention service to help them with urgent problems. In Mittelman's study, the caregivers who received the intervention were less depressed and physically healthier than were those that did not, and AD patients were able to remain at home for almost a year longer than they were in the control group. The savings in nursing home costs were several times the cost of the interventions. This study can serve as a model for other family intervention programs. Similar types of family support should be a part of the treatment of all patients and families with AD and other dementias. Many books, guides, support groups, and Web sites are available for elders and caregivers (see Refs. 28–29 and the appendix) and can provide valuable information and support for these families, especially when more comprehensive programs are not available.

Care of the elderly, especially as their physical or mental health begins to deteriorate, can be a challenge to the healthiest and most resourceful of families. Many more housebound and bedridden elderly live at home as live in an institution. These patients require responsible, attentive care from family members and from community supports. The balance between the patient's and family caregivers' needs can be difficult to achieve successfully. The following example is, unfortunately, not so rare.

> Mrs. Houser told Dr. P. she did not know what to do. Her mother had managed her father's blindness and other health needs with seeming ease, by solely devoting herself to him. Since her mother's death and her father's moving in to their home, however, Mrs. Houser's life had been a shambles. Her volunteer work at the museum had been the first to go, then she had had to get neighbors to take the children to their piano lessons. There was no time for friends and less and less socializing for the Housers as a couple. Her father, on the other hand, seemed pleased with the arrangement. He did not seem to notice his son-in-law's irritation when he visited with him while the younger man worked at his hobby of woodworking. Today, Mrs. Houser reported, her husband had said: "That's it. This can't go on. Either he goes or I do." Dr. P. suggested Mr. and Mrs. Houser and her father come in together to discuss the current living arrangement, and each person's satisfactions and dissatisfactions with it. At the meeting, Mrs. Houser's father agreed to become involved in a nearby senior citizen's center.

Family caregivers are essential members of the health care team. They provide clinical observation, direct care, case management, and a range of other services. In chronic illnesses (e.g., AD) these caregivers may devote years of their own lives to caring for a loved one. Our current healthcare system unfortunately offers more of a patchwork of services than it does a comprehensive, integrated system providing care and support for aging families. Managed care has shifted many of the burdens of caregiving from professionals in the hospital and other institutions to family members at home. As hospital stays have shortened, elderly patients are being discharged home "sicker and quicker," with more healthcare needs than in the past. Hospitals have reduced the number of social workers and discharge planners.

In the United States home services are not well-coordinated or fully covered by Medicare, and clinicians are not adequately reimbursed for home visits or for what can be the very time-consuming task of coordinating services. Insufficient respite care is available for those families who need a break from caregiving. The lack of respite care can encourage an all-or-nothing mentality for families taking care of their sick loved ones so that the family may push themselves to exhaustion and then demand urgent placement for the patient. The patient's status may not have changed, but the caregiver clearly says, "I can't take it anymore." This is one of the circumstances in which elder abuse may be more likely. It is important that clinicians provide emotional support and connect the family with any available home services and community support groups to help prevent caregiver burnout. Table 15.2 lists some national organizations that provide services and advocacy for family caregiving.

TABLE 15.2. Useful Web sites of national organizations for elders or family caregivers

Alzheimer's Association, www.alz.org
Comprehensive services for Alzheimer's patients, including a nationwide registration and identification program that assists individuals who wander and have gotten lost.

American Self-Help Clearinghouse, www.selfhelpgroup.org
Serves as a clearinghouse for various self-help groups and provides information on how to start a support group.

Eldercare Online, www.ec-online.net
A comprehensive source of information, books support, and links.

Family Caregiver Alliance, www.caregiver.org
Information center on long-term care. FCA serves as a public voice for caregivers through education, services, research, and advocacy.

National Alliance for Caregiving, www.caregiving.org
Conducts research, develops national projects, and increases public awareness of family caregiving issues.

National Family Caregivers Association, www.nfcacares.org
Grassroots organization that educates, supports, empowers, and advocates for family caregives.

Well Spouse Foundation, www.wellspouse.org
Membership organization that gives support to spouses and partners of the chronically ill and disabled.

Family-oriented clinicians need to monitor patients and their caregivers to assess and reduce the burden of caregiving. Caregivers themselves need to be evaluated for symptoms of depression, fatigue, somatization, and illness, especially those with heavy responsibilities for patients that require long-term care. The possibility of elder abuse by caregivers or other family members should also be considered; this may be a result of burnout, alcoholism, prior experienced abuse, or longstanding conflictual relations (see Ref. 31 and Chap. 22). The clinician can help the patient and family assess the adequacy and the burden of caregiving along several important dimensions outlined in the Protocol at the end of the chapter.

Many of the challenges of family caregiving should be explored during routine visits before an acute health event creates a crisis. For example, knowing a family's financial status and their ability to afford medications may help in planning for care after a hospital stay. Knowing who helps an older patient with shopping or who brings the patient to the doctor may help in identifying who might be available if a patient breaks a hip.

Understanding a family's dynamics may also help when a family is struggling to accept their mother's dementia.

> Mrs. Towner, a 66-year-old African-American woman, came for her first visit with Dr. U. accompanied by her youngest daughter, Miss Green. The daughter related the following story: Mrs. Towner, twice a widow, had worked for 25 years as a legal secretary in a prestigious law firm. She had always been bright, witty, practical, and much respected. Over the last 3 years her behavior had become more erratic; her work performance began to fall off noticeably, so that no important matters were entrusted to her anymore at her firm. In the previous week, a senior partner had called Miss Green and insisted that her mother see a doctor or face outright dismissal.
>
> A full evaluation strongly suggested Alzheimer's disease. Dr. U. convened a family meeting including Mrs. Towner and several of her children. The children were skeptical and asked many pointed questions: "How can you be sure? Is there a test for Alzheimer's? Are you a neurologist?" Dr U. answered these, then asked: "How do you think we should proceed?" The children offered many alternative options, with the eldest strongly urging a thorough evaluation at Johns Hopkins. Dr. U. then asked Mrs. Towner what she thought about all this: "What do you see as the problem? What do you think would be best?" Mrs. Towner, who had remained silent through most of the meeting, smiled blandly for a moment, then said: "Well, my memory's just no good anymore. I think they should just take me out and shoot me." After a wave of reassurance and genuine avowals of her importance to them, the eldest exchanged pointed glances with her youngest sister and said: "Well, we'll never put her in a nursing home no matter what you say she has."

In this case, the patient's feeling of being abandoned, the family's reluctance to accept her diagnosis, and the daughters' potential disagreement over placement indicate that the family may have difficulty responding to their mother's cognitive decline. Intensive support and intervention may be required with this family before a successful plan is achieved.

Family caregiving is rarely shared equally among family members. One family member, most often the patient's wife or a daughter, assumes the role of the primary caregiver and provides the majority of care. This may create resentment and conflict between the caregiver and other family members, often replicating earlier family dynamics. An uninvolved son or daughter may appear suddenly on the scene to "take charge" and insist on more aggressive medical evaluation or treatment (31). In these cases, it is particularly important for the clinician to meet with as many family members as possible to explore what roles each member has taken, and to see if a consensus about medical decisions can be reached.

Working with Elderly Patients and Their Families About Nursing Home Placement

Despite widespread guilt and ambivalence about nursing home placement in our culture, nursing homes can be a solution for some serious health problems. Placement can result in positive consequences for both the patient and the patient's family (32). Although only a small proportion of all elderly live in institutions at any given time, the numbers become substantial with increasing age. This option can be an important one for patients with serious impairments and for families who are not able to provide care for their loved one. Even so, the decision to make such a placement is often fraught with emotions (e.g., guilt, anger, rejection, or depression) for both the patient and for responsible family members. Many nursing home residents are 85 years or older, so these decisions are often made by the "old old" and their aging children.

The decision for placement of an elderly person in an institution should be made by reviewing the fit between the patient's health needs and personal desires, and the family's resources, abilities, and desires. Patients and families should make these decisions, balancing the needs of the patient and the family, in consultation with their primary care clinician. Multiple options are available: The elder may live alone and receive home services ranging from public health nurse visits to a live-in home health aide; the elder may receive services while living with a family member; or the elder may need to move to an alternate setting. The level of care and support can range from little in an adult-care facility to very high in skilled nursing facilities/nursing homes. Different levels of care match different family and patient needs. When assessing the level of care needed, the question is: How can the patient and family needs be met in the most effective way by the available institutional supports?

One hopeful development is the growing number of alternatives for elder housing. Skilled nursing facilities (SNFs) are no longer the only choice for families. "NORCs" (naturally occurring residential communities) are apartment complexes whose mainly older populations have encouraged them to organize helpful supports and social programs for their residents. Such innovative assisted living programs as PACE (Program for All-inclusive Care for the Elderly, based on the successful On-Lok experiment in San Francisco's Chinatown) are designed to keep persons needing SNF-level care in the community. Medical or social day care services can help alleviate the burden of working relatives. Assisted living sites can provide some support and supervision for elders retaining adequate activities of daily living (ADL) function, whereas Continuing Care Retirements Communities (CCRCs) offer a continuum of care with linked apartments, assisted and nursing home levels, usually requiring an initial, often substantial, entry fee. For those who can afford it, this option allows elders to address future declines in function in a more planned way.

Aside from PACE, most of these alternatives unfortunately involve significant out-of-pocket expense. Payment issues, reimbursement for care, and labor shortages for elder care are unresolved and growing problems. Long-term care insurance, which is one possible solution, still provides incomplete coverage, can vary greatly, and is not yet widely utilized. Another critical challenge without adequate resolution is the generally poor range of options for convenient and affordable transportation when driving is no longer safe (33).

Assessing the Need for Placement

Given the problems regarding determination of placement, the clinician should consider the following questions before making any recommendations (34):

Who thinks the elder needs to move to alternative living arrangements and why?
Why is the issue being raised now?
What are the patient's and family's expectations for the alternative housing?
What needs would be met that cannot be met by the current living arrangements?
What pressures are the patient and family experiencing?

It is ideal for primary care clinicians to discuss issues about long-term care with their older patients before the need arises. One such question might be: "What are your plans for the future should you become sick and need help, or not be able to care for yourself?" These early discussions can be diagnostic: Some patients and families will discuss the issue and implement their decision should the need arise, others may be unwilling to consider the possibility or may make an entirely different decision when faced with the reality of ill health. When an older person starts to have functional difficulties, it is certainly important to discuss the possibility of increased care needs in the future. It may be helpful to have office copies of the planning guides and workbooks mentioned earlier (25–27), or some others, available for review by your patients.

Patients and families vary in their decisions regarding the level of care they desire. Some families jump to nursing home placement early in an illness; others go to great lengths to keep their loved one in a family home. Many families use a range of caregiving services. Let us return to the example of Mrs. Towner (see Fig. 15.1):

> Over the year after her diagnosis, Mrs. Towner's Alzheimer's disease became progressively worse. She resigned from her job after numerous problems and complaints by her employers at the law firm. Her family became increasingly concerned that she was unsafe living alone, that she might leave the gas on, or that she might have some other accident. After several months of discussion, the oldest daughter, Mrs. Centre, invited her mother to move into her family home with her husband and two children.
>
> Over the next 6 months, Dr. U. saw Mrs. Centre twice for what seemed to be stress-related headaches. After the second visit, he asked

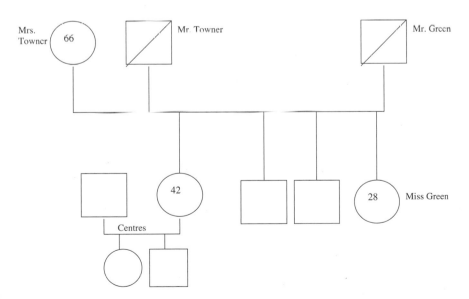

Figure 15.1. Genogram of the Towner family.

how she was handling her mother's illness. Mrs. Centre became teary and said she either had to devote herself to her mother or to her husband and children. She currently felt she was no good to either. She said her sister had been pushing the idea of a nursing home "for everyone's good." Mrs. Centre said she had told herself she would never do such a thing to her mother. Dr. U. suggested Mrs. Centre and her husband and children come in with Mrs. Towner for a family conference to discuss how Mrs. Towner was doing.

At this conference, Dr. U. saw that Mrs. Towner's function had further declined, that Mr. Centre was quite perturbed by her frequent lapses of memory, and that Mrs. Centre felt stuck in the middle. With a knowledgeable social worker present, he discussed the possibility of a day-treatment program, which would give Mrs. Towner the daily activities she had enjoyed when she was a busy person living on her own. The social worker also informed the family of a support group composed of other families going through similar experiences with their loved ones with Alzheimer's. Everyone seemed pleased with the arrangement for day treatment. Mrs. Towner looked forward to having "something to do," and the strain eased on Mrs. Centre's face.

Mrs. Towner did well in the day program for about 1 year, but her continuing deterioration and other family concerns led her family to consider placement. Mrs. Centre called Dr. U. about her mother becoming more irritable and combative, and wandering in the middle of the night. She said she was afraid her mother and her husband were going to come to blows. After examining and talking with Mrs. Towner, Dr. U. met with the family to discuss the alternatives, including nursing home placement. Mr. Centre and Miss Green favored placement. Mrs. Centre seemed to favor placement as well, and was worried about how all this was affecting her children. Mrs. Towner's sons suggested that they go out and visit several nursing homes to see the possibilities first hand.

Within 3 months, Mrs. Towner was placed in a local nursing home. Dr. U. helped her and the family adjust to the changes the placement brought. After an initial depressive period, Mrs. Towner adjusted well to the social life at the nursing home and did well there until the last 6 months of her life, when she became bedridden, unresponsive, and died.

As with the Towner family, a family conference is a useful format for discussing the advantages and disadvantages of placement with many patients and their families (see Chap. 7 for the specifics of conducting a family conference). Once the patient, family, and clinician agree that placement is desirable, the clinician can help guide the family to local resources they can use to select the nursing home or other setting that best meets their needs (see Table 15.2 for resource list). Such explorations undertaken by the family, although often difficult, can help unite them as they all work together to find what is best for their relative.

Facilitating an assessment of the patient's financial resources is an important step in the process. Financial considerations have become such a complex, often overwhelming burden that referral to a social worker, private case manager, and/or financial counselor skilled in this area is often a tremendous relief for the family. It is helpful to become familiar with a few case managers, social workers, attorneys, and agencies who specialize in elder-care issues.

Through family conferences and primary care counseling, Dr. U. was able to help the Towner family make decisions along the way about increasing Mrs. Towner's care. Some families with more serious difficulties warrant a meeting with a family therapist either for consultation or referral (see Chap. 25 on referral to a family therapist). As with other situations, the clinician needs to be alert to signs of serious family stress or dysfunction around questions of caregiving or placement for the elder. Signs of stress may include serious family conflicts, threatened elder abuse, family overinvolvement, threats of abandonment directed at the elder, or overutilizing medical services by any member of the family.

Once an older patient has been accepted and placed in a nursing home, the primary care clinician needs to define what his or her role will be to the patient and the family postplacement. Most large nursing homes, especially in urban areas, have their own medical staff, and there may be limited opportunities for the primary care clinician to retain clinical responsibility for the patient. The present-day demands of primary care practice also make this more challenging; however, it is important to recognize the family's ongoing need for support, and to facilitate communication between the family and nursing home staff. Successful adjustment to either nursing home or home care during the period of chronic illness and physical deterioration may help all parties in facing the next stage—that of the future death of the patient and grieving for the family.

Conclusion

Caring for elderly patients and their families offers unique opportunities for family-oriented clinicians. The increasing interdependency of family members as they age makes a family orientation especially important. Elders need clinical and emotional support to balance autonomy, meaning, changing relationships, and loss as they age. Family caregivers often experience considerable physical and emotional burdens that need to be recognized and addressed by their clinicians. Most families will confront difficult decisions at this stage of the life cycle, including who the family caregivers will be, what kind and level of care does their family member need, whether the elder needs to be placed in an institution, and who will make these decisions, including the final ones at the end of life. This last issue will be addressed in the next chapter.

References

1. Brummel-Smith K: Geriatrics in family medicine. In: Saultz JW (Ed): *Textbook of Family Medicine*. New York: McGrow-Hill, 2000.
2. Administration on Aging: *A Profile of Older American*: 2001 (http://www.aoa.dhhs.gov/aoa/stats/profile/2001/1.html).
3. Jackson S: The epidemiology of aging. In: Hazzard WR (Ed): *Principles of Geriatric Medicine and Gerontology, Fourth ed*. New York: McGraw-Hill, 1999: p. 203.
4. Lustbader W: *What's Worth Knowing*. New York: Tarcher/Putnam, 2001.
4. Zopf PE: *American's Older Population*. Houston: Cap and Gown Press, 1986.
5. Smallegan M: There was nothing else to do: needs for care before nursing home admission. *Gerontologist* 1985;**25**(4):364–369.
6. Brody E: Parent care as a normative family stress. *Gerontologist* 1985;**26**:19–29.
7. Maddox G, Glass TA: The sociology of aging. In: Hazzard WR (Ed): *Principles of Geriatric Medicine and Gerontology, Fourth ed*. New York: McGraw-Hill, 1999.
8. Karlawish JH, Cassarett D, Klocinski J, & Clark CM: The relationship between caregivers' global ratings of Alzheimer's disease patients' quality of life, disease severity, and the caregiving experience. *J Am Geriatr Soc* 2001;**49**:1066–1070.
9. Wei J, Levkoff S: *Aging Well: The Complete Guide to Physical and Emotional Health*. New York: Wiley, 2001.
10. Rowe J, Kahn R: *Successful Aging*. New York: Pantheon Books, 1998.
11. Coleman D, Gurin J (Eds): *Mind Body Medicine, How to Use Your Mind for Better Health*. Yonkers, NY: Consumers Union, 1993.
12. Solomon R, Peterson M: Successful aging: how to help your patients cope with change. *Geriatrics* 1994;**49**(4):41–47.
13. Uncapher H, Arean PA: Physicians are less willing to treat suicidal ideation in older patients. *J Am Geriatr Soc* 2000;**48**:188–192.
14. Stillman et al: Are critically ill older patients treated differently than similarly ill younger patients? *Western J Med* 1998;**169**(3):162–165.
15. Bouman WP, Arcelus J: Are psychiatrists guilty of "ageism" when it comes to taking a sexual history? *Int J Geriatr Psychiatr* 2001;**16**(1):27–31.
16. Ivey DC, Wieling E, & Harris SM: Save the young—the elderly have lived their lives: ageism in marriage and family therapy. *Fam Proc* 2000;**39**(2):163–175.
17. Hausdorff JM, Levy BR, & Wei JY: The power of ageism on physical function of older persons: reversibility of age-related gait changes. *J Am Geriatr Soc* 1999; **47**(11):1346–1349.
18. Medalie JH, Zyzanski SJ, Langa D, & Stange KC: The family in family practice: is it a reality? *J Fam Pract* 1998;**46**(5):390–396.
19. Adelman RD, Greene MG, & Ory MG: Communications between older patients and their physicians. *Clin Geriatr Med* 2000;**16**(1):1–24.
20. Giordano JA: Effective communication and counseling with older adults. *Int J Aging Hum Devel* 2000;**51**(4):315–324.
21. Messinger-Rapport BJ, Rader E: High risk on the highway. How to identify and treat the impaired older driver. *Geriatrics* 2000;**55**(10):32–42.
22. Medalie J, Borkan J, Reis S, Steinmetz D, et al.: *Patients and Doctors: Life Changing Stories from Primary Care*. Madison, WI: University of Wisconsin Press, 1999.

23. Schultz R, Beach SR, Lind B, et al.: Involvement in caregiving and adjustment to death of a spouse: finding from the caregiver health effects study. *JAMA* 2001;**285**(24):3123–3129.

24. McLeod BW: *Caregiving: The Spiritual Journey of Love, Loss, and Renewal*. New York: Wiley, 2000.

25. Schacter-Shalomi Z, Miller R: *From Age-ing to Sage-ing: A Profound New Vision of Growing Older*. New York: Warner Books, 1995.

26. Mittelman MS, Ferris SH, Shulman E, Steinberg G, & Levin B: A family intervention to delay nursing home placement of patients with Alzheimer disease. A randomized controlled trial *JAMA* 1996;**276**:1725–1731.

27. Morris V: *How to Care for Aging Parents*. New York: Workman Publishing, 1996.

28. Loverde J: *The Complete Eldercare Planner: Where to Start, Which Questions to Ask, and How to Find Help, Second ed.* New York: Times Books, 2000.

29. Scileppi KP: *Caring for the Parents Who Cared for You, What to Do When and Aging Parent Needs You.* Secaucus, NJ: Carol Publishing, 1996.

30. Reay AM, Browne KD: Risk Factor Characteristics in Carers who Physically Abuse or Neglect their Elderly Dependents. *Aging Mental Health* 2001;**5**(1): 56–62.

31. Molloy DW, Clarnette RM, Braun EA, et al.: Decision making in the incompetent elderly: "the daughter from California syndrome." *J Am Geriatr Soc* 1991; **39**(4):396–399.

32. Smith KF, Bengtson VL: Positive consequences of institutionalization: solidarity between elderly parents and their middle-aged children. *Gerontologist* 1979; **19**:438–447.

33. Rosenbloom S: Transportation needs of the elderly population. *Clin Geriatr Med* 1994;**9**(2):297–322.

34. Herr JJ, Weakland JH: *Counseling Elders and their Families*. New York: Springer Publishing Co., 1979.

35. Houlihan JP: Families caring for frail and demented elderly: a review of selected findings. *Fam Syst Med* 1987;**5**:344–356.

Protocol: Predictors of Caregiver Burden

The following checklist is an adaptation of factors found to increase care-giver burden (35) and can be used to evaluate or monitor a patient and his or her caregivers. No one factor should be seen necessarily as determining an unmanageable situation, but taken together the factors may be able to assess or predict degree of burden.

The Patient

* Is demented and/or disruptive.
* Is highly dependent on the caregiver.

The Caregiver

* Feels guilty about anger and resentment toward the patient.
* Had a conflictual relationship with the patient before the illness.
* Does not understand much about the patient's problems or condition.
* Has his or her own illness and/or disability.
* Is depressed, isolated, or lonely.
* Has poor relationships with other family members.
* Has little personal time away from caregiving.

The Family

* Denies the patient's diagnosis.
* Leaves most of the caregiving to one person.
* Is in conflict.
* Has few financial resources.
* Has conflictual relationships with the medical providers.

Community Does Not Have

* Adult day care programs or respite care.
* Family psychoeducation and support groups.
* Psychological and family therapy services.

16
Looking Death in the Eye: Facilitating End-of-Life Care and the Grieving Process

The death of a patient presents the primary care clinician with one of the most challenging situations in the practice of medicine. Negotiating the process of dying can also be one of the most rewarding parts of practice because it brings about an emotional intensity for the patient, the family, and professional caregivers that can be moving and healing for all who participate. The knowledge of impending death can facilitate resolution of personal and interpersonal conflicts rooted in previous life cycle stages. Of course, that same emotional intensity also can prove traumatic or bring about long-lasting dysfunction for those families who experience unanticipated death or the death of a young person, or who are unable to resolve the challenges raised by the loss of one of their members.

In the West, there is increasing interest in confronting issues about death and dying. Our society is now beginning to provide institutional support for patients and families facing these changes, with such services as hospice care and bereavement groups for family and friends after the death. On the whole, however, we are a culture that denies the reality of death (1). In the healthcare community, death is an event to be prevented, not accepted (2), and health professionals may seek emotional distance from the dying patient and the patient's family. The death of a patient can be seen as a failure of the clinician's skills whether overtly or covertly. This aspect of traditional professional socialization makes it difficult to facilitate a healthy dying process for our patients or to encourage constructive grieving for their families, and for ourselves. In this chapter we will challenge our culture's tendency to deny death. We support training for health professionals on death and dying, and will provide a model for productive interaction among the healthcare system, the dying patient, and the family. The chapter begins by making practical suggestions about communicating a terminal diagnosis to a patient and family, then turns to treatment planning and making any decisions to limit treatment, end-of-life care, notifying a family of a death, examining clinician issues after a death, and counseling the family about grief issues.

"I Believe You May Die from This Illness"

Even though a terminal diagnosis is sometimes provided by a specialist, the primary care clinician is uniquely suited to communicate this information because of his or her long-standing relationship with the patient and understanding of the family's particular issues and needs. In Western culture, communicating the diagnosis of a terminal illness to a patient and family ideally involves clear, direct statements transmitted in a calm, empathic way (3); however, in some Asian, African, Latin American, and Eastern European cultures with more focus on family (communion) than individual autonomy (agency), many patients prefer that serious diagnoses be communicated to the family rather than to themselves. In these cultures, it is considered cruel and disrespectful rather than empowering to communicate a terminal diagnosis directly to a patient. In these situations, communication occurs with the family; and the family takes charge of the patient and the decision making (4). Recognizing these individual and cultural differences, it is important to clarify prior to delivering bad news, to whom the patient wishes the information to be transmitted, and in what forum. Guidelines for clear communication about a terminal illness include the following:

- When a serious illness is suspected, ask the patient at the time the test is ordered how he or she wishes the results to be communicated: with family, without family, or even to the family only.
- At the time of delivering bad news, first tell the participants that you need to have a serious discussion about the illness.
- First find out what the patient already knows. Begin the discussion from the point of the patient's understanding.
- Communicate directly to the patient about the diagnosis, the treatment, and the prognosis of the illness (e.g., "We don't believe your disease is curable").
- Use clear, simple language. Avoid overmedicalizing or intellectualizing the information.
- Be honest and straightforward about the information as you know it, acknowledging areas of medical uncertainty. Avoid giving an overly optimistic or overly pessimistic prognosis.
- Look the patient, or family member, in the eye and speak calmly. Repeat the basic message several times.
- Wait for the patient or family to absorb the information, providing details as requested. Patients and families often cannot absorb the details at the same time they first hear bad news.
- Once the information is transmitted, sit silently and make space for the patient and family to react as needed.
- Avoid arguments over the diagnosis, or other diversions from the main message.
- Ask the patient or family for any questions.

- Allow people their sadness or anger, rather than trying to reassure them or brighten their mood. In this situation, anger is understandable and sadness can signal healthy anticipatory grieving. These are processes that need encouragement rather than suppression.
- Allow patients some hope. Be humble about predicting how long a patient may survive.
- Say "I wish things were different" rather than "I'm sorry," which can be misunderstood as guilt feelings over a mistake or failure (5).
- Emphasize that you will continue to care for and support the patient throughout his or her illness.
- If the patient chose to receive the information alone, suggest that the process be repeated with the family present. Create a safe atmosphere during the family conference for people to express their feelings honestly and directly if they so desire.
- Recognize that family members are likely to accept the diagnosis at differing points in time. It is as if some members of the family deny the illness and advocate for life to go on, and others accept the diagnosis early and organize to care for the illness. Make space for each person's way of coping, and keep communication channels open for all members of the family and healthcare team.
- Make a follow-up appointment to answer the questions that will inevitably arise when the initial reaction wears off.

Many health professionals find themselves having a tendency to withdraw during the terminal phase, after biomedical intervention is no longer curative. Avoid any temptations to withdraw. Instead, plan for a good death by meeting regularly with the patient and family to discuss medical care, prognosis, and individuals' emotional reactions, even when the medical care is being managed by a specialist. Encourage children in the family to be involved in at least some of these meetings.

Dying patients force us to face our own mortality and that of those we love. Facing these personal issues can help us be calm and straightforward when communicating a terminal diagnosis to a patient, or accept a family member's anger on hearing about the death of a loved one (6). With very difficult or upsetting cases, discussion with a trusted colleague can be invaluable, both for the medical consultation and for the emotional support (7).

After hearing about a terminal diagnosis, the families of dying patients experience a period of high stress that can be manifested by anger, depression, interpersonal conflict, and psychosomatic problems. Holmes and Rahe found the death of a spouse to be the single most stressful life event an individual encounters. Death of another family member ranked fourth, after divorce and separation (8). Primary care clinicians can do much in the way of prevention by spending a relatively brief amount of time attending to family members' reactions and functioning during the terminal illness phase. A "health check" for the spouse or other significant family members of a dying patient is frequently very useful (9). This appointment allows the clinician to address this person's physical and emotional concerns and to raise questions about such sensitive areas as sexuality and finances. Some of these issues are best discussed with the couple together.

The medical care of terminally ill patients is often shared among a number of specialists. The primary care clinician is well-positioned to coordinate the care of the patient among the specialists and between the medical system and the family. Communicating regularly with the specialists involved can avoid the fragmentation of medical care that is so common with complex or terminal cases. Without someone coordinating services, families can receive differing or contradictory messages about a terminal illness.

> Dr. E. had taken care of the large, Italian-American Termillo family for more than 20 years. Mr. Termillo, the patriarch of the family, had always been in relatively good health, although neither Dr. E. nor his family had ever been successful in getting him to stop smoking. Mr. Termillo was recently found to have a lung mass on chest X-ray done when he presented with a cough. A chest surgeon biopsied the mass, which proved to be malignant. After this diagnosis, Mr. Termillo began to see an oncologist and the surgeon on a regular basis, rarely seeing Dr. E. Both specialists confirmed a diagnosis of lung cancer, but the family did not feel they could talk with these physicians about the prognosis. Although Dr. E. thought of Mr. Termillo often, he was actually relieved during this difficult period to be able to distance from this man who reminded him of a favorite uncle.
>
> When Dr. E. received the specialists' reports on Mr. Termillo, he found the surgeon and oncologist presented very different prognoses for this patient. Soon after reading these reports, Dr. E. received a call from, Marcia, one of Mr. Termillo's adult children, pleading with him to make sense out of what the doctors were telling her stepmother about the prognosis. Dr. E. suggested that Marcia convene a family conference at his office in the next week, allowing him time to communicate directly with the specialists involved in Mr. Termillo's care. When he did so, he found that the surgeon's view was that Mr. Termillo had several months to live, if that long, whereas the oncologist was not yet ready to label the patient terminal, saying, "There's always hope." Dr. E. told the specialists of the family's request for more specific information and his own suggestion for a family conference. He invited the specialists to attend. When both declined, he asked them if they had any special message they would like transmitted to the patient or family. Both reiterated the prognosis as they saw it. Dr. E. promised to present both points of view to the family.
>
> Mr. and Mrs. Termillo and three of Mr. Termillo's four adult children attended the family conference. Mrs. Termillo said she was relieved to be meeting with Dr. E., who she trusted and had known for a long time. Marcia, who had requested the meeting, appeared nervous and quickly got to her point: "We're having trouble with the specialists because they

won't tell us what's really going on with our father." Dr. E. asked Mr. Termillo for his understanding of his illness. In a quiet, passive voice, he said, "I don't know." Dr. E. then asked for others' understanding of Mr. Termillo's prognosis. Mrs. Termillo said she understood her husband was going to die, but she did not know how soon. The other adult children split on whether they believed there was any hope. One in particular turned to her father and said she was "not going to sit there and just let him die."

Dr. E. said, "I wish things were different," and spent the rest of the conference reviewing the reports from both specialists, presenting their differing points of view, as well as the available statistics for the particular stage of Mr. Termillo's cancer. As everyone was encouraged to air their feelings, it became more clear that much of the pent-up frustration and anger about Mr. Termillo's illness was being directed at the medical system. At this point, Mr. Termillo asked, "Dr. E., do you think I will die from this?" Dr. E said, "Given the reports from the specialists and the statistics from others with your disease, in all likelihood I believe you will. Whether that will be in 6 months or in several years, we do not know right now."

Dr. E. then talked about the difficulty of dealing with an uncertain prognosis and how important it was for the family to continue to support and communicate with each other during this time. Dr. E. offered to more actively coordinate Mr. Termillo's care, and rescheduled a follow-up appointment for Mr. and Mrs. Termillo for the next month. Mrs. Termillo agreed to be the primary person to dispense information coming from Dr. E.; however, it was clear that the adult children did not entirely trust their stepmother to communicate all the information to them. Dr. E. encouraged all the conference participants to communicate directly with him if they had questions that went unanswered. Dr. E. said another family conference might be useful sometime in the future, and suggested that anyone at this conference could call and request it. Mr. Termillo appeared visibly relieved and thanked Dr. E. for meeting with his family as he left the office (see Fig. 16.1.).

Ongoing family dynamics and unresolved issues are frequently highlighted around a terminal diagnosis. Having a shortage of time with a loved one can result in people wanting some resolution to long-term feelings or problems. As a primary care clinician, facilitating this kind of resolution can be very meaningful for the patient and the family. For example, in the follow-up session with Dr. E., Mrs. Termillo complained that her husband would not speak with her about his feelings. It turned out that this was a long-standing complaint of Mrs. Termillo's, and one she felt desperate to change in their final months together. By providing some support and communication guidelines, Dr. E. was able to help the Termillos speak with each other about Mr. Termillo's illness. The couple then reported feeling closer to each other than they had in years.

This was a case where primary care counseling was appropriate and effective. In addition, Marcia and her siblings each, in their own way, had

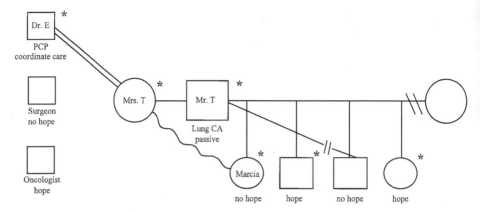

FIGURE 16.1. The case of Mr. Termillo. An asterisk indicates someone who attended the family conference.

unresolved issues about their father leaving their mother and marrying his current wife. Even though this happened 20 years before the diagnosis, Mr Termillo was cut off from his youngest son and his children had never fully accepted his second wife. Referral to a family therapist resulted in a series of sessions that helped the family come to some closure regarding some of these long-standing problems. When conflict is severe, long-standing, and/or jeopardizes the medical treatment of the patient, this sort of referral to a family therapist may be useful. In these more severe cases, the goal may be to help the family pull together enough to work through the issues involving the dying person.

"I Think We Should Talk About What Kind of Medical Care You Would Like, Should You Become Extremely Ill"

Treatment planning with patients and families about a terminal illness allows everyone to confront the reality of an impending death and to participate in and feel some control over the medical care process. Issues range from whether patients prefer another round of chemotherapy or surgery, to questions of hospice care or whether they wish to be resuscitated if they arrest in the hospital. Decisions made to limit medical treatment most often occur because further treatment is viewed as futile. These decisions can involve weighing the risk of premature death against the risk of prolonged, painful life. These choices should often be understood as more ethical (i.e., driven by patient values) than medical (10, 11). Decisions should be made by the patient in consultation with family members.

Negotiations about treatment planning are easiest to accomplish when the clinician has had a previous relationship with the patient and family. These discussions tend to be sensitive and emotionally charged. The clinician can be most effective when he or she can draw on knowledge of the patient and family's history prior to any crisis. In an acute medical crisis, conflicts between the clinician and family regarding decisions to limit treatment can occur when the family cannot process the medical facts because: they are too distraught; they are in denial, guilty, or grieving; the clinician used too much jargon or is unclear (12); the clinician has avoided direct conversation about prognosis; or the clinician sounded as if he or she will abandon the patient.

Prior to any serious illness the clinician has ideally discussed with the patient his or her wishes regarding medical care should a catastrophic accident or illness occur (6, 7). Although these discussions are useful with any patient, they are especially important with elderly patients, patients with chronic illness, or patients facing serious surgery. From an ethical perspective, any decision to limit treatment is best made by the patient rather than by the family or the clinician; hence, the value of the patient having a "living will." It is also important that the patient name a healthcare proxy (i.e., someone he or she trusts to make decisions should the patient lose capacity to do so). Despite the compelling reasons to have such discussions with healthy patients, it is rarely done. This reluctance may reflect such clinician factors as: time constraints in a busy practice, the clinician's own denial and avoidance of death, or fear of causing depression or anxiety in patients. Clinicians may feel at other times that they have not been trained to have the skills for such sensitive discussions (13). It is possible that having such a discussion will result in the patient becoming depressed, anxious, or resistant, so sensitivity, timing, and support are crucial to a successful interaction of this sort. The following are suggestions to facilitate the discussion of terminal treatment guidelines in the ambulatory setting:

1. While taking a routine genogram, ask, "Who in your family do you turn to for support?" Follow up by asking, "Should you become seriously ill or injured, would that be the person you would like me to consult regarding treatment decisions?" (14) Encourage the patient to designate this person his or her healthcare proxy, as in #5.

2. Ask about the patient's values and then his or her wishes for treatment: "Although you are healthy now, it would be helpful to know what your wishes are about your medical care should something catastrophic happen and you were unable to tell me what your wishes were at that time. Let's begin by you telling me the things you value most in life, and under what circumstances life would no longer be worth living for you." (11)

3. Be as specific as possible: "If your lung disease worsened so that I thought you would never be able to breathe on your own again, would

you want to be on a respirator?" "If your heart stopped beating or you stopped breathing, would you want us to start your heart again or put you on a machine to breathe for you?"

4. Encourage the patient to discuss his or her wishes with family members and other loved ones: "It is very important that you discuss these issues with your family while you are healthy and well. If you need any help with this, let me know."

5. Introduce the idea of a "living will." "Some people feel so strongly about what they do and do not want done for them in the event that they cannot make decisions, they have written living wills. Do you feel strongly about this?" If so, suggest a written living will, which should:

a. Be as specific as possible regarding such possibilities as respiratory support, nutritional support, antibiotics, and resuscitation.

b. Name a healthcare proxy who can have final authority, in consultation with other family members to make unforeseen treatment decisions . [Healthcare Proxies have legal authority in several states, and are usually honored in others (11).] The job of the healthcare proxy is to decide what the patient would want if he or she could communicate, not what the proxy wants him- or herself.

c. Contain the signatures of two witnesses (a lawyer's participation is not required).

d. Be updated yearly and/or prior to any hospitalization.

e. Be copied and given to family members, with a copy in the chart (15).

Knowing a patient's preferences is in everyone's best interest. One study asked healthy elderly people whether they wished their preferences about terminal medical care (maximal vs. comfort care) to be recorded in their charts. These researchers found that, whereas not all patients could render a decision, the majority did have a preference: They wish to be recorded (16).

> Mr. Rione was a 36-year-old French Canadian man with a homosexual lifestyle who had been diagnosed HIV positive. Mr. Rione decided with some difficulty to inform his family of his health status. Even though he was reluctant, he also hoped to address some hard feelings that had lingered for more than 10 years since he had revealed his sexual preference. Mr. Rione used his primary care clinician, Dr. Z., as a support and a sounding board during this period of time. As part of the process of discussing the uncertain course of this potential illness, Dr. Z. also discussed how Mr. Rione, his lover, Mr. James, and Mr Rione's family could participate in treatment planning should he become symptomatic or seriously ill. Mr. Rione named Mr. James as his healthcare proxy. In a family meeting with Mr Rione's partner, siblings, and mother, Dr. Z. described some of the potential treatments that are available for people who develop HIV syndromes, and solicited questions and concerns from Mr.

Rione and his family. Even though some tension existed in the family meeting, the group was able to come together around the issue of Mr Rione's illness and the decisions he may face in the future. Dr. Z. emphasized that he was currently not symptomatic, may remain well indefinitely, and that research is very active in this area so that new treatments are likely to develop that are unknown now. Mr Rione's brother ended the family session on a poignant note, noting that the family now had a goal to improve all of their relationships, since being reminded of the finite nature of their lives.

"We Need to Decide Together How to Make You Comfortable, and Give You the Best Quality of Life in the Time You Have Remaining"

Once a patient becomes terminally ill, the hypothetical issues about treatment guidelines become a reality that must be faced. Basic palliative care interventions include: controlling pain and other distressing physical symptoms, providing an empathic presence, and working to alleviate psychosocial problems (e.g., loneliness, financial difficulties, and family conflict). Hospice care is often very useful. It is important to work to increase both agency and communion by helping the patient re-establish a sense of purpose, value, efficacy, and self-worth. These goals may be achieved through individual counseling sessions with the primary care clinician, a spiritual leader, or a mental health professional. Guidelines for patients in these sessions are to:

- Set attainable goals.
- Reminisce about life; emphasize accomplishments and positive memories.
- Identify valued personal characteristics.
- Let go of unfinished business.
- Participate in decision making about treatment; let go of the need to control what cannot be controlled.
- Forgive oneself, and ask for forgiveness.
- Express love directly to loved ones.
- Discuss beliefs about spirituality, the meaning of his or her life, in particular, any afterlife.
- Make use of meaningful religious rites and rituals.

In addition, the clinician should:

- Assess for clinical depression (vs. grieving), and suicidality; consider antidepressants if warranted (17).

In addition to individual counseling, family counseling may also be appropriate to help the patient express difficult feelings or resolve long-standing problems. Home visits are an important part of terminal treatment, and allow for meetings with patients and important family members. It is especially important to hold a family conference to discuss terminal treatment planning (see Chap. 7 for basic guidelines for a family conference). The following guidelines are specific to terminal treatment planning:

1. Ask the patient or family if they want their priest, minister, rabbi, or other religious support to attend the meeting.

2. Begin the conference by asking about less difficult issues (e.g., the current medical treatment), then move on to more highly charged issues (e.g., new prognostic information or questions about life-prolonging care).

3. Address the relevant medical issues, such as:
• What are the treatment options?
• What does the treatment offer the patient?
• What are the probabilities of success and failure?
• Will the treatment cause additional illness? (18)

4. Solicit questions to help decide how much and what kind of medical information the patient and family want. It is easy to present medical information in a way that heavily influences the outcome of a patient or family's treatment decisions in order to be as straightforward as possible and acknowledge any personal biases that may affect the way the information is given. Be careful not to medicalize what are actually ethical issues.

5. Describe and encourage the use of hospice care.

6. Help the patient and/or family weigh potentially good outcomes against potentially undesirable ones.

7. Help both patient and family stay focused on the patient's personal goals as primary in this process.

8. Work on being as nonanxious as possible in the room. Speak slowly. These discussions are most frequently highly emotional for the participants, and benefit from facilitation by someone who is clear and calm.

9. Use clear, jargon-free language. Be a supportive, active listener. Track others' communications and clarify confusing statements made by any participant. Care needs to be taken to attend to communication issues in general because the likelihood of someone misinterpreting another's statements or intentions in this emotionally charged situation is high.

10. Model an ability to tolerate the ambiguity and uncertainty that accompanies all these decisions. Do not rush the decisions if it is not necessary. The patient and family may need time to decide.

11. Communicate a willingness to sustain contact with the patient and the family regardless of their treatment decisions. Ask the patient and family how they would like information distributed, who should be called, and when. Be sure to gather the important phone numbers.

Many people are reluctant to limit medical therapy because they equate it with limiting care for the patient. Assure the patient and the family that all supportive care by the staff will be appropriately aggressive, including providing adequate pain control, attending to bladder and bowel function, discontinuing unnecessary treatments, allowing lengthy or unlimited visiting hours, providing opportunities for the patient to talk (or be silent), and generally showing a high level of patient care (13). Miles suggests that patients or families that respond to discussions around treatment planning with "Do everything!" should be understood as saying "Slow down, give us more time to understand what you are saying," or, "Show us that you care and won't abandon us at this time when our options are so profoundly limited" (18). Regardless of the decisions that are made concerning treatment, it is important to let family members know that their clinician will stand by them and will not withdraw during their difficult time.

To summarize, the best situation occurs when a patient, in conjunction with family members, is able to express his or her preferences regarding treatment decisions. If the patient is unable to communicate and has not previously made his or her wishes known, the burden of responsibility falls almost completely to the family members. In one study 86% of families of incompetent patients made these decisions (19). Treatment decisions can be difficult for families to negotiate without considerable support and information from the medical staff. The clinician may wish to keep in mind the following principles that guide a family conference for terminal treatment planning in which a patient is unable to participate:

1. Keep the care, comfort, and concern for the patient primary.
2. Include all available family members in the conference.
3. Hold the conference at the patient's bedside. Even if the patient is comatose, having the discussion with the patient there makes the decisions more real and diminishes family members' sense of guilt about having to decide about their loved one's treatment.
4. Remind the family (or healthcare proxy) that their job is to decide what the patient would wish to have done, rather than what they themselves would want.
5. Recognize the family's pain, and acknowledge the difficulty of the process.

Patients and families can respond to these discussions about limiting treatment in one of several ways. Bedell et al. found that families were most likely to choose to limit treatment, especially in writing a Do Not Resuscitate (DNR) order, under the following conditions: when the patient was in a coma or brain dead; when clinicians and staff supported and reassured them that this was the appropriate decision; when they were assured that the staff would maintain the patient's medical care and comfort; when the patient had expressed a previous wish to the family regarding care; and when they were told the orders could be changed (19). The age of the patient, severity of the illness, and degree of patient suffering did not predict these family members' decisions.

Some family members clearly and unambivalently want "everything" done to keep their loved one alive. Others appear to be ambivalent, but are unable to decide to limit treatment because they seem to view any restriction as abandonment or even murder. These family members may try very hard to get the medical staff to make these decisions for them or they may demand aggressive treatment because of their own feelings of sadness, denial, fear, anger, guilt, or abandonment. Many of these reactions change over time with a focus on making the patient's needs primary, so it is important to have discussions periodically both to update family members on any new medical information and to allow people to express changes that have occurred in their own thinking.

> Mrs. Katz, an 82-year-old Lithuanian Jewish woman, had been hospitalized for 10 days, but her fevers were still uncontrolled. This was her fourth hospitalization in the last 6 months. With dementia and parkinsonism, complete incontinence, recurrent infections, and deep decubitous ulcers unsuccessfully treated with surgery, death seemed inevitable to her clinician and hospital staff. Dr. S. initiated a discussion of limiting treatment with the patients' two daughters at their mother's bedside. Adele, the younger daughter, had been unusually attentive and involved. She was always available, left two or three phone numbers, visited daily, and made lists of questions and suggestions about her mother's treatment. Observing this painful daily decline, she reluctantly came to accept her mother's impending death as a certainty and favored writing DNR orders. Her sister, Robin, was a much less frequent visitor and was often unreachable because of her long and unpredictable work hours. Her ideas were relayed to Dr. S. by Adele, accompanied by barely disguised anger, because Robin maintained that she could not "give up on Mom."
>
> When Dr. S. finally met with Robin and Adele, Robin expressed bitter frustration at a previous clinician's lack of consideration in never consulting her about her father's care the previous year, when he was "allowed to just die." Until Dr. S. could have a family conference and meet with these daughters together, he was unable to resolve the issues around treatment planning for their mother. By encouraging them to talk together about what their mother would have wanted and what was in her best interest, Robin slowly agreed that limiting treatment was the best option available. Dr S. encouraged both daughters to visit their mother frequently and reassured them she would get the best available care from the staff.

"I Need to Inform You That Your Loved One Has Died"

Notifying family members about the death of a loved one is a difficult, stressful task. Direct, sensitive communication makes it more likely family members will hear the message clearly. Prior discussions with a family about an expected death make this situation generally easier to deal with than an unexpected death. The following are suggestions for notifying the family about a death:

1. Encourage the family to be present at the time of death if at all possible. One study demonstrated that a majority of family members were grateful to be present during a resuscitation attempt for their relative (20). Any action that helps family members participate in and acknowledge their loved one's death may be useful.

2. When the family is expecting the death of one of its members, ask how they would prefer to be notified if they are not present.

3. Notify the family immediately at the time of death.

a. With an expected death, call on the family as previously agreed upon.

b. With an unexpected death, ask the family as a whole to come to the hospital and discuss the events leading up to the death.

4. Think about what you want to say before making the call. Many people remember the exact words spoken by whoever told them of a death.

5. While being sympathetic and sensitive, avoid euphemisms. Use the words "death, dying, and dead" rather than "passed away" or other colloquial sayings.

6. Say, "You have my sympathy," rather than, "I am sorry," which can be construed as an apology.

7. Give the family the opportunity to view the body and say their goodbyes.

a. Arrange for the viewing to occur in a private room.

b. Make sure the body has been cleaned and prepared, so that wounds have been dressed, blood stains removed, and the body draped and placed in an appropriate position.

c. Offer to have a member of the healthcare team stay with the family, especially if only one family member is present.

d. Allow them to remain with the deceased as long as they wish (21, 22).

8. Meet with the family.

a. This may occur before or after the viewing. Either way, it is an important step in showing concern and facilitating a healthy early grieving process.

b. Provide information about the cause of death. Solicit and answer any questions.

c. Answer any questions about autopsy or organ donations.

d. Use active listening skills. Expect and tolerate expressions of intense emotions, especially with a family who learns of an unexpected death. Do not exclude family members who become very upset or emotional. Avoid psychotropic medications, unless someone has serious difficulty sleeping in the weeks after the news.

e. Make yourself available as a support for the family. Suggest a follow-up meeting to discuss autopsy results or questions about the deceased that are likely to arise in the future.

f. Remind the family to call their funeral director.

g. Encourage the family to include children, especially those more than 5 years old, in the funeral and other family gatherings.

9. With an unanticipated or traumatic death, consider making a home visit soon after the death. These families may benefit from support and structure during the early period of shock. With an anticipated death, the primary care clinician may send a sympathy card to the family. If the connection has been a strong or complicated one, attending the wake or calling hours can be very useful. Family members are almost universally appreciative, and it allows the clinician to pay respects to the deceased and to support the surviving family members at a critical time in the life of the family. Attending a funeral may be more difficult in terms of schedule, and may not allow for much direct contact with the family; however, it may be helpful to the clinician for him- or herself.

10. With an anticipated death, telephone the family 1–2 weeks after the death to inquire about their well-being, answer any questions, and schedule a follow-up appointment. With complicated or unexpected deaths (e.g., a car accident, suicide, or homicide), offer the family an appointment soon after the funeral (see the later section on Primary Care Grief Counseling). These situations also warrant referral to and collaboration with a family-oriented mental health professional.

"What Did I Do Wrong?"

One of the most difficult aspects of dealing with a patient's death is the clinician's own feelings. Though in a different and much less intimate role than that of a family member, the healthcare professional may also experience feelings of sadness, loss, anger, or guilt. In addition to facilitating the grief process for the family, the clinician also needs to attend to his or her own grief and difficult feelings. Such rituals as saying goodbye to the deceased and attending the funeral when possible (23) allow for the emotional side of being a doctor to be nourished and utilized. "What did I do wrong?" is an almost universal response after an unexpected or difficult death, certainly for physicians in training. With an unexpected death or the death of a young person, the clinician usually examines the patient's history and course of treatment to determine any professional mistakes on his or her part. This process can be important and useful if it is seen as an opportunity to learn from the careful examination of a case rather than to perpetuate perfectionist, superhuman standards for providing medical care. At those times when mistakes have been made, it is important to face them squarely and to create opportunities for confession and forgiveness (23). Discussing the case with trusted colleagues, or in a Balint-style support group (see Chap. 26) can be both educational and cathartic, especially if uncertainty and guilt remain prominent feelings over a period of time after a patient death (7).

"To Feel Pain and Sadness At This Time is a Normal, Healthy Response"

Primary care grief counseling offers significant opportunities for medical providers to encourage healthy grieving and to prevent pathological or unresolved grief reactions. In the event of sudden, unexpected death, the supportive role of the primary care clinician can be especially important (24). Even in these cases, the usual grief response is time-limited and somewhat predictable in its phases. Normal grieving is characterized by intellectual and emotional awareness of the loss and feelings of guilt, stress, pain, anger, and hostility (25). There is tremendous cultural variability in how and whether these feelings are expressed, from some Greek cultures where widows wear black from the rest of their lives after their husbands die, to British-Americans who may never show visible grieving (26). Grief is typically a cyclical process in which all these feelings may be present at any time, but certain feelings may dominate at different points in the cycle. The *acute phase* begins with the notification of death and is characterized by emotional shock. In Western culture, this phase typically lasts for up to 2 weeks. Depression and somatic symptoms are common and persist into the *second phase*, characterized by rumination over memories of the deceased. During this phase, people may withdraw and become introverted as they examine what the recent death means for their own life. This process typically takes from 3 to 6 months. The third and final phase is the *resolution phase*. At this time, somatic symptoms and preoccupation with the deceased lessen. Bereaved family members begin to plan for the future and to participate again in activities that were an important part of their lives prior to the death. The resolution phase is punctuated by the anniversary of the loved one's death. After this period, which often involves a temporary increase in grief or symptomatology, most people are able to move on.

The following are principles for primary care grief counseling:

1. With a traumatic death, schedule an office visit soon after the funeral. With an anticipated death, schedule an office visit within 1 month after the loss for interested family members to review the death and the autopsy results.

2. Encourage family members to talk about the circumstances surrounding the death, recall memories, and openly discuss feelings of sadness, anger, and guilt. Give them permission to grieve.

3. Inquire about any significant changes in financial status. Settling an estate, the loss of income, and the lack of experience managing money can intensify the grieving process.

4. Normalize signs of grieving (e.g., crying spells, lack of energy, and preoccupation with the deceased). Tell the family that normal or uncomplicated grief typically takes at least 1 year for the active phase to resolve.

5. Avoid the use of such psychotropic medication as sedatives or hypnotics, except in unusual circumstances, or when a family member is unable to sleep. A sedated person at a funeral may not be able to participate or even remember this important time. Starting antidepressant, antianxiety, or antipsychotic medications are typically not indicated during bereavement.

6. Monitor the medical status of the recently bereaved closely as research indicates that the bereaved are at higher risk of serious illness and death (see Chap. 2). Encourage family members to come in for a health evaluation at 6 months to assess any increased risk for illness or delayed difficulties with grieving.

7. Refer interested family members to community-based self-help support groups, such as the Widow-to-Widow group, the group for parents of sudden infant death syndrome (SIDS) children, or any of the many other bereavement support groups. Support and information from those who have experienced a similar loss themselves can be extremely helpful to the bereaved.

8. Monitor family members for signs of unresolved grief reaction; (25,27,28) (see Table 16.1). Refer if necessary.

Prolonged and extreme reactions to grief are themselves dangerous and necessitate referral to a specialist. Such a referral is best made to both the person with the symptoms and that person's family. Referral may be made for evaluation, bereavement counseling, psychiatric treatment, or family therapy, as is appropriate.

The following example describes a close, married couple from the time of the acute phase of the husband's illness to the year after his death.

Mrs. Stowe, a 75-year-old German-American woman, had cared for her older husband for more than 20 years. He was blind and suffered from Alzheimer's disease. Over the previous year he had become increasingly difficult to care for: He became incontinent and began wandering at night. His normally cheerful mood changed gradually as he became more irritable and resisted any assistance. After being struck by him on several occasions, Mrs. Stowe decided she could no longer care for him at home. She had kept him with her in their small apartment with few

TABLE 16.1. Signs and symptoms of an unresolved grief reaction

1. Prolonged, severe clinical depression (i.e., a pervasive sense of worthlessness and self-blame lasting longer than 12–18 months)
2. Prolonged social isolation, withdrawal, or alienation
3. Emotional numbing in which the patient largely denies an emotional reaction to the loss, resulting in a kind of wooden or flat emotional presentation
4. An inability to cry
5. Talking as if the dead person were still alive
6. Persistent compulsive overactivity without a sense of loss
7. Persistence of a variety of physical complaints (e.g., headaches, fatigue, dizziness, or multiple injuries)
8. Profound identification with the deceased and prolonged acquisition of symptoms belonging to the illness of that person
9. Extreme, persistent anger (may be directed at the clinician)
10. Alcohol or drug abuse, persistent requests for sedative or narcotic medications
11. Marital or family problems
12. Work or school problems

services long past the point when most families would have placed a demented elderly member. At 84 years old, the physical and emotional stress of caring for her husband was beginning to affect her health. Her three children had been encouraging her for several years to arrange for placement.

Because the couple had significant savings, Mr. Stowe was placed in a nearby nursing home within a month of Mrs. Stowe's decision. She became quite depressed shortly after he left home. Their family clinician, Dr. C., encouraged her to visit him regularly and express her feelings. She spent most of her day with her husband in the nursing home, but continued to feel she had betrayed him. She now felt she had nothing worthwhile to do with herself.

Several months after his admission, Mr. Stowe suffered a massive stroke and died within a week. Mrs. Stowe became increasingly depressed over the next 6 months, grieving over his death and feeling that her life, which had been spent caring first for her children and then for her husband, was now worthless. Her family tried to cheer her up, which only made her feel that they did not understand her grief. Efforts to get her involved in social activities in the apartment house where she lived were unsuccessful because she viewed any social activities as "a waste of time."

A month after Mr. Stowe's death, Dr. C. met with Mrs. Stowe, her children and several of her grandchildren, who were concerned about Mrs. Stowe's emotional state. Dr. C. explained that the intensity of Mrs. Stowe's grief was testimony to what a special relationship the couple had, and that to give up that grief too soon would seem to Mrs. Stowe to be dishonoring her husband. He encouraged Mrs. Stowe's children to share their memories of their father and how much they also missed him with their mother.

> Dr. C. met with Mrs. Stowe every 3 months for the first year
> of bereavement. At 6 months, he began to encourage her to get involved
> in volunteer work where she could help and care for other people.
> A year after her husband's death, Mrs. Stowe's grief and depression
> had begun to lift. She was doing some volunteer work at a local
> hospital and felt she had found some meaning in her life. Her
> spirits were improved though she continued to miss her husband
> deeply.

Grief typically sends "shock waves" throughout a family system (29). One
of the goals of primary care management of terminal illness, death, and
grieving is to channel these shock waves so they can have a restorative
effect, and to monitor their influence to prevent future disruption or
symptomatology.

References

1. Becker E: *The Denial of Death*. New York: Macmillan, 1973.
2. The Support Investigators: A controlled trial to improve care for seriously ill hospitalized patients. *JAMA* 1995;**274**:1591–1598.
3. Ptacek JT, Eberhardt TL: Breaking bad news: a review of the literature. *JAMA* 1996;**276**:496–502.
4. Candib L: Truth-telling about cancer and end-of-life issues in the multicultural setting: reconsidering autonomy, families and health conference. San Diego, CA, March 4, 2000.
5. Quill TE, Arnold R, & Platt F: "I wish things were different": expressing wishes in response to loss, futility, and unrealistic hopes. *Ann Intern Med* 2001; **135**:551–555.
6. Servalli EP: The dying patient, the clinician, and the fear of death. *N Engl J Med* 1988;**319**:1728–1730.
7. McDaniel SH, Bank J, Campbell T, Mancini J, & Shore B: Using a group as a consultant. In: Wynne LC, McDaniel SH, & Weber T (Eds): *Systems Consultation*. New York: Guilford Press, 1986.
8. Holmes TH, Rahe RH: The social readjustment scale. *J Psychosom Res* 1967;**11**:213–218.
9. Fuller RL, Geis S: Communicating with the grieving family. *J Fam Prac* 1985; **21**:139–144.
10. Schneiderman LJ, Arias JD: Counseling patients to counsel clinicians on future care in the event of patient incompetence. *Ann Intern Med* 1985;**102**:693–698.
11. McCann RM, Chodosh J, Frankel RM, Katz PR, Naumburg EH, & Hall WJ. *Advance Directives and End of Life Discussions: A Manual for Instructors* Rochester NY: University of Rochester School of Medicine and Dentistry, 1997 (unpublished manual).
12. Goold SD, Williams B, & Arnold RM: Conflicts regarding decisions to limit treatment: a differential diagnosis. *JAMA* 2000;**283**:909–914.
13. Lo B, Jonsen AR: Clinical decisions to limit treatment. *Ann Intern Med* 1980;**93**:764–768.

14. Maher E: Establishing treatment guidelines in geriatric patients. In: *Family Medicine Grand Rounds*. Rochester, NY: University of Rochester School of Medicine, March 31, 1988.
15. Concern for Dying: *A Living Will*. New York, Concern for Dying, 1983.
16. Snow RM, Atwood K: probable death: perspective of the elderly. *South Med J* 1985;**78**:851–853.
17. Miles SH: The limited treatment plan. Part II: planning with patients and their families. *Clin Rep Aging* 1987;**1**:14–16.
18. Block SD: Assessing and managing depression in the terminally ill patient. *Ann Intern Med* 2000;**132**:209–218.
19. Bedell SE, Pelle D, Maher PL, & Clearly PD: Do Not Resuscitate orders for critically ill patients in the hospital: how are they used and what is their impact? *JAMA* 1986;**256**:233–237.
20. Doyle CJ, Post H, Burney RE, Malno J, Keefe M, & Rhee KJ: Family participation during resuscitation: an option. *Ann Emerg Med* 1987;**16**:673–675.
21. Tolle S, Elliot D, & Girard D: How to manage patient death and care for the bereaved. *Postgrad Med* 1985;**78**(2):87–95.
22. Engel GL: Grief and grieving. In: Schwartz LH, Schwartz JL (Eds): *The Psychodynamics of Patient Care*. New York: Prentice Hall, 1972.
23. Irvine P: The attending at the funeral. *N Engl J Med* 1985;**315**(26):120.
24. Wadland WC, Keller B, Jones W, & Chapados J: Sudden, unexpected death and the role of the family clinician. *Fam Syst Med* 1988;**6**(2):176–187.
25. Lindemann E: Symptomatology and management of acute grief. *Am J Psychiatr* 1944;**101**:141.
26. McGoldrick M, Almeida R, Hines PM, Rosen E, Garcia-Preto N, & Lee E: Mourning in different cultures. In: Walsh F, McGoldrick M: *Living Beyond Loss: Death in the Family* New York: WW Norton, 1991; pp, 176–206.
27. Brown JT, Stoudemire GA: Normal and pathological grief. *JAMA* 1983; **250**(3):378–382.
28. Pasnau RO, Fawzy FI, & Fawzy N: Role of the physician in bereavement. *Psychiatr Clin N Am* 1987;**10**(1):109–120.
29. Bowen M: Family reaction to death. In: Guerin P (ed): *Family Therapy*. New York: Gardner Press, 1976.

Protocol: Talking to Patients and Families About Terminal Illness, Treatment Planning, and Grief

Communicating a Terminal Diagnosis

1. When a serious illness is suspected, ask the patient at the time the test is ordered about how he or she wishes the results to be communicated: with family, without family, or even to the family only.
2. At the time of delivering bad news, first tell the participants that you need to have a serious discussion about the illness.
3. Find out what the patient already knows: Begin the discussion from the point of the patient's understanding.
4. Communicate directly to the patient about the diagnosis, the treatment, and the prognosis of the illness.
5. Use clear, simple language: Avoid overmedicalizing or intellectualizing.
6. Be honest and straightforward, acknowledging areas of medical uncertainty: Avoid giving an overly optimistic or overly pessimistic prognosis.
7. Look the patient or family member in the eye and speak calmly: Repeat the basic message several times.
8. Wait for the patient and family to absorb the information, providing details as requested.
9. Sit silently and make space for the patient and family to react as needed.
10. Avoid arguments over the diagnosis, or other diversions.
11. Ask what questions the patient or family has.
12. Allow people their sadness or anger.
13. Say "I wish things were different" rather than "I'm sorry".
14. Allow patients some hope: Be humble about predicting how long a patient may survive.
15. Emphasize that you will continue to care for and support the patient throughout his or her illness.
16. If the patient chose to talk alone, suggest that the process be repeated with the family.
17. Recognize that family members are likely to accept the diagnosis at differing points in time. Make space for each person's way of coping, and keep communication channels open for all members of the family and healthcare team.
18. Make a follow-up appointment.
19. Avoid any tendency to withdraw during the terminal phase: Meet regularly with the patient and family. Encourage children in the family to be involved.

Treatment Planning for a Terminal Illness

Discussing Terminal Treatment Guidelines in the Ambulatory Setting

1. While taking a routine genogram, ask, "Who in your family do you turn to for support?" Follow up by asking, "Should you become seriously ill or injured, would that be the person you would like me to consult regarding treatment decisions?"
2. Ask about the patient's values, and then his or her wishes for treatment.
3. Be as specific as possible.
4. Encourage the patient to discuss his or her wishes with family members.
5. Introduce the idea of a "living will," which should:
    a. Consider specific possibilities, such as respiratory support, nutritional support, antibiotics, and resuscitation.
    b. Name a healthcare proxy who can have final authority, in consultation with other family members, to make unforeseen treatment decisions.
    c. Contain the signatures of two witnesses.
    d. Be updated yearly and/or prior to any hospitalization.
    e. Be copied and given to family members, with a copy in the chart (15).

Guidelines for Terminal Treatment Planning with the Patient

1. Set attainable goals
2. Help the patient:
    a. Reminisce about life; emphasize accomplishments and positive memories.
    b. Identify valued personal characteristics.
    c. Let go of unfinished business.
    d. Participate in decision making about treatment; let go of the need to control what cannot be controlled.
    e. Forgive oneself, and ask for forgiveness.
    f. Express love directly to loved ones.
    g. Discuss beliefs about spirituality, the meaning of his or her life, in particular, any afterlife.
3. Encourage the use of meaningful religious rites and rituals.
4. Assess for clinical depression (vs grieving), and suicidality; consider antidepressants if warranted

Guidelines for Terminal Tre.atment Planning at a Family Conference

1. Ask the patient or family if they want their priest, minister, or rabbi to attend the meeting.
2. Begin the conference by asking about less-difficult issues, then move on to more highly charged issues.
3. Address such relevant medical issues as:

- What are the treatment options?
- What does the treatment offer the patient?
- What are the probabilities of success and failure?
- Will the treatment cause additional illness?

4. Solicit questions to help decide how much and what kind of medical information the patient and family want. Be as straightforward as possible and acknowledge any personal biases. Be careful not to medicalize what are actually ethical issues.
5. Describe and encourage the use of hospice care.
6. Help the patient and/or family weigh potentially good outcomes against potentially undesirable ones.
7. Help both patient and family stay focused on the patient's personal goals as primary.
8. Be as nonanxious as possible.
9. Use clear, jargon-free language. Be a supportive, active listener. Track others' communications and clarify confusing statements made by any participant.
10. Model an ability to tolerate the ambiguity and uncertainty that accompanies all these decisions.
11. Communicate a willingness to sustain contact with the patient and the family regardless of their treatment decisions.

Principles for Terminal Treatment Planning at a Family Conference in Which a Patient Is Unable to Participate

1. Keep the care, comfort, and concern for the patient primary.
2. Include all available family in the conference.
3. Hold the conference at the patient's bedside.
4. Remind the family that their job is to decide what the patient would wish to have done, rather than what they themselves would want.
5. Recognize the family's pain, and acknowledge the difficulty of the process.

Notifying the Family About a Death

1. Encourage the family to be present at the time of death, if at all possible.
2. When the family is expecting the death of one of its members, ask how they would prefer to be notified if they are not present.
3. Notify the family immediately at the time of death:
   - With an expected death, call on the family as previously agreed.
   - With an unexpected death, ask the family as a whole to come to the hospital and discuss the events leading up to the death.
4. Think about what you want to say before making the call: Many people remember the exact words spoken by whoever told them of the death.

5. While being sympathetic and sensitive, avoid euphemisms: Use the words "death, dying, and dead."
6. Say, "You have my sympathy," rather than, "I am sorry," which could be construed as an apology.
7. Give the family the opportunity to view the body and say their goodbyes.
   a. Arrange for the viewing to occur in a private room.
   b. Make sure the body has been cleaned and prepared.
   c. Offer to have a member of the healthcare team stay with the family.
   d. Allow them to remain with the deceased as long as they wish.
8. Meet with the family.
   a. Before or after the viewing to show concern and facilitate a healthy early grieving process.
   b. Provide information about the cause of death: Solicit and answer any questions.
   c. Answer any questions about autopsy or organ donations.
   d. Use active listening skills: Expect expressions of intense emotions.
   e. Make yourself available as a support for the family: Offer to have follow-up meetings, either to discuss autopsy results or questions about the deceased that will likely arise in the future.
   f. Remind the family to call their funeral director.
   g. Encourage the family to include children, especially those older than 5 years, in the funeral and other family gatherings.
9. With an unanticipated or traumatic death, consider making a home visit soon thereafter: With an anticipated death, send a sympathy card to the family and/or attend the calling hours or funeral.
10. With an anticipated death, telephone the family 1–2 weeks after the death to inquire about them, answer any questions, and encourage any necessary follow up.

Primary Care Grief Counseling

1. With a traumatic death, schedule an office visit soon after the funeral, and consider rapid referral to a family therapist: With an anticipated death, schedule an office visit at within 1 month with interested family members to review the death and the autopsy results.
2. Encourage family members to talk about the circumstances surrounding the death, recall memories, and openly discuss feelings of sadness, anger, and guilt.
3. Inquire about any significant changes in financial status.
4. Normalize signs of grieving during the first year (e.g., crying spells, lack of energy, and preoccupation with the deceased).
5. Avoid the use of such psychotropic medication as sedatives or hypnotics, except when previously prescribed or when a family has a serious sleep disturbance.

6. Monitor the medical status of the recently bereaved: Encourage family members to come in for a health evaluation at 6 months to evaluate any increased risk for illness or delayed difficulties with grieving.
7. Refer interested family members to community-based self-help support groups.
8. Monitor family members for signs of unresolved grief reaction; refer if necessary.

17
Genetic Screening, Testing, and Families

> "I'll never understand why my mother chose to put her faith
> in God rather than her geneticist."
> —little boy in the 1997 film, *Gattaca*

Even before scientists focused on cracking the human genetic code, our cultural expectations and fears about a Genetic Revolution were depicted in stories, films, and other media, raising such questions as:

What is the essence of being human?

How much will we try to control the sex, the temperament, and the genetic heritage of our children?

Popular reactions to the advances in genomics and the expanding realities of genetic testing will seriously affect primary care at both the individual and the family levels. Obtaining a family history will now more specifically include genetic screening for every patient. As a result, many patients will at least consider genetic testing especially as more genetic tests become available. For these patients, primary care clinicians will need to provide some form of genetic counseling.

> Genetic testing refers to the examination of a person's DNA or biochemical products of the DNA to gain information about the current or future health status of that person or his or her relatives. Genetic testing may be used to predict whether a person will develop or is at increased risk of developing symptoms of a particular disorder or if a person is at increased risk for having children with a particular disease. Prenatal genetic testing is used to determine if an unborn child will have a genetic condition. Testing may also be used to confirm a diagnosis. (1)

Testing is now available for many single gene-dominant disorders like Huntington's disease and those illnesses traditionally thought of as "genetic." Tests are also rapidly becoming available for mutations implicated in such illnesses as breast and colon cancer. Many illnesses involve some combination of genetic and environmental influences, with variable levels of certainty about when and how the illness will be expressed. These gene mutations represent "susceptibility genes" that will allow clinicians to focus on medical and behavioral prevention. With the ability to know which illnesses a patient is at risk for developing, the hope is that diagnosis and treatment can be rendered more sensitive, specific, effective, and safe (2); however as Frances Collins, the Director of the Human Genome Project, said, ". . . premature introduction of predictive tests, before the value of the information has been established, actually can be quite harmful" (3).

The rapid developments in genomic science have indeed far outpaced our understanding of their concomitant psychosocial, ethical, and legal implications. As with every scientific advance, clinicians attempt to apply a rational process for evaluating the value and appropriate role of these technological achievements for each patient in his or her family and community context. For some patients, genetic counseling and testing brings relief, and hope for prevention. Testing can reduce anxiety and improve the accuracy of perceived risk (4). For a minority of patients, test results may be informative, but distressing over time (5). *Genotype* implies permanence and immutability. Patients may believe that these tests will allow them certainty and prediction about their life course that is actually far from our grasp. Adding to the complexity, genetic concerns are inevitably both an individual and a family issue. What one individual thinks is right for him or her may conflict with what other family members think is in their best interest.

This chapter will take into account the multiplicity of scientific, psychological, and cultural issues involved, and lay out some guiding principles for primary care assessment and counseling that can be adapted to each individual situation as new scientific developments enter mainstream healthcare. We will divide the chapter into four chronological phases: risk assessment and genetic screening, pretest counseling, posttest counseling, and long-term follow up.

Raising the Possibility: Risk Assessment and Genetic Screening

Primary care clinicians presently often undertake the first steps in genetic screening, though that initiative may shift to the patient as more information penetrates mainstream culture. Patients themselves may raise questions about their risk for inherited illness at points of life transition, such as the decision to marry or to have a child. Being the first line of assessment requires that primary care clinicians educate themselves so as not to under- or overstate risk for any particular genetic illness (6). Genetic factors exist for most common chronic, serious disorders, including coronary artery disease and cancer, but their precise influence remains unclear. Heredity also affects susceptibility to many familiar, less lethal disorders (e.g., glaucoma, migraine, osteoporosis, peptic ulcer, and rheumatoid arthritis). Certain psychiatric or behavioral problems (e.g., depression or alcoholism) appear to have a genetic connection.

Clinicians should consider a hereditary influence when they learn about a disease that has an unusually early age of onset, occurs in multiple family members, and develops in otherwise low-risk people, among other factors. In many cases, however, nongenetic factors like social or environmental forces may be more important than genetic ones in the development of a disorder.

The genogram (or "pedigree," as geneticists refer to it) provides the basic template for all individualized genetic risk assessment (as opposed to generalized population screening) (see Chap. 3 for how to draw a genogram). (7) A thorough three-generation genogram that includes diseases with a genetic connection is a traditional component of the medical history. Ethnic origin should be recorded because it is important for many conditions (e.g., hemoglobinopathics, breast cancer, etc). Age and cause of death should be included for relatives who have died. For significant illnesses, record age at diagnosis (in live and deceased relatives) because this information can help to establish a possible genetic connection. Ask particularly about any congenital problems in biologically related relatives, because these details are relevant to a pedigree and are not often offered spontaneously (8). Some organizations and programs now offer a service that guides the patient through a computer-generated family history questionnaire (e.g., see the University of Virginia Web site).

> Jeanine and Al Murphy, both of northern European heritage, just moved to town and were thinking about having children. Jeanine made an appointment for a routine physical with her new physician. The office sent a health history form to Jeanine prior to her appointment. The physician then asked further questions from the form during her first visit, and learned that Jeanine's mother and grandmother died of breast cancer in their fifties. Jeanine's mother's sister was diagnosed with breast cancer in her thirties; she was treated and survived.

These histories, often taken before a patient is symptomatic or worried, allow the clinician to develop a risk profile. A conversation naturally ensues from this information:

> Dr. M.: There is a lot of breast cancer in your family. What does that mean to you?
> Jeanine: It concerns me a lot. When my mother was first diagnosed, she was only 42, and after the surgery they thought they got it all. But, 8 years later the cancer returned and they tried everything, including chemotherapy. It was horrible.

Dr. M.: Horrible?
Jeanine: She lost her hair, lost a lot of weight, and had all these sores
    in her mouth. She was pretty miserable.
Dr. M.: I imagine you don't want the same thing to happen to you.
Jeanine: I think that's unlikely. Since the time I was born, everyone has
    said I look more like my father, so it has always seemed to me that
    I would not inherit this problem of my mother's.

A few simple exploratory questions will often reveal a wealth of information about what the illness means to the patient. Clinicians need to be wary of making assumptions. Each patient will have a unique and idiosyncratic understanding of the implications of genetically linked disease based on his or her own personal background, experience, education, personality, and disposition. In this particular case, the patient, although concerned, was convinced that because she did not look like her mother she was unlikely to have an inherited genetic predisposition toward breast cancer. As a result, she was disinclined to perform any increased surveillance activities and found the thought of earlier mammograms or breast self-exams at odds with her self-image.

The physician realized that Jeanine's belief could be based on misinformation; it also could be hopeful denial. Either way, education was needed to help Jeanine accurately evaluate her statistical or calculated risk, as opposed to her perceived risk, and commit to basic surveillance activities. Large discrepancies between perceived risk and calculated risk can lead to decisions based more on emotional precedent than scientific rationale. Part of family-oriented primary care practice involves negotiating a plan based on science that takes the patient's and the family's health beliefs and emotional context into account.

Another strategy for understanding how patients think about their risk is to ask family members for their thoughts about the family illness history. If they are not present, ask the patient what he or she knows about how others in the family think.

Dr. M: What does your husband think about your risk for breast cancer?
Jeanine: He never met my mother, but agrees from the pictures that I
    don't look much like her. I have talked to him quite a bit about
    how the illness and how her death affected me.

Family-oriented questions can illuminate the meaning of the illness in the family. This woman has constructed a potentially problematic way to cope with the possibility of her increased risk. Her husband is involved and plays a role in helping his wife interpret the information and make her decisions. Research provides evidence that family members influence a patient's decisions and emotional response to genetic information (1,9). Family environment also influences risk modification behaviors (10).

Raising the possibility of genetic testing does not come without consequences. When a clinician introduces the possibility of a genetic test to a patient, the event necessarily brings the patient to a decision point. To most patients, this is not as simple as deciding whether to go along with the recommendation to have their cholesterol checked. Finding a mutation carries a different stigma, and more direct concern about morbidity and mortality. Just considering the possibility can frighten some patients and their families. Some have concerns about maintaining insurance coverage. This all means that the clinician must seriously consider the consequences of raising the possibility of genetic testing. One important issue to consider when bringing up genetic testing is whether preventive or treatment measures exist if a mutation is discovered.

John Rolland has identified three phases for people who test positive for genetic mutation, but are yet to be symptomatic: a precrisis phase, a crisis phase, and a chronic phase. The *precrisis phase* is the time when the patient is blissfully ignorant of the possibilities. The *crisis phase* begins after the possibility of genetic testing has been raised and extends through an acute period after a mutation has been discovered. The *chronic phase* then begins and extends until the time symptoms develop. Each individual and family will handle each phase differently. (11)

In Jeanine's case, the clinician's exploration did not reveal any knowledge of BRCA 1 and 2 testing, so the clinician has to decide if, when, and how to raise the topic.

Dr. M.: To what extent are you aware of the recommendations for women in your situation?

Jeanine: Well, I sometimes do breast exams, and my previous doctor talked to me about getting a mammogram, but I was very busy, and then we moved, and I just never got around to it. I think I should probably get a baseline.

D. M.: That's a good idea and I'd be happy to arrange it. I do encourage all women to do regular monthly breast exams and I'm glad to hear you do them, at least some of the time. I also want to mention the possibility of genetic testing. It's not a standard recommendation, but I thought that you might have heard about it?

Jeanine: Yes, I had a friend who knew of someone who had it done.

Dr. M.: It's complicated and I can give you some more information about it to take home. I think you should probably talk to your husband about it, too. There are several genetic mutations that are associated with breast cancer. There is a blood test that looks for these mutations that can be passed on in families. If the mutation is present, those women have a higher likelihood of getting breast cancer than women who do not have the mutation. You should also know that if you don't have the mutation it does not necessarily mean you won't get breast cancer. It is recommended that someone in the family who has had breast cancer be tested for the mutation first.

Jeanine: Really?

Dr. M.: Has anyone in your family had the testing done?

Jeanine: I don't think so. My aunt mentioned something about testing once, but I'm pretty sure she never had the test.

Dr. M.: If you like, I can give you some information on it and we could talk some more, say in a month. The test is expensive, somewhere close to several thousand dollars. If you wish, we could enroll you in a research study at the University where the test will be free and the process comprehensive and standardized.

Jeanine: Okay.

For many patients, the decision to have genetic testing is one that takes place over time. They need to absorb the information and become educated about what the test does and does not reveal about risk. The limits and expense of the test(s) need to be discussed in detail. For some, this process may take years.

There are some situations in which the clinician may decide to put off the discussion of genetic testing (e.g., with children or because a patient is under severe stress of some other kind and the delay is unlikely to affect outcome). For their part, patients refuse the test because there is no treatment currently available. Huntington's disease is such a disorder. In situations where no treatment is known, the advantage to testing is psychosocial rather than biomedical. A patient may wish to have testing in order to deal with anticipatory anxiety, plan whether or not to have children, or how to organize family finances. These circumstances are difficult and may benefit from collaborative care with a family therapist. The burden of knowledge of a mutation must be weighed against the ongoing worry over the ambiguity of the situation for the patient and the family.

Dr. T. saw Joe at age 38 for the first time, after his mother was diagnosed with Huntington's disease. His mother's sister and brother each had the disease and the family realized that was probably the case with their grandmother as well (see Fig. 17.1). Both Joe and Jill, his wife, were worried. Joe had a tremor in his hand that had developed over the past several years. Jill followed Dr. T. down the hall while Joe undressed for the exam and told him that Joe had been having memory lapses for the past year or so. She was so worried that this was a sign of Huntington disease that she did not tell her husband after the first several episodes. Dr. T. had helped this couple adopt two children when they were unable to conceive themselves. Jill mentioned how relieved she was that their children could not have the illness. She said she found herself paying careful attention to their financial situation and mentally assuming that she would have to make decisions about their young children's college, for example, by herself. Dr. T. realized in talking to these patients individually that anxiety over this anticipated illness was driving a wedge between this previously close couple. He suggested the couple see one of his family therapy colleagues, and they both agreed (see Fig. 17.1).

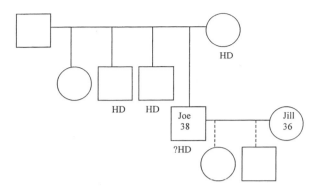

FIGURE 17.1. A couple facing Huntington disease.

Huntington disease is a single gene, dominant disorder. Penetrance for the gene is 100%, so if one has the mutation and lives to middle age, that person will almost certainly get the disease. Still, exactly when and how the disease will unfold is unknown. More common, multifactorial genetic disorders are ambiguous, complex, and riddled with the potential for misunderstanding. The clinician must be especially wary of genetic determinism (e.g., "If you have the gene then you get the disease; if you do not have the gene then you do not get the disease") with multifactorial disorders. In these circumstances, patients can misunderstand and exaggerate the implications of genetic testing, not understanding that environmental or behavioral factors (e.g., diet, stress, or exercise) may play a role in the final expression of the disease. In any case, it is important to help each person feel a sense of agency about what he or she does have control over and work toward acceptance of what he or she does not. A person may be able to alter their environment, diet, or exercise behavior. They may seek preemptive treatment (e.g., having prophylactic bilateral mastectomies or taking tamoxifen before breast cancer is diagnosed) if they have a genetic mutation.

With multifactorial disorders, patients may overestimate the contribution of genetics to their overall risk profile. Prior to genetic education, they may believe they have a significant family history when in fact they do not. For example, a relative dying of a cancer of any type may be perceived by a patient as increasing his or her risk for *all* cancers. Primary care clinicians can make a significant contribution by providing education and reassurance, and avoiding unnecessary anxiety and referral. Primary care clinicians need to educate themselves about the nuances of genetic screening and testing (12), Clinicians need to know which illnesses have a genetic connection (see Table 17.1) (13), what tests are available, and which diseases can be affected by advance knowledge. In one study (14), GPs in England tended to overestimate genetic risk. These physicians acknowledged the dif-

TABLE 17.1. Common disorders with significant genetic components

Single Gene Disorders
Cystic fibrosis
Huntington's
Sickle Cell
Thalassemia
G6PD deficiency
Hemochromatosis
Hemophilia
Hypercholesterolemia
Neurofibromatosis

Multifactorial Disorders
Alzheimers
Asthma
Blood clot or pulmonary embolism
Cancers
Coronary artery disease or myocardial infarction before age 60
Depression
Diabetes
Essential hypertension

Multifactorial Conditions
Diabetes
Asthma
Epilepsy
Alcoholism or drug abuse
Birth defects
Mental retardation
Suicide

Adapted and expanded from reference 16. Used with permission.

ficulty in calculating and communicating risk to patients, and as a result were disinclined to do it. A computerized risk assessment was proposed as a solution (see the Harvard Cancer Risk, University of Texas Southwestern Medical Center CancerGene, and Cambridge University Family Genetic Web sites).

Preparing the Patient with Information: Pretest Counseling

Once the primary care clinician has screened the patient and the decision has been made to proceed with genetic testing, the next step is to provide pretest counseling. In some cases, the reason for genetic testing is to further delineate the diagnosis (e.g., breast and colon cancer) and to guide future treatment. In other cases, the purpose of testing may be to identify carrier states. In all instances, appropriate pretest counseling must preceed genetic testing. For patients living in an urban area with a strong family history and knowledge of the genetic illness, initial counseling regarding genetic screening may occur with a genetic counselor.[1] For most patients, some pretest counseling will first occur in a primary care clinician's office. For example, in providing routine prenatal genetic counseling to a couple who is not at increased risk (e.g., Bill and Sandy) the clinician may first wish to establish the usefulness of the information to the couple.

> Dr. C.: There are several rare, but serious, conditions for which we can screen in pregnancy. These problems can cause mental retardation, paralysis, shortened lifespan, and even the death of your baby. These problems include Down's syndrome, cystic fibrosis, and neural tube defects. I can explain each to you, if you'd like. But first, it's helpful for me to know ahead of time whether you would consider terminating your pregnancy if your baby had one of these conditions?

Some couples who do not want to terminate their pregnancies under any circumstances may still want testing and information. In these cases, it is important to provide patients with pamphlets and written information about the disorder. It is also worth saying:

> Dr. C.: Some parents are interested in knowing whether their baby has one of these conditions, even if they would not choose to terminate the pregnancy. Something medical can sometimes be done to improve the outcome.

Although it usually does not require extensive discussion, prenatal genetic counseling is too often rushed with comments like, "this is just a routine test." For example, a newly pregnant couple may ask a question about the purpose of maternal serum α-fetoprotein testing. If the test is negative, the clinician may manage with a "routine test" comment; however, this comment is clearly problematic when it becomes necessary to explain an abnormal test result. All patients deserve to be educated about any genetic test that is proposed for them.

Explaining the limits and capabilities of the testing process to patients can be challenging. Many patients are understandably reluctant to learn the details of false positives and false negatives, pretest probability, and variable penetrance. Clinicians may be reluctant to take the time to explain these complex concepts; however, now that the National Institutes of Health, American College of Obstetricians and Gynecologists, and American College of Medical Genetics recommend offering cystic fibrosis (CF)

---

[1] The names of certified genetics counselors may be found at www.nsgc.org.

testing to all Caucasians who are pregnant or considering conception, clinicians are required to describe at least the basics of these concepts.

> David and Alice had been living together for 3 years and had talked about having children, but did not feel quite ready. It came as a surprise when Alice's pregnancy test was positive, but the couple was happy nonetheless. They had several friends with healthy young children and had little idea what could possibly go wrong. When their clinician offered prenatal testing for cystic fibrosis at the first visit, they were shocked out of their idyllic dream of parenthood into the sober reality that something could go awry. They discovered they had quite different approaches to this stress. Alice was a "come what may" kind of person, whereas David was much more interested in information and the potential for changing a situation that was unacceptable to him. To complicate matters, Alice had a cousin with CF. In addition, the physician himself was ambivalent about the new testing guidelines. He thought the test was of low utility and unnecessarily worried parents. Explaining the test took time out of his busy schedule. His mixed feelings were communicated to David and Alice and increased their conflict. Consultation with colleagues, and a Web-based CME course, allowed this physician to help this couple understand more clearly and decide about testing in their next visit.

A difficult public health lesson was learned from sickle cell screening in the 1960s when adequate pre- and posttest counseling was not accomplished. This is a particular risk with generalized population screening. A well-intentioned push for universal screening for sickle cell anemia, fueled by tremendous excitement for the new simple technology, brought sickle cell testing to every African-American community. Virtually no pretest counseling was done, unfortunately, with little more than a short pamphlet provided. It was assumed that people who were tested would be able to understand the difference between sickle cell trait and sickle cell disease, and that many who were positive for the trait, but did not have the disease, were left desperately confused by not understanding this important difference.

The test for Tay-Sachs was developed shortly thereafter, and because of the mistakes with sickle cell testing, a concerted and extensive effort was made to ensure that adequate pretest counseling was done. Before the test was carried out, people had to demonstrate comprehension of the meaning and implications of the test. The results of this testing process were much more satisfying, with a dramatic reduction in the amount of misunderstanding that took place. The history of testing within different ethnic groups may influence the response of any given patient to the suggestion of genetic testing. In addition to cultural factors, family response can have a powerful influence on the patient's decision and experience of genetic testing. In the pretest counseling visit, it is important to ask patients to predict what their own and others' response will be to test results, whereas understanding it may be a different story when the actual result arrives. Emotions are hard to predict and the intensity is usually greater than anticipated. Genetic testing may stimulate a poignant existential awareness, and the clinician must be prepared to witness these strong sentiments in patients and family members (see Table 17.2 for the important elements involved in pretest counseling).

Genetic testing centers traditionally provide sophisticated pretest counseling. As testing becomes commonplace, however, more and more of this may occur in the primary care clinician's office, which is not unlike HIV testing. Even when the actual genetic testing takes place outside the primary care clinician's office, patients can benefit from the advance education and preparation given by the primary care clinician. Some patients may need encouragement to write down questions to bring to the genetics counselor. Taking along a family member or friend who is not biologically implicated is recommended. These companions will often remember details that the patient may not because they are less overwhelmed by the emotion of the experience.

Education about the process promotes realistic expectations and can reduce anxiety. For example, it may be helpful for patients to know that genetic testing centers usually send out an extensive precounseling questionnaire, and that the first visit takes 1–2 hours. It is rare to have testing done at that first visit (unless prenatal), and there is usually only one posttest visit. Prior to entering the testing process, patients may want to review their life and disability insurance. Multiple studies across various illnesses now show that the psychological risk posed by most genetic testing is not great (15). Collaborative care with a family therapist, however, is important early in the process for individuals or families with a history of affective disorder or other emotional or relational difficulties, or for those with an unusual amount of anxiety or ambivalence about the testing.

All results come to the patient in writing, but not necessarily to the primary care clinician, so it is important to gain patient permission to estab-

TABLE 17.2. Elements of primary care pretest genetic counseling

- Provide an explanation of false positives, false negatives, inconclusive results, and general probabilities.
- Explain the implications of a positive test result.
- Describe the potential benefits, risks, and limitations of testing.
- Ask the patient to make a prediction of how he or she will feel about positive or negative results.
- Ask the patient to make a prediction of what he or she will do depending on the results of the test, listening carefully for problematic blame and guilt.
- Ask who the patient intends to tell the results and ask for predictions about how they will react.
- Discuss confidentiality and its potential limits.
- Review alternatives to testing.
- Assess the coping styles of the patient and the family system.

lish professional lines of communication early in the process. Individuals found to be at increased risk, even if they ultimately choose not to proceed with testing, should be encouraged to enroll in clinical research programs where they are most likely to get state-of-the-art care that is frequently free.

> To return to the Murphy case, Jeanine brought Al in to see Dr. M. to discuss further whether she should proceed with BRCA testing.
>
> Dr. M.: Hello Al, good to meet you. Your being here is a nice support to Jeanine.
>
> Al: Thank you. I love Jeanine and this seems pretty important.
>
> Dr. M.: Have you all had enough time to read through the materials that I gave you?
>
> Jeanine: Yes, thank you, they were very informative. We also found some good stuff on the Internet. I didn't realize how controversial this is.
>
> Dr. M.: Maybe we should begin by you telling me what you have learned so far?
>
> Jeanine did most of the talking, but Al was clearly very involved, holding her hand, nodding, and adding various clarifications for emphasis. The imprecision of the testing, the persistence of considerable ambiguity, and the possibility of inconclusive results irritated them. They were also worried about upsetting Jeanine's aunt by asking her to take the test first.
>
> Dr. M.: You two have done an impressive job of research and frankly I feel you know about as much as I do about the testing. If you like, I can direct you to some other educational resources, including the University genetic testing center. How would you like to proceed?
>
> Jeanine (looks at Al): I think we have pretty much decided to go ahead with testing. It sounds like the University is the place to go.
>
> Dr. M.: It is. Let me tell you about how the whole process works, and I'll give you my routine advice about how to get the most out of seeing a specialist. You probably have thought about most of this already, but I want to be sure I do everything I can to be helpful. We can talk about approaching your aunt, and I should also ask about your siblings.

The pretest counseling phase is often when family members become more involved: spouses for support and extended family members to gain information about their own risk. Patterns of family rules and boundaries, along with personal beliefs about sharing medical information, will heavily influence this process. For example, some people still prefer not to disclose a history of mental illness or cancer. There may be considerable diversity in the way various family members cope with the need to know and the dispersal of information. Confidentiality in these contacts can be a delicate balance between the pursuit of reliable information and respecting the identified patient's need for privacy and autonomy. Patients in the United States have the right to confidentiality with any genetic testing. In a random survey of the populace, the vast majority (97%) stated they want to inform at-risk family members, especially when the disease may be preventable;

however, a very small number (18%) believe that physicians should inform at-risk family members against a patient's wishes (16). From the legal perspective, the clinician's "duty to warn" potentially affected family members has not fully been developed in the U.S. legal systems. Legal experts and medical ethicists debate the individual right to privacy versus the family member's right to knowledge about their own risk (ASHG Social Issues Subcommittee on Familial Disclosure) (17).

Anticipating disclosure issues should be part of pretest counseling. Whether done by a primary care clinician or a collaborating family therapist, it can take a considerable amount of coaching and discussion to decide who in the family will be involved and how any test results will be communicated. Part of pretest counseling is anticipating whom the patient will tell, and who might be affected and want to know.

> Kathy had breast cancer at age 28, just after the birth of her second child. Given her young age, Kathy decided to undergo genetic testing and found that she did have the BRCA1 mutation. This result shocked both her and her husband, and they decided to take a year to adjust before telling her extended family. Toward the end of that time, her first cousin was diagnosed with breast cancer. Kathy immediately told her cousin of her own test results. The cousin was infuriated, blaming Kathy for her cancer, and saying that if she had known perhaps she could have undergone some preventive procedures. This was unlikely given the time frame but the tension created in the family from lack of disclosure led Kathy to write a long and descriptive letter that she photocopied and sent to every family member of whom she knew.

Some physicians advocate that a family meeting be held to negotiate a "family covenant" when faced with a patient who plans to undergo genetic screening/testing (18). With the patient's agreement, this covenant allows the clinician to facilitate discussion about which family members wish to be informed about test results, and which opt out, before any screening is undertaken. The covenant is then placed in the patient's chart.

Posttest Counseling

Most test results will be delivered at a genetic testing center in tertiary care; however, those primary care clinicians who order testing are responsible for delivering test information. This section will discuss the elements of primary care posttest counseling. Even for those patients who receive the news at a testing center, some aspects of this conversation may occur at follow up soon after in primary care. Anticipating the results of genetic testing tries the patience of every patient and their family. The experience is often loaded with anxiety, trepidation, and expectation. Many variations of the anticipated conversation will have been mentally rehearsed prior to the visit. From the moment the patient arrives, he or she will be searching for clues about the result. From the receptionist, to the nurse, to the moment the clinician walks in the room, the patient wonders who knows the news. Given the anticipation, a short greeting, and perhaps a brief introduction is all that is necessary before delivering the news.

> Francisca and Julio Jiminez arrived for the posttest counseling visit frazzled and at their wit's end. Dealing with traffic and parking had been difficult and Julio was disturbed by what he thought was Francisca's strange complacence. She was certain that she would be positive for one of the BRCA mutations and this did not seem to bother her. Julio was desperately afraid of losing her and could not understand why she was not more nervous.
>
> Dr. S. (smiling): Francisca . . . Julio, nice to see you.
>
> Francisca and Julio (together): Good to see you, too.
>
> Dr. S: I have good news. The test was normal. There is no evidence for any mutation.
>
> Julio (beaming): Oh, thank you, God!
>
> Francisca (stunned and speaking slowly): Are you certain?
>
> Dr. S. (puzzled): Yes, I'm quite certain. As we discussed previously, this does not necessarily mean that you will not get breast cancer. We should still do the standard screening for someone with the high-risk family history you have.
>
> Julio: I am so happy. Thank you, doctor.
>
> Francisca (looking down and away): I. . . I. . . I. . . don't what to say.
>
> Dr. S. (concerned): Francisca, you seem pretty stunned by the news and I'm guessing that maybe you were expecting something different?
>
> Francisca: I was certain I would be positive for the mutation. My mother had breast cancer and was found to have the mutation, my aunt had breast cancer, and one of my sisters has already had breast cancer. I have thought for years that I would eventually get the disease, sooner rather than later, and have lived my life with that expectation. I guess I still feel that way. . . am certain of it. . . and I guess the result really doesn't change my thinking about this. (long pause) I would still like to go ahead with a mastectomy. I was thinking that being positive for the mutation would just make my decision easier on everyone else.

Even a negative test that brings apparent good news can be stressful to a vulnerable patient. The clinician must be sensitive to each individual's perspective and mindset. In this particular case, because of family history, Francisca had organized her self-concept around the notion that she was eventually going to get breast cancer. Her expectation was that the test would confirm her belief. The negative result would seem to require a reorganization of her self-concept. Despite the findings, however, she still maintained her desire for mastectomy to minimize the chances of contracting breast cancer. In fact, if a women's family history is strongly positive for breast cancer, being BRCA negative may only slightly decrease the likelihood that she will get breast cancer. Francisca wanted to get the test, more to help convince others of the sanity of her desire for prophylactic mastectomy, and not so much for her. The negative result ultimately did not alter her self-image, but it did leave her with less rationale to convince others, and it was about this that she was most distressed. Another example illustrates the role testing can play at times of developmental transition.

> Dick and Kathy had been dating for 2 years and were engaged to be married in 6 months. Two of Kathy's sisters had been treated for breast cancer and the third one had just been diagnosed. Kathy had previously considered BRCA testing, but eventually called it off. Her previous boyfriend, Don, had become so anxious about the prospect of Kathy getting breast cancer that he left her. In contrast, Dick understood from the beginning about Kathy's risk profile and wanted to marry her, for better or worse. "We're all at risk for something," he said.

Long-Term Follow Up

Because genetic testing centers typically offer a single posttest counseling visit, responsibility for long-term follow-up of patients falls to the primary care clinician. Because of this, primary care clinicians need to have good communication with testing centers. This means obtaining the results of genetic testing and asking to be informed as new technology and information becomes available. Most patients assume this communication will occur; however, some may be very concerned about the potential impact of having the results in the medical chart. Fears about insurance and job discrimination are widespread, although very few documented cases of discrimination have yet been reported.

In the long term, despite education during the acute testing phase, some patients do drift back to their previous perception of risk. In one study of women with family patterns of inherited breast cancer, the percentage of women with an accurate perception of their own risk went up after counseling to 31% from a baseline of 9%. One year later, the percentage of women with a correct assessment of their risk had dropped again by half, suggesting that in the absence of further counseling these women reverted to their old, inaccurate perceptions (19). As with any chronic illness, when the patient who tests positive is in the presymptomatic phase, the clinician needs to attend to the patient's changing perception and need for information, support, and guidance, even though no disease process is yet manifest. Continuity with the patient and the family will provide a continuously available resource that the patient and family can access as they need. Both the kind of help and the pace with which it is needed will vary from patient to patient, family to family, and illness to illness.

Conclusion

Genetic screening, testing, and counseling for hereditary illness is the quintessential argument for a biopsychosocial paradigm encompassing the most basic units of biology to human behavior, family, society, and the environment. Complex legal and ethical consequences need to be considered. Early in the twenty-first century, we stand at the beginning of a long process of understanding genetic factors in illness and the mainstream application of this knowledge in primary care practice. Many scientific and psychosocial issues are not yet resolved. It is difficult to keep up with new tests as they become available. There is a lag between when genetic tests make the news and when they are available through local labs and hospitals. There is also an understandable fear that the time required for adequate communication will not be available. Even so, decoding the human genome and deriving clinical applications are underway and will have far-reaching effects. A streamlined and bidirectional flow of information from cutting-edge research to geneticists to primary care clinicians to patients and their families will ensure sensible application of this new health technology.

References

1. Davidson ME, Weingarten K, Pollin TI, Wilson MA, Wilker N, & Hsu N, et al.: Consumer perspectives on genetic testing: Implications for building family-centered public policies. *Fam Syst Health* 2000;**18**(2):217–235.
2. McKusick VA: The anatomy of the human genome: a neo-vesalian basis for medicine in the 21st century. *JAMA* 2001;**286**:2289–2295.
3. Collins FS, Guttmacher AE: Genetics moves into the medical mainstream. *JAMA* 2001;**286**:2322–2324.
4. Meiser B, Halliday JL: What is the impact of genetic counseling in women at increased risk of developing hereditary breast cancer? A meta-analytic view. *Soc Sci Med* 2002;**54**:1463–1470.
5. Speice J, McDaniel SH, Rowley P, & Loader S: A family-oriented psychoeducation group for women who test positive for the BRCA1/2 mutations. *Clin Gen* 2002;**62**:121–127.
6. Cornfeld M, Miller S, Ross E, & Schneider D: Accuracy of cancer-risk assessment in primary care practice. *J Cancer Ed* 2001;**16**:92–97.
7. Bennett R: *The Practical Guide to the Genetic Family History*. New York: Wiley-Liss, 1999.
8. Rose P, Emery J: Assessment and management of genetic risk. In: *Oxford Textbook of Primary care*. Oxford, England: Oxford University Press, (In Press).
9. Coyne J, Anderson K: Marital status, marital satisfaction, and support processes among women at high risk for breast cancer. *J Fam Psychol* 1999;**13**:629–641.
10. Wyman PA, Cowen EL, Work WC, Hoyt-Myers L, & Magnus KB: Caregiving and developmental factors differentiating young at-risk urban children showing resilient versus stress-affected outcomes: a replication and extension. *Child Devel* 1999;**70**:645–659.

11. Rolland J: Families and genetic fate: a millennial challenge. In: McDaniel SH, Campbell TL (Eds): Special issue on genetic testing and the family. *Fam Syst Health* 1999;**17**(1):123–132.

12. Primary care Faculty Development: Family medicine, general internal medicine & general pediatrics. *Genetics in Primary care Training Program Curriculum Materials*. Washington DC, HRSA Contract #240-98-0020, 2001.

13. Acheson L: Managing genetic information in families, Society for Teachers of Family Medicine Annual Family in Family Medicine Meeting. San Diego, March 1, 2002.

14. Fry A, Campbell H, & Gudmundsdottir H, et al.: General practitioners views on their role in cancer genetics and current practice, *Fam Prac.*

15. Lerman C, Croyle RT, Tercyak K, & Hamann H: Genetic testing: Psychological aspects and implications. *J Clin Consult Psychol* 2002;**70**:784–797.

16. Lehmann LS, Weeks JC, Klar N, Biener L, & Garber JE: Disclosure of familial genetic information: perceptions of the duty to inform. *Am J Med* 2001;**109**: 705–711.

17. American Social of Human Genetics, Social Issues Subcommittee on Familial Disclosure: Professional disclosure of familial genetic information, 1999.

18. Doukas D, Berg J: The family covenant. *Am J Bioethics* 2001;**1**:3:2–10.

19. Emery J, Watson E, Rose P, & Andermann A: A systematic review of the literature exploring the role of primary care in genetic services. *Fam Prac* 1999;**16**(4):426–445.

Protocol

Raising the Possibility: Risk Assessment and Genetic Screening (Primary Care Clinician)

- Use genogram to track hereditary illnesses.
- Understand the meaning of the illness to the patient.
- If interested or concerned, encourage the patient to gather information about the disease and the test.
- Invite the patient to bring a significant other or other family members to discuss possibility of genetic testing.
- If appropriate, refer to a tertiary-care genetic testing center.

Preparing the Patient with Information: Pretest Counseling (Primary Care Clinician or Genetics Counselor, Mental Health Professional Also Occasionally Needed)

- Explain false positives, false negatives, and inconclusive tests and specific details of how these concepts apply to the testing under consideration.
- Understand how these concepts apply in the individual's context (i.e., pretest probability and positive predictive value of a test).
- Discuss the implications of a positive test.
- Discuss the potential benefits, risks, and limitations of testing.
- Ask patients to predict, as much as possible, how they will feel about the results of the test.
- Ask patients to predict, as much as possible, what they will do depending on the results of the test. Listen carefully for problematic issues of blame and guilt.
- Ask patients who will be told about the results and to speculate about how these people will react.
- Discuss confidentiality and its potential limits.
- Review alternatives to testing.
- Schedule for testing if patient decides to follow through.

Posttest Counseling (Primary Care Clinician Or Genetics Counselor, Mental Health Professional Also Occasionally Needed)

- Deliver results in writing.
- Have patient accompanied by a significant other that is not at risk.
- Give patient a full explanation of results in writing.
- Provide emotional support.

- Discuss alternatives directed toward early detection and/or prevention.
- Provide information concerning testing of other family members.
- Assess how the patient and family are coping with the information.
- If positive for a mutation, refer to relevant specialists, including mental health.
- If positive, check in a few days later by phone.

Long-Term Follow Up (Primary Care Clinician)

- Review results again. If relevant, review report from testing center. Provide updated information.
- Discuss the meaning of the illness and the results to the patient, partner, and family.

Appendix 1: Selected Genetic Testing Web Sites

American Medical Association: www.ama-assn.org
Centers for Disease Control: www.cdc.gov/genetics
National Newborn Screening and Genetics Resource Center: genes-r-us.uthscsa.edu. Contains Genetics in Primary Care Curriculum and web links.
National Institutes of Health: www.nih.gov
Genetic Alliance: www.geneticalliance.org. An international coalition of individuals, professionals, and genetic support organizations that work together to enhance the lives of people affected by genetic conditions.
The Genetic Resource Center: www.pitt.edu/~edugene/resource/. An online resource for genetic counseling information.
Gene Clinics: www.geneclinics.org. A clinical information resource that relates genetic testing to diagnosis, management, and counseling for inherited disorders.
Gene Tests: www.genetests.org. A genetic testing resource funded by the National Library of Medicine. Includes an introduction to genetic counseling and testing concepts.
The Genome Action Coalition: www.tgac.org. Comprised of patient advocacy, professional, research, pharmaceutical, and biotechnology organizations and companies that come together to promote genome research.
National Coalition for Health Professional Education in Genetics: www.nchpeg.org. Promotes health professional education and access to information about advances in human genetics to all health professionals.
National Center For Biotechnology Information: www.ncbi.nlm.nih.gov. Lists hereditary conditions.
National Society of Genetic Counselors, Inc.: www.nsgc.org. Lists genetic counselors.

18
The Developmental Challenges of Chronic Illness: Helping Patients and Families Cope

Families, not healthcare providers, are the primary caretakers for patients with chronic illness. They are the ones that help most with the physical demands of an illness, ranging from preparing special meals for a family member with heart disease, to assisting with insulin administration for a diabetic, to running a home dialysis machine. Families are also the primary sources of emotional and social support: the ones with whom to share the frustrations, discouragements, and despair of living with chronic illness. Families are certainly stressed by these experiences, but they can also be resources that are often overlooked. How well each family adapts to chronic illness can influence the course of the illness, as well as the relationship between patients and their clinicians. This chapter will present a comprehensive psychosocial approach to working with families with chronic physical illness, by establishing a partnership with the families and supporting them as co-providers of care.

Since the 1980s, a growing body of family research has demonstrated how family relationships have a powerful influence on the course and outcome of many chronic illnesses (1). After suffering a myocardial infarction, women who have few emotional supports have two to three times the mortality rate of other women (2). Family criticism or hostility has been shown to predict poor outcomes from diabetes, asthma, migraine headaches, and weight loss (1). The quality of the marriage of a chronically ill person has predicted survival in several chronic illnesses. Marital stress and negativity worsens survival in coronary heart disease (3) and end-stage renal disease (4). Women with breast cancer who cannot confide in their spouse have higher recurrence rates than do those who are in a confiding marriage (5). Family researcher James Coyne (6) demonstrated that marital quality is a stronger predictor of mortality in congestive heart failure than any biomedical marker, including ejection fraction.

Family relationships can influence both the physiology as well as the daily management of the chronic illnesses. Family criticism, hostility, and nagging can undermine patient's efforts to adhere to medical recommendations and make lifestyle changes. Unhappily married persons have poorer immune function than do happily married persons (7). In congestive heart failure, chronic marital conflict may result in persistent adrenergic stimulation, which has been shown to be detrimental to the heart.

Although family interventions have been shown to improve outcomes in chronic illnesses in childhood and the elderly, there are few family intervention trials in adult chronic illness (1). Diabetic control has been improved by couples or marital interventions. Gonzales, Steinglass, and Reiss (8) have developed an innovative multifamily psychoeducational group intervention for family with chronic medical illnesses and are testing it with several different illnesses. Overall, this research suggests that primary care clinicians should assess and address the quality of family relationships when caring for patients with chronic illness because these relationships have a strong influence on the course and outcomes of these illnesses.

Chronic illness affects all aspects of family life. Old and familiar patterns of family life are changed forever, shared activities are given up, and family roles and responsibilities must often change. Even though it is stressful, many families successfully care for their ill family members, while managing the other emotional, social, and functional tasks of family life. This requires that families negotiate a balance between the person with the illness and the needs of the rest of the family. Primary care clinicians can support families by discussing this balance, the stresses involved, and possible solutions to facilitate management of multiple responsibilities and care. Clinicians can also monitor families to recognize when imbalance occurs, such that the needs of the ill person, the caregivers, or other family members are not being met. The following example illustrates some family challenges of coping with a serious chronic illness.

Jim Prusky was a 33-year-old machinist of Russian descent. He had not felt well since his mid-twenties, but it was not until age 32 and he had some vision loss in one eye that the diagnosis of multiple sclerosis was made. He had attributed his chronic fatigue and depression to dissatisfaction and stress from working on the assembly line. His primary care physician initially diagnosed his leg weakness and gait disturbance as a herniated lumbar disc. He and his 30-year-old wife, Harriet, had undergone sex therapy for his erectile dysfunction. Although therapy helped their sexual relationship, his erections did not return, despite his use of Viagara. Their 4- and 6-year-old boys did not understand what was happening to their father, who no longer wrestled with them after work or carried them around on his shoulders. Timmy, the youngest, began having behavior problems at nursery school.

Jim and Harriet's relief about knowing what was "wrong" was balanced by a lack of effective treatment and poor prognosis. Over the next few years, Jim was in and out of the hospital with acute exacerbations of the illness. He initially recovered from each new neurological deficit, and he and his family maintained hope that he would stabilize; however, he gradually became more disabled and had to quit his job when he could no longer safely work on the assembly line. Harriet returned to work as a librarian, and Jim cared for the children after school.

With time, family life revolved more and more around Jim's illness. There was no longer time or money for going out to movies or restaurants, and many of their friends stopped asking them over for meals. Jim was self-conscious about using a walker in public and stopped going out to the grocery store or to the children's school. Harriet worried constantly about Jim's health and encouraged him to rest as much as possible. At the same time she resented how little housework he did, and felt physically and emotionally burdened by all of her responsibilities. She began developing migraine headaches that occasionally incapacitated her.

For most people in good health, their bodies are a given. For people with a chronic illness, their bodies, and therefore their illnesses, are always with them (9). How is it that some people carry their illnesses in the forefront at all times, such that their illnesses fully define themselves and their interactions, whereas others acknowledge their illness, but also engage fully in other aspects of life? There are unfortunately no individual personality factors or family coping experiences that easily predict how people will cope. Each patient and family requires a careful assessment.

Assessment occurs over many visits, but usually requires convening the family, perhaps around the initial diagnosis, or during an acute initial hospitalization (see Chaps. 7 and 24). Meeting with the household is also helpful after the initial crisis, when the family has settled into the day-to-day demands of living with chronic illness. Family meetings allow opportunities for education, as well as assessment about the psychosocial stresses of the particular illness, and the family's experience, beliefs, stressors, and strengths. Each of these illness and family characteristics should be components of family assessment.

Family Assessment

Illness Characteristics

It is critical to recognize that every illness produces unique stresses. Rolland (10) has developed a psychosocial typology of chronic illness that delineates how the following illness characteristics influence the specific kinds of adaptations that families will have to make.

1. Onset: Did the illness begin suddenly or gradually?

Illnesses with acute onset (e.g., strokes or spinal cord injuries) require rapid mobilization of resources and put enormous acute stress on a family.

Illnesses with gradual onset (e.g., lupus or arthritis) allow families more time to adapt, but may create great uncertainty and anxiety.

2. Course: Is the illness progressive, constant, or relapsing?

For slowly progressive diseases (e.g., chronic obstructive pulmonary disease or AIDS), the patient has gradually increasing needs for assistance, with corresponding increases in family role changes. A different family experience occurs with constant course illnesses (e.g., strokes or amputations) in which the family learns to cope with a stable change. A third pattern occurs with relapsing illnesses (e.g., hemophilia or asthma) in which families shift back and forth from crisis orientation to chronic adaptation. These illnesses demand the most flexibility.

3. Prognosis: Is the illness rapidly fatal, does it shorten lifespan, or is there a risk of sudden death?

Fatal illnesses (e.g., amyotrophic lateral sclerosis or terminal cancer) require that the family cope with impending death. Illnesses with a risk of sudden death (e.g., coronary artery disease) add an additional stress of unpredictability and constant vigilance.

4. Disability: What are the physical or mental limitations associated with the illness?

The degree to which the disability affects the roles and responsibilities of the patient will influence family stress and adaptation. A physically disabling illness in a man who works as a laborer will be much more difficult for both the patient and family than a similar disability in a school teacher. Loss of cognitive abilities (e.g., in dementia or some strokes) is often one of the most difficult burdens for families (11).

Medical knowledge of disease course and prognosis allows clinicians to consider the likely stresses and demands facing a family. The often gradual onset of multiple sclerosis (MS), for example, may result in initial confusion, anxiety, and sometimes denial. There can often be a paradoxical sense of relief when the diagnosis is finally made, although the challenge of unpredictability remains. The stepwise decline is recognized each time that a new limitation occurs, and family members may experience a repeat crisis. A clinician should be able to educate families about the unique stresses for any illness and help anticipate how they will need to cope with those specific demands.

Family Developmental Stage

The hopeful expectation for most people is that they will become ill, if at all, only near the end of their life. There are certain times in the life cycle when illness and disability are expected and more easily integrated. The clinician can assess and educate families by helping families think about how illness stressors are related to their family life cycle (10,12).

1. What is the current stage of the family life cycle?

Illnesses that are completely unexpected or "out of phase" (e.g., cancer in children or multiple sclerosis in young adults) are usually more disruptive than are gradual progressive illnesses in an older adult. The impact of a parent's serious illness will similarly be very different if the children are very young, adolescent, or adult.

2. How are family developmental tasks impacted by the illness?

Chapter 3 described how family developmental stages either pull for more family connectedness ("centripetal") as during the childbearing years, or pull apart ("centrifugal"), as when children are leaving home (13, see Fig. 3.1). If a chronic illness occurs during a centripetal phase of development (e.g., severe childhood illness), the family may respond by pulling toward one another rather than moving toward greater individuation. Minuchin and colleagues (14) have described psychosomatic families of children with diabetes, asthma, and anorexia nervosa, in which an extreme form of this pattern of overinvolvement may exacerbate the illness. In a scenario more common to primary care, a father may not allow his daughter with asthma to visit other children's homes. From the father's perspective, he worries about animal hair or mold and a possible asthma attack. From an outside perspective, the family looks overly protective. The likelihood is that most parents have reason to be very protective when their children have significant illness, and may appear to be overly protective. The challenge is to recognize the tendency for overinvolvement and help families work to balance the need for illness care with growth of all family members.

The centripetal forces of the illness can be particularly disruptive when chronic illness occurs in a centrifugal period (e.g., adolescence). The adolescent may be pushing for autonomy in all aspects of life, including illness care, whereas the parents want reassurance that the illness is being controlled. Houser (15) has described diabetes, with its demands for strict adherence to diet, exercise, and insulin injects, as an "anti-adolescent" illness because the care needed for the illness is in contrast to the spontaneity desired by adolescents.

> Dr. K., a family physician, had cared for the Prusky family for 10 years, and had delivered their two children. He knew this couple had a strong marital relationship prior to having children, but initially had some problems parenting their first child. Jim was very strict about discipline, just as his father had been, and Harriet tried to compensate by being lenient. With some brief primary care counseling, they had been able to assume more balanced roles in disciplining.

With Jim and Harriet's preoccupation after Jim's diagnosis of MS, their youngest son, Timmy, began to have behavioral problems both at nursery school and at home. Jim again felt that Harriet was too lenient with Timmy and became very strict and authoritarian. The couple noticed their increased conflict, the worsening of Timmy's behavior, and brought him to Dr. K. for help. In one session, Dr. K. helped the parents find ways to pay special attention to both children in the midst of all the illness-related stresses. This reduced the need for either child to resort to misbehavior to get their parents' attention.

Family Health Beliefs

Physician and anthropologist Arthur Kleinman (16) has made an important distinction between illness and disease. Disease describes the medical condition, whereas the illness experience includes "how the sick person and members of the family or wider social network perceive, live with, and respond to symptoms and disability" (p. 3). The perception of illness includes the appraisal of severity, and the meaning that the disease has for the patient and family. This attention to meaning is a significant component of medical family therapy treatments of families with health problems (10,12). Nursing researchers Wright, Watson, and Bell (17), have written about how family members can recognize and modify their implicit and explicit health beliefs. Discussing family health beliefs is a natural extension of primary care, in which any history of a patient's symptoms usually includes questions about patient perceptions. Family assistance includes assessing the agreement and variety of health beliefs among family members.

1. What does each family member think caused the illness?

Health beliefs usually reflect a combination of knowledge about disease (e.g., an understanding of cardiac risk factors), personal views of health and illness, and religious and cultural beliefs. Health beliefs may be quite idiosyncratic and not internally consistent. A woman may believe that illness in general is largely a matter of chance, but that her husband developed heart disease because of stress at work. It is clarifying to identify the unique views held by each family member about health in general and about this particular illness episode. Some common beliefs about the etiology of illness include:

Fate or bad luck.
Blame for inadequate self-care (e.g., smoking, lack of exercise).
Blame for past misdeeds (e.g., an illegitimate birth, divorce).
Blaming other family members (e.g., "Your drinking made me ill," or, "I get chest pain whenever we fight").
Genetics (e.g., "Cancer runs in our family").
Medical maltreatment (e.g., "I got lung cancer after my endoscopy").
Religion (e.g., "It's God's will").

2. What do family members believe they or others can do to improve the patient's health?

A family's sense of control about an illness may be quite different than their beliefs about its etiology. A family may believe that the illness is the result of past misdeeds, but that there is nothing they can do to control the illness; or that the disease occurred by chance, but the individual is responsible for maintaining the best health possible. *Agency* (18, 19, 12) or self-efficacy is the sense of active involvement one can have in their own health care. These terms are preferable to "control" because chronic illness has many aspects that cannot be controlled.

3. How do family members believe that the clinician can be helpful?

Families will have different beliefs about how much influence the clinician or medicine in general has on the illness. This is the area in which personal and cultural beliefs about illness and treatment are significant. Some families will expect the clinician to be responsible for illness care and even blame the clinician when the illness is diagnosed or worsens.

> After his diagnosis, Jim read extensively about MS, especially its etiology and treatment. He became especially concerned about whether he had been exposed to heavy metals in his job. When a co-worker also developed MS, he solicited Dr. K.'s help in getting an occupational health expert to study their plant.
>
> Harriet became interested in dietary treatments for MS. Jim tried a gluten-free diet for 6 months. Although it was time consuming, expensive, and not always very tasty, the couple felt that at least they were doing something to try to get better. Although Dr. K. informed them that there was no solid evidence that such a diet would help, he told them it could do no harm and was worth a try.

Multigenerational Patterns of Coping with Illness

The ways in which individuals and families cope with chronic illness are often passed down from one generation to another. There may be family myths, expectations, or rituals that surround illness and go back many years. An understanding of how previous generations have dealt with illness may help predict future adaptations.

- How have previous generations responded to serious chronic physical or mental illness?

This information can be elicited by obtaining a family genogram. Ask about illnesses in the family going back at least three generations, and some brief ideas about how different family members coped. Look for repeating patterns (e.g., denial of the illness, over- or under-functioning of the ill person, and family coalitions that developed around the illness). Although this can be done with the patient alone, family input and corroboration is usually more efficient and valuable.

> The Pruskys' genogram (Figure 18.1) revealed little information about Jim's family history. His father and mother had both come to the United States from Poland, and their parents had been hard-working people who died of "natural causes" in their sixties and seventies. Jim's father was nearing retirement, and his mother was healthy. Harriet's maternal grandfather had suffered a severe stroke in his early thirties and her grandmother was his caretaker for more than 20 years. Harriet's mother, Emily, had an excessively close relationship with her mother, and only left home and married after her father died. Harriet feared that Jim would become similarly dependent upon her, and she did not want to become a martyr like her grandmother and mother. She also worried about the impact of Jim's illness on their children's development.

Other Stress and Demands on the Family

• What other kinds of stressor strains are occurring for the family?

A chronic illness is a major stress on families, but families commonly face numerous stresses simultaneously. Additional stressful life events will influence the family's ability to cope with the chronic illness. Ask about specific stressors, including:

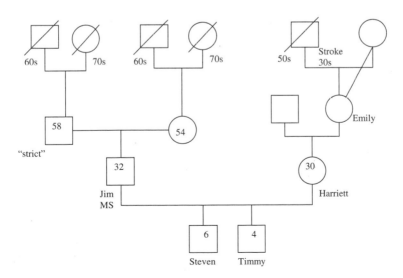

FIGURE 18.1. The Prusky family.

- recent deaths, hospitalizations, other serious illness
- marital distress or recent divorce
- financial or work problems, especially unemployment or the threat of unemployment.

Even positive life events or normal life cycle changes can be quite stressful, including:

- a new baby
- a recent marriage
- a job promotion.

> Shortly before Jim's MS was diagnosed, he was promoted to a supervisor on the assembly line. Although the job provided more income, it involved more responsibilities and required that he walk up and down the line, troubleshooting any problems that arose. As his illness progressed, his job became more stressful and exhausting, until he could no longer safely do his work. There were unfortunately no sedentary jobs he could transfer to, so he was considered disabled and laid off from work.

Family Strengths and Supports

Assessments all too often focus on deficits and neglect strengths. Identifying family strengths and resources makes care plans more relevant. The process of discussing strengths also reinforces a family's sense of competence and hope.

1. What are the family's strengths and sources of support?

Strengths and resources include people, patterns of coping, material, and spiritual support. Who and what does the family turn to for support? Does the family feel pride in its ability to solve problems and access resources?

2. What has helped the family cope with crises in the past?

Reviewing past crises helps identify what kinds of coping strategies have been used before. It can remind families of what they can do with this new crisis.

3. How adaptable is the family to change?

Has the family been able to make the necessary changes in role functioning with this illness? What are the signs of their ability to do so? Can they think of other changes that they may need for the near future?

4. Does the family accept outsiders, especially healthcare providers, into the family to help?

Some families close ranks around an ill member and are suspicious of healthcare providers, whereas other families can become excessively dependent upon the healthcare system. This style may represent the family's way of accepting help or dealing with outsiders, or it may be the result of a previous experience with the healthcare system that either did not respond to the family's needs or assumed too much responsibility for their problems.

> Dr. K. met with the Pruskys every 3 or 4 months to review Jim's medical condition and see how the family was doing. During an early session, Dr. K. had the family list and discuss their strengths. These strengths were:
>
> - a loving and caring marital relationship
> - equal sharing of family responsibilities
> - flexibility in family roles
> - a small group of close friends
> - a supportive extended family, many of whom lived in the area
> - a good working relationship with health care professionals.
>
> Dr. K. encouraged them to draw upon these strengths and support when they developed difficulties.

Primary care clinicians monitor these family concerns over time. Families will vary over time in their coping abilities, but an ongoing assessment provides a window to observe caregiving stress. The following characteristic warning signs for families with chronic illness may indicate that a family can benefit from primary care counseling.

1. The illness and its demands tend to dominate family life, and other family needs are neglected.

When a new illness occurs or when a crisis erupts with an ongoing illness, it is expected and adaptive for families to focus on the crisis. When illnesses become chronic, however, families should move from this crisis mode to a long-term adaptation that allows them to handle the demands of all family members.

2. There are inappropriate family coalitions between the patient and one or more family members, or previous coalitions are intensified by the chronic illness.

This can happen, for example, if a mother becomes excessively involved in the personal life of her adolescent son who has diabetes, whereas the father may withdraw or be excluded (9).

3. The family's coping response often becomes rigid.

The family fears that any change may adversely affect the family and their current adjustment. This is particularly likely when the illness experience includes unpredictable crises. For example, a wife whose husband has been coping well with MS for 2 years may not visit family out of state because she fears that could set off a change in her husband's condition.

4. The family is increasingly isolated from friends and extended family.

Families can get tired of making explanations about the illness to others. They may not want to bother others with their problems, or they may not feel that others can fully understand their difficulties. It may be easier to interact less frequently with others, and a pattern of increasing isolation can spiral.

Helping Families Cope with Chronic Illness

A primary care family-oriented approach to chronic illness shares some principles from the clinical approaches of psychoeducation (20) and medical family therapy (12). These models assume that patients and their families do their best to cope with the demands of chronic illness and have many, perhaps untapped, resources. Families are viewed as informed partners in the treatment process. Key elements of this approach are support and education. Psychological and social support is a significant benefit of the family–clinician relationship. Supportive relationships provide empathy, an opportunity to share feelings, and an assessment of how the family is coping, including referrals, if necessary, to mental health professionals.

Families with chronic illness often feel blamed by themselves, friends, or even health professionals for difficulties they experience. A primary care clinician can remind families that they have been "hit by lightning," and that they are coping with losses, new patterns of activity, and uncertainty that makes old family patterns ineffective. When families feel that they are not coping well, a suggestion that they could use counseling can feel like further failure. A primary care approach can be framed as an additional resource that most families coping with illness can use. In this approach, families should know they are part of the solution, rather than part of the problem. Specific strategies for education and support follow.

Provide Education and Help with Problem Solving

Clinicians should help patients and their families become experts on the illness, and partners in the treatment process. Studies have shown that family members want more information about illness in their family (21) and that having knowledge about an illness gives patients and families a better sense of agency about how to manage the illness. Families can be encouraged to shift from a passive to a more active stance in dealing with the illness. The active stance can be reinforced by helping families discuss specific plans and possibilities.

For some illnesses, the clinician may not have the time or the knowledge to educate families fully about the illness. The clinician can instead point to sources of reliable information, including other specialists, readings, Web sites, classes, or consumer groups. Suggestions of further information are best made when the clinician has learned what the patient and family already know, and the family's preferred methods of education.

Understanding how behaviors are symptoms of the disease can be very helpful for families. In MS, for example, a patient's irritability or forgetfulness may be interpreted as willful and negative behavior. Families may then respond in unhelpful or angry ways that perpetuate conflict and negative patterns. Knowing that these behaviors may be characteristics of the illness may help families respond in more empathic and helpful ways.

> Dr. K. learned that Jim and Harriet had read extensively and were quite knowledgeable about MS. In addition to answering their questions, he referred them to the local MS association. There they joined a monthly support group and met other couples and families who were dealing with different stages of the illness. They were able to share their frustrations and sorrow and learn very specific and practical coping skills. From other patients with MS, they learned that Jim's difficulty concentrating and his sensitivity to temperature changes were common in the illness.

Help Remove Blame, and Accept Unacceptable Feelings

Patients and family members go through stages of dealing with chronic illness that are often similar to those dealing with death: shock, denial, anger, bargaining, grief, and acceptance. Each person, however, may be at different stages in dealing with or accepting the illness. Some may deny aspects of the illness or be angry, whereas others are grieving, and a family member may go back and forth between stages. Because of the personal demands of illness the patient is often ahead of the rest of the family in dealing with the illness, which can create conflicts.

Family members will rarely initiate discussion of these concerns, but can be reassured when a clinician states that these are normal responses and invites discussion:

> "Many families who are coping with illness find themselves feeling resentful about other people who seem to have no health problems. Does that ever happen to you all?"

Initiating these conversations allows discussion of things that are usually unacceptable for conversation. These comments also let families know that they can bring up other concerns that are not easily discussed.

> For the Pruskys, Harriet's efforts to get Jim to look at the bright side of this illness were partly because she was still trying to deny the seriousness of the illness, whereas Jim was grieving the loss of his health. Dr. K. was able to help Jim and Harriet realize that both views were helpful at different times, and that they could share their views without trying to convince one another about who was correct.

Blame is one of the stages that deserves special attention. As discussed in the section on health beliefs, patients and family members often feel blame about what caused the illness. This can extend to blame about why the patient is not coping better with the illness. There is important work about how people's attitudes can impact their disease. Bernie Siegel's work (22) has especially given patients hope in the face of terrible diagnoses. This work taken to extreme, however, can elicit blame—that the person has not had a sufficiently strong will or made enough changes to make a difference. It can be shared among family members who can feel that they have not been strong enough, supportive enough, or decreased stresses sufficiently to make it possible for the person to be coping better with their illness.

Normalize Common Family Responses to Illness

Families are reassured to learn that their responses and feelings are "normal." Some information about family life cycle and illness response can help parents understand why their adolescent seems so unwilling to take her asthma medicine regularly. Listing the multiple family demands and stressors that a family is experiencing helps families think that they are doing well in the face of difficulties. Discussion about "ambiguous loss" (23) helps families realize that it is expected that they will mourn some aspects of their previous life. This "normalizing function" is one of the benefits of support groups and internet support groups of others experiencing the same or similar illnesses.

1. Encourage the family to openly discuss the illness and their emotional responses.

Most families do not often talk about the chronic illness, except the most pragmatic aspects of day-to-day coping (8). It is common for families to feel overwhelmed, angry, and depressed about the illness, but to be reluctant to share those feelings, fearing that it will put more burdens on the patient. Encouraging the honest discussion of feelings at a family conference can have a very powerful and therapeutic effect upon the patient and family. A single experience of sharing feelings in a safe environment sometimes allows families to open up and communicate emotional reactions that have been suppressed for years. Families can be referred for medical family therapy if family conflict or significant negative affect occurs. Some ways to facilitate family communication include the following points.

2. Ask directly about their experience.

"What has it been like for all of you to deal with your mother's illness day after day and week after week?"

3. Elicit and empathize with feelings associated with the family's specific problems concerning the illness.

When a family member describes a problem, ask, "That sounds pretty tough, how do you feel about having to face that every day?"

4. Inquire about common emotional responses.

"Jim, do you ever get angry at Harriet for being healthy and able to do the things you cannot?" or "Harriet, how often do you feel guilty about being healthy when your husband has been so ill?"

5. Ask the patient or a family member what kind of feelings they have seen in other family members.

"Jim, how has Harriet dealt with your illness?" or "Who in this family is the most upset about Jim's illness?"

6. Help family members accept the patient's feelings.

It is natural to want to help patients to feel better. Attempts to cheer people up or distract them can be helpful, but they can also be well-intentioned but complicated. Attempts to cheer someone up who is discouraged or depressed can sometimes make that person feel misunderstood and more alone and depressed.

> Jim: I am so discouraged! None of these treatments seem to help at all, and I keep getting weaker and weaker. Sometimes I just want to give up and stop everything.
> Harriet: Don't say that, Jim. You haven't had as many relapses since you've been on Cytoxan, and your vision seems a bit better.
> Dr. K.: Harriet, it sounds like it's difficult for you to hear how discouraged Jim is at times about his illness.

Enhance the Family's Sense of Agency: Help the Family Determine What Can Be Changed and Accept What They Cannot Control

Illness is always an out-of-control condition. Many respond to this by either trying to increase control over aspects of their life; others experience anxiety, powerlessness, and uncertainty in multiple aspects of their life. Agency is the personal sense that one can make choices in dealing with illness and the healthcare system even in the face of uncertainty (12, 18). Enhancing agency means things like increasing involvement in one's care, or setting limits on a family member's "helpfulness." Education, making choices about treatment, or specific involvement of others enhances sense of agency.

Help the Family Become Effective Advocates

Most serious chronic illnesses involved extended and repeated contact with multiple medical specialists and community agencies. The primary care clinician can help the family work effectively within the healthcare system and become empowered and assertive, without being overly demanding or alienating providers. When the patient or family encounter roadblocks or problems in getting information or appropriate medical care, it is most helpful for the primary care physician to suggest ways that the family can proceed, rather than directly intervening to solve the problem. If the family is able to solve the problem, their self-confidence will increase and they will be able to deal more effectively with similar problems in the future. For example, if the family does not feel they have received sufficient information from a surgeon about a planned operation, the primary care physician should encourage the family to call the surgeon and explain that they need this information before proceeding further. This will be more helpful than having the primary care clinician become the go-between with the specialist and the family. Advocacy can also be enhanced through family contact with professional organizations, their websites, and family discussion groups.

> Through the MS association, the Pruskys learned of an experimental treatment for MS being studied at a medical center 150 miles from their town. They sent for information on the treatment and reviewed it with Dr. K. They visited the medical center and learned the details of the study from the investigators. Finally, Jim decided not to enter the study because the treatment seemed too risky, without enough promise for success, and required frequent and inconvenient trips to the medical center.

Facilitate the Family's Involvement in the Care of the Patient Through Negotiations with the Patient

Most families would like to assist the patient in the care of his or her illness, but sometimes have difficulty negotiating an optimal plan. Clinicians can discourage family conflict by helping family members be available for assistance while respecting the patient's right for autonomy. This is done in two ways:

1. Encourage all appropriate family members to learn specific skills involved in the care of the patient.

A patient can teach others how to do certain tasks (e.g., drawing up insulin syringes or giving injections if the patient is sick or begins to lose vision). Even when the family members will not be responsible for a task, learning about specific procedures (e.g., how to change the colostomy bag) can help normalize the disability.

2. Have the patient tell other family members how they can help.

Patients should remain in charge of their illnesses, except when they are incompetent. Problems arise when family members try to decide what is best for the patient or try to help in ways that feel intrusive to the patient. Negotiating how the family can help can reinforce the members' interests in helping as well as the patient's autonomy.

> Dr. K.: Jim, it sounds like getting dressed in the morning can be quite difficult. Would you like Harriet's help with any of it?
> Jim: Yeah, I guess so.
> Harriet: Well I try to help him every morning, and he just snaps at me.
> Jim: Well, I'm not an invalid!
> Dr. K.: Jim, could you tell Harriett what kind of things you want her to help you with?
> Jim: She could start by not treating me like I'm an invalid. . .
> Dr. K.: Well—this often happens when spouses want to help each other, but they don't want to make the other feel badly. Could you think about specific things that you'd like help with?
> Jim: The one thing I have trouble with is putting on my ankle brace.
> Dr. K.: Is there anything else you'd like her to help with?
> Jim: No, I can handle the rest.
> Dr. K.: Are there things you would prefer that Harriet not do for you?
> Jim: Yes, I don't like her hovering around me asking if she can help me get dressed.
> Dr. K.: Harriet, what do you think about all of that?
> Harriet: I don't mean to hover. I really just want to help when it looks so difficult.
> Dr. K.: That makes a lot of sense. It's really important that you two feel comfortable checking with one another because things can change. But right now, Jim, you'd prefer to get dressed yourself no matter how long that takes you, correct?
> Jim: That's right. I appreciate this, Harriet.

Help the Family Balance the Demands of the Illness and the Needs of Family Members

Encourage the family to normalize family life as much as possible, by only changing those aspects of family life that must be altered. From discussion groups with families with chronic illness, Gonzalez, Steinglass, and Reiss (8) describe the importance of "putting the illness in it's place." This powerful image is a way of stating that the patient's illness is only one aspect of family life, and that other aspects should be encouraged. This allows a creative and often light-hearted discussion of ways to maintain family routines and rituals, and encourage family activities with recognition, but in spite, of the illness.

Family members will often view this as being selfish (i.e., "How can I think about myself when he/she is so sick?"). It can be explained that taking care of one's own needs is necessary in order to be able to care for the ill family member. A focus on family activities other than illness is helpful for family members and for the person with illness. The challenge for the family is to find an appropriate balance between caring for the illness and caring for the family. This balance requires ongoing reassessment.

> Dr. K: Jim, in the process of helping you with your illness, do you think Harriet is taking good care of herself?
>
> Jim: No, and I worry about that. She used to have lunch with her friends every Wednesday, and now she comes home to check on me. I wish she wouldn't sacrifice those lunches.

Encourage Connections with Others

As families move from acute illness crisis to the chronic care stage, they can become increasingly isolated from others. They may tire of not being able to make plans, or feel that it is too much trouble to arrange contact with others. Other friends and family may want to help but do not know how, so they may call or visit less frequently. McDaniel, Hepworth, and Doherty describe the importance of enhancing communion (12, 19), the emotional connections to others that are frayed by the demands of illness. The primary care clinician can ask about contacts with others, and encourage families to maintain relationships, and accept the resources that others are willing to provide.

Identify Families Requiring Referral for Medical Family Therapy

Because of the enormous changes required, most families dealing with serious chronic illness can benefit from supportive family counseling at some point during the illness course. Clinicians can offer this to all families as a possible resource rather than a statement that they are not doing well and need therapy. Some families, however, should be strongly encouraged to seek specialized mental health treatment (see Chap. 25). Specific indications for referral include:

Poor management or complications of the illness.
The development of any serious psychiatric disorder (e.g., severe anxiety, depression, or suicidal thinking).
Illness or symptoms in other family members.
Emotional disturbance in other family members (e.g., depression, anxiety, school or work problems, chronic insomnia).
Family, marital, or sexual problems.

Jim became withdrawn and depressed 2 years after diagnosis, and Harriet's migraine headaches became incapacitating. Despite Dr. K.'s counseling during office visits, the couple fought more about Harriet's attempts to help Jim, which only made him more angry and withdrawn. Dr. K. suggested that they might benefit from seeing a counselor on a more regular basis to deal with the tremendous stresses related to the illness. The couple agreed and sought treatment with a medical family therapist for several months. Throughout that time, they continued to see Dr. K. for medication management and support. They recognized that their living situation had not drastically changed, but they were better able to support one another and their children.

Chronic illness is increasingly an expected part of the life course of families. It is often a crisis that severely stresses families and threatens to disrupt them. The shared experience of coping with chronic illness is also an opportunity for growth; to become closer and develop new and healthier patterns of interaction. As family members face their fears and uncertainties, they can also discover the importance of one another, and the valued aspects of their lives. A clinician is one of the few who can intimately share this journey with patients and families. A clinician who is willing to listen, to talk honestly, and to provide needed information and support to both patients and their families, can make this journey easier for all.

References

1. Campbell TL: Family interventions in physical disorder. In: Sprenkle D (Ed): *Effectiveness Research in Marriage and Family Therapy.* Alexandria, VA: American Association of Marriage and Family Therapy, 2002.
2. Berkman LF, Leo Summers L, & Horwitz RI: Emotional support and survival after myocardial infarction. A prospective, population-based study of the elderly. *Ann Intern Med* 1992;**117**:1003–1009.
3. Orth-Gomer K, Wamala SP, Horsten M, Schenck-Gustafsson K, Schneiderman N, & Mittleman MA: Marital stress worsens prognosis in women with coronary heart disease: the Stockholm Female Coronary Risk Study. *JAMA* 2000;**284**: 3008–3014.
4. Kimmel PL, Peterson RA, Weihs KL, Shidler N, Simmens SJ, Alleyne S, et al.: Dyadic relationship conflict, gender, and mortality in urban hemodialysis patients. *J Am Soc Nephrol* 2000;**11**:1518–1525.
5. Weihs KL, Enright TM, Simmens SJ, & Reiss D: Negative affectivity, restriction of emotions, and site of metastases predict mortality in recurrent breast cancer. *J Psychosom Res* 2000;**49**:59–68.
6. Coyne JC, Rohrbaugh MJ, Shoham V, Sonnega JS, Nicklas JM, & Cranford JA: Prognostic importance of marital quality for survival of congestive heart failure. *Am J Cardiol* 2001;**88**:526–529.
7. Kiecolt-Glaser JK, Newton TL: Marriage and health: his and hers. *Psychol Bull* 2001;**127**:472–503.
8. Gonzalez S, Steinglass P, & Reiss D: Putting the illness in its place: discussion groups for families with chronic medical illnesses. *Fam Proc* 1989;**28**:69–87.

9. Shuman R: *The Psychology of Chronic Illness: The Healing Work of Patients, Therapists and Families*. New York: Basic Books, 1996.
10. Rolland J: *Families, Illness and Disability: An Integrative Treatment Model*. New York: Basic Books, 1994.
11. Houlihan JP: Families caring for frail and demented elderly: a review of selected findings. *Fam Syst Med* 1987;**5**:344–356.
12. McDaniel SH, Doherty WJ, & Hepworth J: *Medical Family Therapy: A Biopsychosocial Approach to Families with Health Problems*. New York: Basic Books, 1992.
13. Combrinck-Graham L: A developmental model for family systems. *Fam Proc* 1985;**24**:139–150.
14. Minuchin S, Rosman BL, & Baker L: *Psychosomatic Families: Anorexia Nervosa in Context*. Cambridge, MA: Harvard University Press, 1978.
15. Houser S: personal communication, Hilton Head, 1988.
16. Kleinman A: *The Illness Narratives: Suffering, Healing and the Human Condition*. New York: Basic Books, 1988.
17. Wright L, Watson W, & Bell J: *Beliefs: The Heart of Healing in Families and Illness*. New York: Basic Books, 1996.
18. Totman R: *Social Causes of Illness*. New York: Pantheon Books, 1979.
19. Bakan D: *The Duality of Human Existence*. Chicago: Rand McNally, 1969.
20. Anderson CM, Reiss DJ, & Hogarty G: *Schizophrenia and the Family*. New York: Guilford Press, 1986.
21. Morisky DE, Levine DM, Green LW, et al.: Five year blood pressure control and mortality following health education for hypertensive patients. *Am J Public Health* 1983;**73**:153–162.
22. Siegel BS: *Love, Medicine and Miracles*. New York: Harper and Row, 1986.
23. Boss P, Caron W, Horbal J, & Mortimer J: Predictors of depression in caregivers of dementia patients: Boundary ambiguity and mastery. *Fam Proc* 1990;**29**: 245–254.

Protocol: Helping Patients and Families Cope with Chronic Illness

Family Assessment

Illness Characteristics

- Onset: Did the illness begin suddenly or, gradually?
- Course: Is the illness progressive, constant, or relapsing?
- Prognosis: Is the illness rapidly fatal, does it shorten lifespan, or is there a risk of sudden death?
- Disability: What are the physical or mental limitations associated with the illness?

Family Developmental Stage

- What is the current stage of the family life cycle?
- How are family developmental tasks impacted by the illness?

Family Health Beliefs

What does each family member think caused the illness?

- Fate or bad luck.
- Blame for inadequate self-care (e.g., smoking, lack of exercise).
- Blame for past misdeeds (e.g., an illegitimate birth, divorce).
- Blaming other family members. "Your drinking made me ill," "I get chest pain whenever we fight."
- Genetics: "Cancer runs in our family."
- Medical maltreatment "I got lung cancer after my endoscopy."
- Religion: "It's God's will."

What do family members believe they or others can do to improve the patient's health? How do family members believe that the clinician can be helpful?

Multigenerational Patterns of Coping with Illness

Other Stress and Demands on the Family

Family Strengths and Supports

What are the family's strengths and sources of support?
What has helped the family cope with crises in the past?
How adaptable is the family to change?
Does the family accept outsiders, especially healthcare providers, into the family to help?

Warning Signs for Families with Chronic Illness

1. The illness and its demands tend to dominate family life and other family needs are neglected.
2. There are inappropriate family coalitions between the patient and one or more family members, or previous coalitions are intensified by the chronic illness.
3. The family's coping response often becomes rigid.
4. The family is increasingly isolated from friends and extended family.

Helping Families Cope

Provide Education and Help with Problem Solving

Help Remove Blame, and Accept Unacceptable Feelings

Normalize Common Family Responses to Illness

Encourage the Family to Discuss the Illness and Their Emotional Responses Openly

- Ask directly about their experience.
- Elicit and empathize with feelings associated with the family's specific problems concerning the illness.
- Inquire about common emotional responses.
- Ask the patient or a family member what kind of feelings they have seen in other family members.
- Help family members accept the patient's feelings.

Enhance the Family's Sense of Agency: Help the Family Determine What Can be Changed and Accept What They Cannot Control

Help the Family Become Effective Advocates

Facilitate the Family's Involvement in the Care of the Patient Through Negotiations with the Patient

- Encourage all appropriate family members to learn specific skills involved in the care of the patient.
- Have the patient tell other family members how they can help.

Help the Family Balance the Demands of the Illness and the Needs of Family Members

Encourage Connections with Others

Identify Families Requiring Referral for Medical Family Therapy

- Poor management or complications of the illness.

- The development of any serious psychiatric disorder (e.g., severe anxiety, depression, or suicidal thinking).
- Illness or symptoms in other family members.
- Emotional disturbance in other family members (e.g., depression, anxiety, school or work problems, or chronic insomnia).
- Family, marital, or sexual problems.

19
Integrating the Mind–Body Split: A Biopsychosocial Approach to Somatic Fixation

SECOND THOUGHTS

It's five o' five
day's almost done.
All the patients seen
but one.

I stand outside
the exam room door,
read the nurse's note
with horror.

"New patient says
teeth itch at night,
stomach aches when shoes
too tight.

"Numbness starting
in the knee.
dizziness
since '63.

"Food goes up
instead of down,
always tired,
lies around. . ."

Tears start to fall,
I just can't hide 'em.
The note goes on
Ad infinitum:

". . .climbing stairs
causes gas,
no sense of smell
When driving fast.

"Left hand hurts
and right hand's weak,
sneeze sends pain
from hands to feet.

"Last week had
a pain in the chest. . ."
Stop! No more!
Can't read the rest!

I think business school
would have been wiser,
'cause they don't have
somaticizers.

—Tillman Farley, M.D. (1, p. 131)

Clinician frustration with somatizing patients is well-documented (2) and has led to labels such as "heartsink" or "crock" for patients that embody their emotions. *Somatic fixation* is a process whereby a physician and/or a patient or family focuses exclusively and inappropriately on the somatic aspects of a complex problem (3). Somatic fixation can occur with diagnoses of somatoform disorders (e.g., hypochondriasis, somatization disorder, conversion, psychogenic pain disorder) and psychosomatic disease, and with any illness, especially chronic illness, when there is a one-sided emphasis on the biomedical aspects of a multifaceted problem. Despite very difficult life situations, somatically fixated patients tend not to present with anxiety, depression, or trouble coping, but with numerous physical symptoms. The number of patients in any family practice with some degree of somatic fixation is high. Another study found somatization disorder in a family practice to be both a prevalent problem as well as an expensive and difficult one. deGruy et al. found that these patients had a 50% higher rate of office visits, 50% higher charges, charts that were close to twice as thick as the average chart, and significantly more diagnoses than matched controls (4). This chapter will advocate for a biopsychosocial approach to somatic fixation, first describing the phenomena and the vicious cycle that clinicians, patients, and families can be drawn into, and then elucidating principles of a successful biopsychosocial approach to the management and treatment of these problems.

Like many primary care problems, somatic fixation ranges in severity from mild to severe, and may cut across diagnostic categories (5). Even though only about 1% of primary care patients meet the criteria for Somatization Disorder, all types occur with more frequency in subsyndromal form. Kroenke, Spitzer, deGruy, et al. (6) propose a new category of "Multisomatoform Disorder" that may be of particular use in primary care. This disorder is defined by three or more current, unexplained symptoms, and a 2-year history of significant disability and marked impairment, as well as a high level of physician frustration. These subthreshold disorders may respond well to a direct question about the emotional component of their symptoms (e.g., "Do you think there's any possibility that these symptoms are related to stress in your life?").

> A young Irish-American college girl was brought in by her nurse practitioner mother because of headaches. After interviewing the girl and her mother together, the clinician asked the stress question with the girl alone. She responded affirmatively, connecting her headaches to particularly difficult school assignments or tests. It was relatively easy to go from this mutually agreeable diagnosis regarding her headache to some psychoeducation about muscle tension coupled with stress management and relaxation techniques that were supported by her mother. The treatment succeeded in reducing the frequency and severity of the girl's headaches.

Somatic symptoms are a prominent part of affective disorders and may be the first indication of a major or minor affective disorder that may benefit from psychotropic and/or psychotherapeutic treatment; however, a depression or "stressed" explanation is likely to be met first with denial. Patients are instead attached to some biomedical explanation, the need for tests, and for biomedical intervention. It is a longer process to negotiate the connection between mind and body, and may benefit from the inclusion of a psychotherapist on the treatment team.

Sarah was a 38-year-old Swiss-American divorced mother of a 10-year-old boy. She compulsively attended aerobics class every day during the week, and came in to her nurse practitioner, Mr. R., reporting fatigue, muscle aches, low back pain, and headaches. Mr. R. knew this patient had recently been through a difficult and painful divorce, and that her mother had moved to Florida in the preceding year as well. After several office visits and a complete physical exam, he developed a mutually agreeable explanation for her symptoms that included the idea that Sarah had always had a "sensitive body" and the fact that she'd recently endured many stressful losses. The treatment plan included starting her on antidepressants to treat her pain and asking her to see Dr. M., a psychologist on their team. Mr. R. said, "We've agreed you have a sensitive body that has endured many recent stresses. I'd like you to see my colleague, Dr. M. She is a psychologist who works with many of my patients who have symptoms that persist, symptoms that we don't completely understand. Her office is next door." After some initial hesitation, Sarah agreed to stop on her way out and make at least one appointment to see if she felt Dr. M. could be a helpful member of her treatment team.

Dr. M. used a symptom diary with Sarah to uncover significant vegetative symptoms of major depression, including sleep disturbance and weight loss. Dr. M. suggested to Mr. R. that he evaluate Sarah for a trial of antidepressants. In the meantime, she conducted 15 psychotherapy sessions with Sarah about her marriage, her divorce, her parenting, her mother's move, and her support network. While discussing these stressors, they also worked on accurately labeling her physical and emotional sensation, and using the sensations and the symptoms as important information to consider in decision making. After 6 months, Sarah had reduced her exercise to four times per week, had a more accurate sense of what symptoms were problematic and what were just helpful cues about her emotional life, and had begun dating again.

Severe somatic fixation can be extremely taxing, both emotionally and financially, for the primary care clinician. The following example illustrates a common course for severe somatic fixation that can occur in association with a serious illness. It represents a mix of somatization disorder, hypochondriasis, major depression and anxiety, and amplification of organically based pathology. These patients with mixed presentations can be very difficult to manage and treat. As with all somatizing behavior, multicausality is the rule rather than the exception, so all aspects of the patient's problem need assessment and attention. Psychosocial information is usually best gathered through asking about the stress associated with having physical symptoms.

Although Mr. Hammer's only biomedical problem was mild hypertension, this German-American man visited his family physician, Dr. E., frequently for numerous concerns about his health. His anxiety could usually be reduced temporarily by a brief physical exam and reassurance by Dr. E. During one of these visits, a prostate nodule unfortunately was detected, causing Mr. Hammer to become extremely fearful and upset.

A biopsy of the nodule revealed cancer, and Mr. Hammer underwent a radical prostatectomy. He and his wife were reassured by the surgeon that he had "gotten it all" immediately after surgery; however, when the final pathology report came back, the surgeon explained that all the malignant cells may not have been removed, and that Mr. Hammer should receive radiation therapy. Mr. Hammer agreed, but had great difficulty dealing with the news that there might be some residual cancer. He became severely depressed and was referred to a psychiatrist who hospitalized him for 1 week. Mr. Hammer improved on antidepressants, and was discharged to Dr. E.'s care. The consulting psychiatrist felt Mr. Hammer should remain on antidepressants, and said he was "not a good candidate for psychotherapy."

During these events Mr. Hammer's level of somatic fixation escalated dramatically. Dr. E. saw him frequently, monitored his physical state carefully, and reassured him liberally. This seemed of only momentary benefit to Mr. Hammer. Mr. Hammer confessed his fears to his wife, who also reassured him, speaking from her own experience of having two episodes of breast cancer and a period of serious depression between the two episodes.

Mr. Hammer worked all his life in construction and had retired several years before this health event. He prided himself in being active and handy around the house. In the several years after his treatment for cancer, he became inactive, withdrawn, and preoccupied with the prospect of a recurrence of his cancer. He reported pain and discomfort in the prostate area, difficulty concentrating, and dry eyes. Every time Mr. Hammer experienced a new symptom, Dr. E. evaluated him, always with negative findings. There were similar results whenever his surgeon evaluated him. Dr. E. was concerned about Mr. Hammer's persistent depression and tried several times to change him to a more effective antidepressant. Each time Mr. Hammer had such difficulty making the change and reported so many side effects that his physician maintained him on the original medication. Mr. Hammer was no longer severely depressed several years postsurgery, but he was quite markedly somatically fixated.

Because of the seriousness of Mr. Hammer's disease, he and his care providers had difficulty pursuing the psychosocial aspects of his adjustment. Mr. Hammer had always been action-oriented rather than emotionally or verbally oriented, so he had little to draw on from his previous life to help him adjust to his new status. In fact, his father had a serious illness late in mid life and had not been able to make a healthy adjustment. He had become reclusive and very difficult to deal with until his death some years later.

In addition to Mr. Hammer's somatic fixation, Dr. E. struggled with her own tendency to panic over her patient's symptoms. She was very fond of Mr. Hammer and felt in some way responsible for not picking up the cancer earlier, so that when he requested more tests to evaluate his symptoms she almost always concurred, with or without strong medical evidence to support the testing.

Table 19.1 illustrates the range of somatic fixation or biopsychosocial attention possible for patients and for clinicians. Patients may range from being comfortable with health, physical, and emotional experience in the middle of the continuum, to amplifying symptoms and worrying over illness or expressing somatic delusions at one extreme, to being hypersensitive to emotions or having psychic delusions at the other. Clinicians may also attend to somatic, psychic, or biopsychosocial issues, ranging from utilizing an integrated, biopsychosocial approach in the center of the spectrum, to treating the biomedical and psychosocial separately or referring out most psychosocial problems, to one extreme of perceiving and treating only biomedical problems. Even though many clinicians overvalue the biomedical contribution to a patient's symptom complex, there are occasions, at the other end of the spectrum, when the biomedical is undervalued and clinicians may attend exclusively to psychosocial issues.

> Dr. J. was the dean of a local junior college and had a particularly bad day. He had the unfortunate task of firing a professor known well to him. He had not eaten all day because of the stress. Later in a meeting, he passed out, sustaining a laceration to his chin. He was noted to be in atrial fibrillation on presentation to the Emergency Department. The resident had been certain it was exclusively due to stress.

Clinicians are ironically particularly vulnerable to overvaluing psychological contributions with patients who are known to somatize. This has led to the cautionary dictum, "Somatizers get sick, too." The goal with all patients is to weight the contribution of all factors in a patient's life properly to provide accurate and comprehensive treatment.

Why is somatic fixation so widespread and so difficult to manage? There are a number of individual, family, cultural, and heath system factors that support the maintenance of somatic symptoms.

TABLE 19.1. Spectrum of attention to biopsychosocial issues by patients and clinicians

Psychic delusions	Hyper-sensitivity to emotions	Healthy and happy	Hypersensitive to bodily sensations	Obsessed by physical symptoms	Somatic delusions
Purely psychosocial	Psychosocial focus, then biomedical	Biopsychosocial model	Assess biomedical then psychosocial	Biomedical focus, refers psychosocial	Purely biomedical

1. Individual factors.

The first relevant individual factor is rooted in the normal human experience of physical sensations. Kellner and Sheffield found that 60–80% of healthy individuals experience some somatic symptoms in any 1 week (7). If even a small proportion of these people saw their clinician, our offices would be flooded with patients. In addition, individuals' perceptions of a symptom are quite variable. It is well documented that the same amount of tissue pathology produces varying degrees of functional impairment and subjective distress in different individuals (8). In the previous case example, Mr. Hammer was very sensitive to any physical sensation in his body (and equally insensitive to emotional cues). After his surgery, he experienced a much greater degree of impairment and distress than most patients with similar disease and treatment.

2. Familial factors.

Many family factors can potentially support or reinforce somatic fixation (9, 10). A subgroup of people are raised in an environment where they receive attention for physical pain, but no attention for emotional pain. These repressed families condition children to experience any need or problem as physical. Physical symptoms become their language for a range of experiences, from physical to emotional. Symptoms become communication, and these patients may learn to amplify their bodily symptoms in an attempt to get their needs met (11). In keeping with this explanation, Katon found that chronic, severe somatizers also tend to have a developmental history of gross neglect and abuse as well as a family history of relatives using somatization or pain behavior as a way of coping or solving problems (9, 12–15). In the prior example, Mr. Hammer's father somatized. His family was emotionally unexpressive and communicated through physical symptoms. Even though he did not report a history of physical abuse, his parents did seem to be stressed and incapable of meeting many of his emotional needs.

3. Cultural factors.

In addition to the individual and family contributions to the development and maintenance of somatic fixation, our culture contributes to the problem by promoting the notion of a mind–body dichotomy. Our language and much of our belief systems encourage patients like Mr. Hammer to conceptualize the physical as apart from and unrelated to the emotional. The notion that a physical symptom must have a primarily organic cause, or that an emotional feeling is determined primarily by some psychological experience, is well-accepted in our society. The idea that mind and body are an integrated, related, communicating whole has only recently, and tentatively, been considered by the wider Western society. Medicine itself focused particularly on biomedicine in the twentieth century, in part because of the many scientific and technological advances that have occurred relatively recently. These advances make it that much more seductive to conclude that biomedicine *is* medicine, rather than it being one very important component of the diagnosis and treatment of a patient.

4. Health system factors.

Barsky points to the medical–industrial complex that promotes a medical ideology and seeks to tranlate it into consumer demand for medical products and services. This medicalization of distress contributes to a growing number of "functional somatic syndromes" whose scientific status and medical basis remain unclear (e.g., problems such as chronic fatigue syndrome, total allergy syndrome, food hypersensitivity, reactive hypoglycemia, systemic yeast infection, fibromyalgia, etc.) (16).

The biopsychosocial approach is a medical model that operationalizes the systemic approach to human suffering. Although it is helpful with any medical problem, it is particularly effective for the management and treatment of somatic fixation. *Every physical symptom has some biologic, some psychologic, and often some social component to it. A clinician needs to be able to assess each of these areas, without exclusively focusing on any one component of the symptom.*

The Battle of the Health Belief Systems

Somatic fixation can also be described as an interactional process that occurs when the health belief system of a patient and/or family does not match that of a clinician. For example, after Mr. Hammer's surgery, Dr. E. believed that Mr. Hammer's symptoms were a result of his fear, depression, and ongoing sensitivity to bodily cues. Mr. Hammer, however, believed that these symptoms indicated a recurrence of his cancer. These differing diagnoses made it difficult for the two individuals to understand each other or to communicate without conflict.

Figure 19.1 illustrates the vicious cycle that can occur in interactions between a somatically fixated patient or family and a clinician who hold differing health-belief systems. This cycle can begin when a patient experiences symptoms and seeks help from a health professional. If we assume that the clinician does not routinely use a biopsychosocial approach, then that clinician might review the patient's symptoms, listen sympathetically, and perhaps order some tests and prescribe some medication. In the next interaction, the tests may come back equivocal or negative. The clinician then experiences relief. At that point, some patients experience some temporary relief, but the cycle starts over again once symptoms recur. Other patients are perplexed and anxious, and continue to pursue diagnosis and treatment.

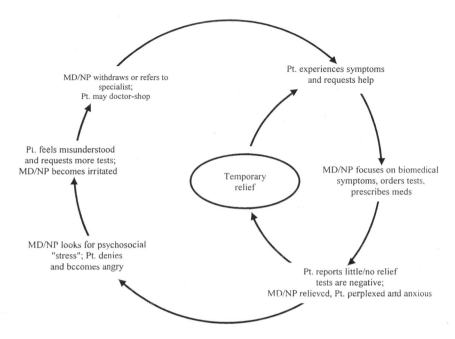

FIGURE 19.1. Somatically fixated clinician–patient interaction.

With no biomedical answers, the clinician turns to a psychosocial evaluation. The patient may then become angry and deny that the problem is "in my head." At this point the patient feels misunderstood and requests more tests, leading the clinician to become irritated.

Concerned family members may heighten the polarization. At this point, the clinician may withdraw from the patient and/or refer out to a specialist, or the patient may drop out of the practice and begin a process of doctor-shopping. Either outcome sets the cycle into motion again as the patient presents his or her symptoms to a new clinician. The lack of a shared belief system can result in a vicious cycle in which both clinician and patient are locked into a battle over the patient's somatic fixation.

The way out of the struggle involves adopting an integrated biopsychosocial approach from the beginning of interaction with the patient. From a broad perspective, treatment consists of slowly educating and demonstrating to the patient the interconnections between biological and psychological systems. At the end of a course of treatment clinician and patient are closer to sharing a common health belief system that recognizes this interdependency.

Twelve Principles for a Biopsychosocial Approach to Somatic Fixation

> Mr. and Mrs. Hunter were well-known to Dr. B. as patients who were extremely sensitive to physical symptoms and tended to worry about illness and disease. They wished to be seen together, except when Mrs. Hunter brought their sons in for care. This couple had many strengths: They were devoted to parenting their three sons, they enjoyed their work, and they were committed to their Lutheran church and their community; however, they were unusually conscious of their bodily cues. They and their sons each had occasional flu, colds, and headaches, which would send them to the office requesting medicine. On each visit Dr. B. would treat the problem, reassure them, and check into other life events that might be stressing the family at the time. Until the last few years, this approach was effective. At that time, Mr. and Mrs. Hunter lost a second daughter to congential heart defects soon after birth. Within a year, Mr. and Mrs. Hunter were making at least monthly visits to Dr. B. with multiple somatic complaints. Reassurance and benign diagnoses no longer were effective in decreasing their anxiety.

Treating such somatically fixated patients as the Hunters requires careful and explicit attention to principles of biopsychosocial medicine:

1. From the beginning, evaluate biomedical and psychosocial elements of the problem concurrently.

The clinician can avoid operationalizing the mind–body split by mixing biomedical and psychosocial questions in the interview, a technique suggested by Doherty and Baird for all primary care interviewing (17). In particular, it is important to avoid working up the patient medically, finding nothing, then turning to a psychosocial evaluation. This dichotomy mimics the patient's belief that the two are separate, unrelated processes. It relegates the psychosocial to a position of lesser importance and leads to the common patient accusation: "You think this is all in my head." Avoid this problem by interspersing questions about disease signs and symptoms with questions about recent stressful life events and family problems from the beginning.

Limit the medical work-up to what seems necessary rather than what is requested, helping the patient and family come to accept the multifaceted nature of the problem and the many costs to unnecessary medical intervention. Screen especially for mental health problems such as depression and anxiety, problems that may benefit from medication and/or psychotherapy.

2. Solicit the patient's symptoms, but do not let the symptoms run the interview.

It is important to respect the patient's somatic defenses: If these patients were able to tolerate direct expressions of emotion or distress, they would not have to somatize. By soliciting symptoms, the clinician is able to speak the patients' language, enter their belief system, and metaphorically gain access to and validate their emotional experience. It is especially important to structure these interviews in such a way that the patient feels his or her concerns are heard and yet does not dominate the interview with long, rambling descriptions of pain and symptomatology. Several techniques can keep the primary care clinician active and prevent the patient from dominating the interview with excessive detail about symptoms:

- Remain active in the interview: Reflect the patient's comments or ask a question after each sentence or two by the patient.
- Interrupt if necessary.
- Assume a curious or perplexed posture rather than a frustrated, intimidated, or weary posture.
- Unusual symptoms call for unusual diagnostic procedures—ask the patient to diagram symptoms, measure their length or intensity, and be active in the diagnostic process.

The primary care professional must be able to persist through what is typically a difficult early period of evaluation and heavy symptom focus by the patient. Requesting a symptom diary, especially one that includes both biomedical and psychosocial information about symptoms, can be useful in allowing patients their concerns about their symptoms, involving them in the diagnostic process, and providing information for the patient and the clinician about the symptoms. The diary may be requested by explaining: "Your body is trying to signal us about something important, unfortunately, we do not understand its signals just yet. We must work together to try and discover what it is telling us."

> Early in treatment with the Hunters, Dr. B. tried but had difficulty discussing the deaths of the couple's two daughters. Attempts to broach psychosocial issues were met with Mr. Hunter complaining that he had a sexually transmitted disease, or that his right testicle was cold, or that his semen were discolored. Mrs. Hunter usually accompanied her husband to see Dr. B. and had her own litany of physical complaints. They included abdominal pain, ear pain, headaches, and unusual vaginal discharge. Mr. and Mrs. Hunter tended to be symptomatic simultaneously. Attention or attempted treatment of one person inevitably led to symptoms and the need for treatment in the other. This couple may have had a chlamydia infection at some time, although no evidence existed of such an infection by the time of the consultations.
>
> Rather than increase the patient's resistance by focusing totally on the emotional, Dr. B. carefully interspersed his psychosocial questions with more biomedical questions about Mr. Hunter's symptoms. Early in treatment, Mr. Hunter rarely answered the questions about stress directly, but continued to complain of various symptoms, including pains that shot up through his chest, being awakened by the sound of bubbles popping in his lungs, and being generally lethargic and unable

to work. Dr. B. asked both members of the couple to keep a symptom diary, and the patients brought in pages of symptoms and complaints, reporting little about their emotional states.

3. Develop a relationship with the patient that is collaborative.

It is important to match clinician style to what the patient and family need. Many patients benefit from structure and a clear diagnosis that is mutually acceptable. Most will resist a strongly authoritarian position. Also, any implication to the patient that a "magic bullet" exists to relieve them of their symptoms is dangerous. Instead, it may be useful to describe the symptoms as mysterious and scientifically baffling; this approach underscores the clinician's inability to treat these problems from a purely biomedical perspective. These attitudes on the part of the professional also underline the importance of the patient's contribution to the diagnosis and treatment of these difficult problems.

4. See the patient at regular intervals, not dictated by symptom occurrence or intensification (2), and discourage visits to other healthcare professionals, except upon specific referral (18).

Regular and frequent appointments with the primary care clinician are important to disconnect the patient's experience of crisis and symptoms resulting in attention and care. Attention and care is instead given liberally without relation to acute symptoms. It is also important that patients be routed through the primary care nurse or physician for all acute and chronic complaints, avoiding Emergency Department visits and referrals to medical specialists unless clearly indicated. Multiple work-ups and dispersal of these patients' care tend to reinforce biomedical fixation. When biomedical referral is necessary, it is important to talk with the consultant beforehand and be specific about the referral question: "I don't think this is a serious physical problem. What do you think?"

> Dr. B. was careful in the early stages to share his concern and confusion with the Hunters over their symptoms. He agreed with them that they deserved to have a "cure," but stated that an easy solution did not seem possible in their case. They would have to work together to manage these difficult and mysterious problems. Dr. B. also underlined his accessibility to the Hunters, telling them to see him every several weeks for the next few months until they began to function a little better. He encouraged then to bring any acute or chronic complaints to him rather than elsewhere. He told them other services (e.g., the emergency room or even other clinicians unfamiliar with their cases) were likely to be ineffective with their problems and cost them more money because they would have to start from ground zero with each new evaluation. The Hunters agreed they did not wish more aggravation than they already had.

5. Negotiate a mutually acceptable diagnosis.

This requires first eliciting the patient and family's diagnoses of the problem. It is important to understand the meaning of the symptom to the patient and family, and to validate their distress rather than disputing any symptoms. Over time, working from their understanding, the clinician then negotiates a mutually acceptable explanation. These explanations may be idiosyncratic (e.g., "We've agreed these headaches are part of your payment in the divorce agreement"), or they may include functional somatic syndrome diagnoses (e.g., chronic fatigue or pervasive environmental allergies) (16). The important point in the negotiation is that the patient and family feel heard and understood, and that the diagnosis points to a plan that addresses both biomedical and psychosocial elements of the problem.

6. Elicit any recent stressful life events, life cycle challenges, or unresolved family problems.

Of particular importance to somatic fixation are such problems as early abuse or deprivation, unresolved grief, alcohol or drug abuse, and workaholism and other forms of overfunctioning. In addition, such questions as, "How do these symptoms affect your day-to-day life?" can help to understand the psychosocial context of the symptom. These questions may be best addressed during a family meeting.

> Both Mr. and Mrs. Hunter initially worried that they had cancer. Mr. Hunter later reported that a friend had suggested perhaps he had AIDS, and Mrs. Hunter continually worried that she had some serious "female problems" or some other life-threatening illness. Testing and physical exams revealed no medical evidence for any of these concerns. Over 2–3 months of visits, the Hunters slowly began discussing the stressful events in their family life, which included long work hours and alcohol abuse by Mr. Hunter, and the difficulties that had occurred after their babies' deaths. The clinician and the couple eventually agreed that their symptoms were likely a result of some mixture of an early chlamydia infection, depression and unresolved grief after their daughters' deaths, alcohol abuse, and marital stress.

7. Invite the family to participate early in treatment.

Including the family is important because symptoms can be maintained or intensified as they come to have meaning to significant others. Symptoms sometimes have such interpersonal effects as eliciting expressions of concern or sympathy and affording relief from responsibilities or work. At a family conference, it is useful to:

a. Request each person's observations, diagnoses, and opinions about the illness and the treatment.
b. Listen for how the illness may have changed the typical roles or balance of power in the family.

c. Try to understand any marital and/or transgenerational meaning for the symptom by asking, "Has anyone else in the family had an illness that in any way resembles this one?"

d. Ask what each person is doing to help the patient with the illness.

e. Ask how family life would be different if the patient's symptoms disappeared or improved.

f. Develop a treatment plan that the group can accept and request each person's help in its implementation.

> Interviewing Mr. and Mrs. Hunter together was both efficient and informative. Both Mr. and Mrs. Hunter reported that their illness had brought them closer together. Mr. Hunter had stopped working, the couple spent all their time together, and their fears of dying helped them readjust their priorities and realize how much they meant to each other. In fact, as Mr. and Mrs. Hunter improved, both worried that complete symptom relief would result in renewed marital stress or at least more distance between them, or another episode of alcohol abuse by Mr. Hunter.
>
> A few months after their treatment began, Dr. B. invited both spouses' parents in to share their concerns about their childrens' illnesses. An in-depth genogram taken in that session revealed that both Mr. and Mrs. Hunter's fathers were alcoholic and their mothers both had chronic medical problems that appeared to fit a pattern of somatic fixation. Both families agreed they had much in common. In this session, they arrived at a plan for the couple's parents to help with the grandchildren so the couple might return to work as their functioning improved.

8. Solicit and constantly return to the patient and family's strengths and areas of competence.

Patients with severe somatic fixation often have a history of deprivation or abuse; support is an important part of their treatment. Also, it is easier to build on strengths than to rectify deficiencies.

9. Avoid psychosocial fixation; continue with an integrated approach.

In addition to the psychological aspects of somatic fixtion, there are frequently biomedical components. Also, somatically fixated patients get sick at times, so it is important to remain fully alert for somatic signs of serious disease.

An ongoing integrated approach is both scientifically sound and an art form in itself. *The best interventions with somatically fixated patients are those that combine the biomedical and the psychosocial (i.e., biomedical interventions that make psychological sense and psychosocial interventions that make biomedical sense).* Explanations about scarring, stress, or a depressed immune system similarly are attempts at integrating these two aspects of the illness. It is often helpful to recommend or prescribe different forms of complementary medicine for these patients, particularly when the treatments fit the patient's belief system. Patients with musculoskeletal pain may respond to chiropractic manipulation, if they believe their body is "out of alignment" or to acupuncture, if they believe their Qi or essential spirit is depleted. Massage therapy has been demonstrated to be effective for patients with chronic low back pain (19). Many alternative practitioners use a biopsychosocial approach and address patients' psychological issues as part of their treatment. Developing collaborative relationships with them can be particularly helpful when treating somatizing patients.

> With the Hunters, continued focus on their devotion to each other and their commitment to good parenting of their children helped to support and balance the treatment. As an outgrowth of the focus on their good parenting, discussion of their daughters' deaths became somewhat easier. One very important intervention occurred when Dr. B. reviewed the Hunters' daughters' autopsy report with them. Although the couple had consistently had difficulty speaking directly about their sorrow, this medical approach facilitated their grieving and allowed them to ask questions that had heretofore not been asked. In addition, Mrs Hunter regularly visited a massage therapist, which she reported was "more helpful than anything else." With her permission, Dr. B. consulted every few months by phone with this masseuse about her care.

10. Find a way to enjoy somatically fixated cases.

These cases are traditionally frustrating and time-consuming for clinicians, as demonstrated by the vicious cycle described in Figure 19.1. These patients and their families often feel frustrated, angry at the medical establishment, and discouraged about the patients' illnesses. Finding a way to enjoy these cases, to turn despair into curiosity, allows one to stay connected to these difficult patients, and to prevent clinician burn-out. Cognitive and emotional strategies for enjoying these patients and their families include:

a. Listen to the patient's symptoms as metaphors for their larger problems.
b. Monitor both the patient's and your own discomfort with uncertainty. Somatic fixation offers many opportunities to rediscover that which we understand or have control over and that which we do not.
c. Discuss the case with a clinician colleague, or invite that person to consult. Frustration with any patient or family is often dissipated when some respected colleague can offer support and another point of view.
d. Refer or collaborate closely with a family therapist or other mental health consultant. Many severe cases of somatic fixation require in-depth experience and expertise in both the biomedical and the psychosocial areas; collaboration offers an avenue of support and shared responsibility for difficult cases; also, collaboration about this disorder can be the most cost-effective approach. Smith and colleagues, in a randomized con-

trolled study that has now been replicated, found that a psychiatric consultation coupled with recommendations for the primary care clinician of patients with somatization disorder reduced these patients' medical costs by 53% (20, 21) (see Chap. 25 for more on collaborating and referring to mental health professionals).

> Although Dr. B. felt he had made considerable progress in helping Mr. and Mrs. Hunter, he remained concerned about lingering grief issues as well as continued signs of marital distress. As in some cases of severe somatic fixation, Dr. B. decided that he needed to consult with a family therapist to provide effective biopsychosocial care to this couple.
>
> The therapist, Dr. T., and the clinician, Dr. B., held a joint meeting with the couple for Dr. B. to introduce Dr. T., make the referral, coordinate treatment with the couple, and lend his support to the new endeavor. Dr. B. and Dr. T. then discussed the session and developed a joint treatment plan. Dr. T. met with the couple 10 times over a 9-month period. The clinician and the therapist met together with the patients several times over that period. Dr. T. was able to take the time to provide Mr. Hunter with the support he needed to discuss his daughters' deaths. In one of the early joint sessions, Mr. and Mrs. Hunter stated they had grown apart during the year after their daughters' deaths and Mr. Hunter revealed that he had increased his drinking behavior and had an affair during this time. Mr. Hunter clearly felt guilty about this experience, although Mrs. Hunter seemed to have forgiven him. It became clear between this issue and the deaths of their daughters why many of their symptoms were either focused on their genitals or were related to pregnancy and reproduction in some way.
>
> As these issues were aired, Dr. B. and Dr. T. recognized the couple's commitment to each other, supported them each as individuals, and simultaneously dealt with their ongoing biomedical concerns. Although Dr. T. usually conducted the interviews around such emotionally sensitive issues as the affair or the couple's sex life, Dr. B. provided support, checked into symptoms that seemed new or concerning, and provided some creative interventions (e.g., reviewing the daughters' autopsy reports with the couple as a way of facilitating their grief work).

11. Judge progress in these patients by monitoring changes in their level of functioning rather than in their symptoms.

Symptom-free living (i.e., a "cure") is unlikely in these patients. Treatment is "care" rather than "cure." More realistic goals involve a decrease in symptoms and an increase in functioning in such areas as work and family relationships. Restraining rapid change and encouraging the patient slowly to adopt a more healthy life style can have a beneficial effect.

12. Terminate the intense phase of treatment slowly.

It is always useful to be cautious with somatically fixated patients about too-rapid improvement in their symptoms. Predicting some symptoms as an inevitable part of healing helps the patient to keep his or her expectations low and to move at his or her own pace. When some improvement has occurred, it is helpful to wonder aloud what problems might emerge if the patient was to recover completely. In addition to a restrained, cautious approach to treatment, the clinician may also realistically predict relapses as improvement occurs. These predictions prevent disappointment and make the typical flare-ups in symptoms part of the course of recovery.

With an increase in the patient's general level of functioning and a decrease in the incapacitating nature of the symptoms, it is useful to slowly lengthen the time between office visits; however, for the success of this process, it is crucial that the patient feel the clinician is available to him or her regardless of symptom status.

> By the end of 9 months, Drs. B. and T. and the patients agreed that Dr. T. no longer needed to meet with the couple. Mr. and Mrs. Hunter were not symptom-free, but the severity and frequency of their symptoms had diminished. Mr. Hunter was now working again, and Mrs. Hunter had a job for the first time since before her pregnancies. The couple reported that their commitment to each other and their family was strong. Dr. B. continued to see his patients, although less frequently, and Dr. T. remained available for consultation if needed.

Figure 19.2 summarizes the biopsychosocial approach to somatic fixation. With this approach, the clinician addresses a patient's complaints with an integrated biomedical and psychosocial evaluation from the beginning. The health professional also solicits help from family members early in the process. When the tests are equivocal or negative, patient, family, and the clinician may be perplexed, and a collaborative relationship is established to manage the patient's mysterious symptoms. The message that the clinician does not fully understand the symptoms, does not have a quick answer or pill that will solve the problem, and is able to tolerate the uncertainty while continuing to work up the various aspects of the patient's problem is of great importance. At this point, the clinician may or may not consult with a medical colleague or a family therapist to share in the evaluation. In either case, the professional should *set limited, concrete goals for treatment and measure outcome by monitoring the patient's functioning* in areas of work, family, and personal life rather than only the patient's symptom picture. As functioning improves and symptoms become less severe, the clinician is cautious about a cure and raises a concern about possible relapse in the patient's symptomatology. When patient functioning has improved adequately, the patient and clinician agree to make sessions more infrequent. The clinician, however, gives a clear message that he or she will continue to remain available to the patient and the family.

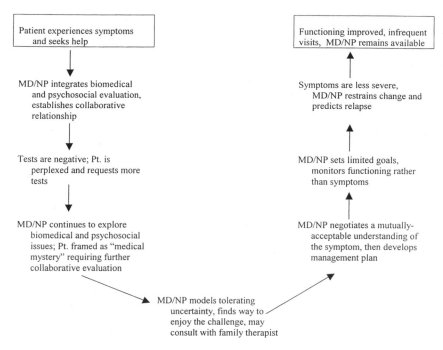

FIGURE 19.2. A biopsychosocial approach to somatic fixation.

This biopsychosocial approach to the management and treatment of somatic fixation offers clinician, patient, and family a way out of the vicious cycle that can develop around this problem. It can offer an effective alternative for treatment, and provide the clinician with a vehicle to enjoy working with this often difficult and frustrating problem.

References

1. McDaniel SH, Hepworth J, & Doherty WJ: *Medical Family Therapy: A Biopsychosocial Approach to Families with Health Problems.* New York: Basic Books, 1992.
2. Quill TE: Somatization disorder: one of medicine's blind spots. *JAMA* 1986; **254**(21):3075–3079.
3. Van Eijk J, Grol R, Huygen F, et al.: The family doctor and the prevention of somatic fixation. *Fam Syst Med* 1983;**1**(2):5–15.
4. deGruy F, Columbia L, Dickinson P: Somatization disorder in a family practice. *J Fam Pract* 1987;**25**(1):45–51.
5. Kirmayer LJ, Robbins JM: Three forms of somatization in primary care: prevalence, co-occurrence, and sociodemographic characteristics. *J Nerv Mental Dis* 1991;**179**:647–655.
6. Kroenke K, Spitzer RL, deGruy F, Hahn SR, Linzer M, Williams JB, et al.: Multisomatoform disorder: An alternative to undifferentiated somatoform dis-

order for the somatizing patients in primary care. *Arch Gen Psychiatr* 1997;**54**:352–358.

7. Kellner R, Sheffield BR: The 1-week prevalence of symptoms in neurotic patients and normals. *Am J Psychiatr* 1973;**130**:102–105.

8. Eisenberg L: Interfaces between medicine and psychiatry. *Comp Psychiatr* 1979; **20**:1–14.

9. Livingston R, Witt A, & Smith GR: Families who somatize. *Develop Behav Pediatr* 1995;**16**:42–46.

10. Wood BL: Beyond the "psychosomatic family": a biobehavioral family model of pediatric illness. *Fam Proc.* 1993;**32**:261–278.

11. Barksy AJ: Patients who amplify bodily sensations. *Ann Intern Med* **91**:63–70.

12. Katon W: Somatization in primary care. *J Fam Pract* 1985;**21**(4):257–258.

13. Pennebaker JW: Traumatic experience and psychosomatic disease: Exploring the roles of behavioural inhibition, obsession, and confiding. *Canadian Psychol* 1985;**26**:82–95.

14. Dickinson L, deGruy F, Dickinson W, & Candib L: Complex PTSD: Evidence from the primary care setting. *Gen Hosp Psychiatr* 1998;**20**:1–11.

15. Dickinson L, deGruy F, Dickinson W, & Candib L: Health-related quality of life and symptom profiles of female survivors of sexual abuse in primary care, Archives of Family Medicine 1999;**8**:35–43.

16. Barsky AJ, Borus JF: Functional somatic syndromes. *Ann Intern Med* 1999; **130**:910–921.

17. Doherty W, Baird M: Forming a therapeutic contract that involves the family. *Family Therapy and Family Medicine.* New York: Guilford Press, 1983.

18. Epstein RM, Quill TE, & McWhinney IR: Somatization reconsidered. *Arch Int Med* 1999;**159**:215–222.

19. Cherkin DC, Eisenberg D, Sherman KJ, Barlow W, Kaptchuk TJ, Street J, et al.: Randomized trial comparing traditional Chinese medical acupuncture, therapeutic massage, and self-care education for chronic low back pain. *Arch Intern Med* 2001;**161**:1081–1088.

20. Smith GR, Monson RA, & Ray DC: Psychiatric consultation in somatization disorder. *N Engl J Med* 1986;**314**(22):1407–1413.

21. Smith GR, Rost K, & Kashner TM: A trial of the effect of a standardized psychiatric consultation on health outcomes and costs in somatizing patients. *Arch Gen Psychiatr* 1995;**52**(3):238–243.

Protocol: Twelve Principles for a Biopsychosocial Approach to Somatic Fixation

1. Use a biopsychosocial approach from the beginning.
   a. Begin by interspersing biomedical and psychosocial questions in the interview.
   b. Do a balanced, reasonable work-up, neither overusing tests nor avoiding the biological aspects of the symptoms.
2. Solicit the patient's symptoms, but do not let the symptoms run the interview.
   a. Reflect or ask a question after each sentence or two by the patient.
   b. Interrupt if necessary.
   c. Assume a curious or perplexed posture rather than a frustrated, intimidated, or weary posture.
   d. With unusual symptoms, use unusual diagnostic procedures that allow you to remain active (e.g., measuring the length or intensity of symptoms).
   e. Keep the patient active in the diagnostic process (e.g., request a symptom diary including both biomedical and psychosocial information about symptoms).
3. Develop a relationship with the patient and family that is collaborative.
   a. Avoid taking a traditional, authoritarian position or promising any easy answers to the patient's symptoms.
   b. Consider framing the patient's symptoms as mysterious and scientifically baffling, requiring the patient, family, and clinician to work together to manage the problem.
4. See the patient at regular intervals and discourage visits to other health providers, except on specific referral.
   a. Schedule regular appointments, not dictated by symptom occurrence or intensification.
   b. Route all acute and chronic patient complaints through the primary care clinician.
   c. Have patients avoid Emergency Department visits, medical specialists, and inpatient treatment, unless specifically recommended by the primary care clinician.
   d. When referral is indicated, be sure to talk with the consultant beforehand and be specific about the referral question(s).
5. Negotiate a mutually acceptable diagnosis
   a. Elicit the patient and family's diagnoses of the problem.
   b. Explore the meaning of the symptom to the patient and family.
   c. Work toward mutually acceptable diagnoses or explanations for the symptoms.
   d. Given their diagnoses, what treatment do they expect will be useful?
   e. Develop a plan that addresses both biomedical and psychosocial aspects of the problem.
   f. When appropriate, collaborate with any nontraditional healers.

6. Elicit any recent stressful life events, life cycle challenges, or unresolved family problems—ask especially about:
   a. A history of early abuse or deprivation.
   b. Unresolved grief.
   c. Alcohol or drug abuse, workaholism, and other forms of overfunctioning.
7. Invite the family to participate in the process early in treatment.
   a. Request each person's observations, diagnoses, and opinions about the illness and the treatment.
   b. Listen for how the illness may have changed the typical roles or balance of power in the family.
   c. Try to understand any marital and/or transgenerational meaning for the symptom by asking: "Has anyone else in the family had an illness that in any way resembles this one?"
   d. Ask what each person is doing to help the patient with the illness.
   e. Ask how family life would be different if the patient was asymptomatic.
   f. Develop a treatment plan that the group can accept and request each person's help in its implementation.
8. Solicit and constantly return to the patient and family's strengths and areas of competence.
9. Avoid psychosocial fixation; continue with an integrated approach.
   a. Use interventions that combine the biomedical and the psychosocial.
   b. Use biomedical explanations that also have psychosocial meanings (e.g., stress, scarring, or depressed immune system).
10. Find a way to enjoy somatically fixated patients.
    a. Listen to the patient's symptoms as metaphors for their larger problems.
    b. Monitor both the patient's and your own discomfort with uncertainty.
    c. Discuss the case with a clinician colleague or invite that person to consult.
    d. Refer or collaborate closely with a family therapist or other mental health consultant.
11. Judge progress in these patients by monitoring changes in their level of functioning rather than in their symptoms.
12. Terminate the intense phase of treatment slowly.
    a. Caution patients from too-rapid improvement.
    b. Keep your own expectations low; set realistic goals.
    c. With some improvement, ask what problems might emerge if the patient were to recover completely?
    d. Predict relapses.
    c. Slowly lengthen the time between office visits when the patient experiences an increase in general level of functioning and a decrease in the incapacitating nature of the symptoms.
    f. Remain available to the patient.

20
Mobilizing Resources: The Assessment and Treatment of Depression in Primary Care

Depression is one of the most common problems seen in primary care and is associated with significant morbidity, mortality, and economic cost. At any one time, between 5 and 9% of primary care patients suffer from major depression, and an equal number have other depressive disorders, including dysthymia and minor depression (1). Depression causes as much disability and impact on quality of life as major chronic medical illnesses (e.g., ischemic heart disease, strokes, or diabetes), and it negatively affects the outcome of most chronic illnesses. Despite its high prevalence and morbidity, depression remains underdiagnosed and undertreated in primary care. It is estimated that up to 50% of depressed patients are undetected in primary care, and those that are detected are often inadequately treated (2). Underdetection results in part because these patients present with somatic rather than psychological symptoms, especially chronic pain, fatigue, and sleep problems. Many patients have co-existing medical problems with symptoms that overlap with depression. The diagnosis of depression is hampered by competing demands faced by primary care clinicians (3). Compounding this, most reimbursement systems create additional challenges by not paying for mental health diagnoses and "carving out" depression treatment to mental health professionals.

Depression is influenced by biological, psychological, and social factors. The family and social factors are often overlooked when assessing and treating depression in primary care. This chapter will provide an overview of the identification, assessment, and treatment of depression in primary care, with a focus on how the primary care clinician can mobilize and integrate individual and interpersonal resources. We will emphasize an interpersonal approach to understanding and treating depression and the link between family relationships and depression.

An Interpersonal Approach to Depression

Family relationships can have a powerful influence on the onset, course, and treatment of depression, and depression has a negative impact on the quality of most family and social relationships. Interpersonal factors, especially marital distress and family criticism, can precipitate depressive episodes and relapse, and worsen depressive symptoms. Individuals in a distressed marriage are three times more likely to develop depression than are those in nondistressed relationships (4). In turn, depression often results in more negative and critical behaviors toward one's spouse or partner, which can further worsen marital distress and depressive symptoms. Stressful marital or family events (e.g., illness or death of a family member, separation, or divorce) often precede the onset of depression (5).

Social and interpersonal stressors that disrupt the patient's normal sources of support and nurturance can trigger depression. When these disruptions occur, the depressed person typically turns to family members to obtain reassurance and support. Although partners and family members initially respond positively, over time family members may feel overburdened, irritated, or "burned out." The patient may then perceive these responses as rejection and feel more needy or depressed. This pattern may spiral over time as family members offer varying degrees of support that the patient experiences as inadequate, and the depressive symptoms are maintained or intensified (6).

Identification and Assessment of Depression

The assessment of depression should simultaneously address three aspects of the system: the depressed person, the partner, and any relationship problems between the two of them. The family-oriented clinician is in an ideal position to conduct such an assessment and to initiate treatment. In the following sections we will discuss guidelines for assessing and treating depressed persons from an interpersonal perspective.

> Mrs. Pulcino, a 36-year-old Italian-American woman, came to see Dr. C. for the fourth time in 2 months. Mrs. Pulcino was married and had two children, one of whom was school aged (see genogram, Fig. 20.1). She worked outside the home as an aide in a nearby nursing home. Mr. Pulcino drove a delivery truck and also maintained a 100-acre farm. Mrs. Pulcino reported symptoms of fatigue, headaches, and diffuse muscle pains. In the previous 3 months, she had also seen Dr. C. for a cold and an intestinal flu.
>
> Mrs. Pulcino told Dr. C. she was afraid there was something seriously wrong with her. None of Dr. C.'s tests revealed any organic causes for her symptoms; however, Mrs. Pulcino was clearly feeling ill.

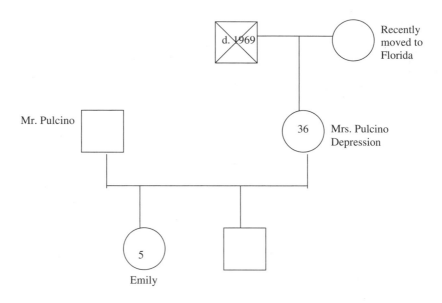

FIGURE 20.1. The Pulcino family.

Some patients talk openly with their clinician about their emotional or interpersonal problems, but others do not. Somatic complaints are often the primary way in which depressive symptoms are presented in a medical setting. The clinician's first task is to recognize the signs that assessment for depression may be necessary. An increase in the number of office visits, functional complaints, infections, and reports of pain and anxiety by the patient are often a harbinger of a depressive episode.

Screening

The U.S. Preventive Services Task Force recommends the routine screening for depression "in clinical practices that have systems in place to assure accurate diagnosis, effective treatment and follow up (7)." This new recommendation is based upon research that clearly demonstrates that early detection and treatment of depression in primary care results in reduced morbidity, especially in settings where there is a systematic approach to assessing and treating depression.

Screening for depression can be accomplished by asking two simple questions during routine office visits:

• Over the past 2 weeks, have you felt down, depressed, or hopeless?
• Over the past 2 weeks, have you felt little interest or pleasure in doing things?

These questions appear to be as effective as longer screening instruments (e.g., Beck Depression Inventory) (8). Whether a more open-ended question (e.g., "How has your mood or spirits been over the past few weeks?") works as well as these yes/no questions has not been studied.

The two preceding questions should be asked routinely of patients who are at increased risk for depression, especially those with a prior history of depression, unexplained somatic symptoms, comorbid psychological conditions (esp. any anxiety disorders), substance abuse, and chronic pain. When a patient screens positive, a more detailed interview is needed to make an accurate diagnosis. The PRIME-MD offers an efficient and validated method for conducting such an assessment (9) (see Table 20.1).

An assessment for depression should focus on the patient in the context of his or her significant relationships. An interpersonal approach helps the clinician gather a broad range of information and develop a treatment team that can include the patient and his or her main supports. Key elements in the assessment process include: evaluating the depressed individual, involving the partner, exploring relationship difficulties, suicide assessment, and measuring the effect of other life stressors.

In preparation for involving significant others in treatment, it is helpful to assess how the patient's symptoms may affect or be affected by his or her relationships with others:

- Who is most concerned about you?
- How do others respond to how you are feeling?
- What do others think is the cause of your depression?
- What do others suggest to remedy the situation?

These questions explore interpersonal factors that may contribute to the patient's depressive symptoms as well as help to alleviate them.

TABLE 20.1. Depression assessment questions (PRIME-MD)

During the past 2 weeks, have you often been bothered by:
Little interest or pleasure in doing things?
Feeling down, depressed, or hopeless?
Trouble falling/staying asleep, sleeping too much?
Feeling tired or having little energy?
Poor appetite or overeating?
Feeling bad about yourself—or that you are a failure?
Trouble concentrating on things (e.g., reading the newspaper)?
Moving or speaking so slowly that other people could have noticed? Or being so fidgety or restless that you have been moving around more than usual?
Thoughts that you would be better off dead or of hurting yourself?

A positive response to five or more of these questions is consistent with depression.

Dr. C. begins the assessment of Mrs. Pulcino with these individual and interpersonal dimensions in mind.

> Dr. C. learned that Mrs. Pulcino had been having difficulty sleeping for almost 4 months and had gained 10 pounds over the same period. At times she felt confused and helpless to change her situation. Mrs. Pulcino often wished it would "all come to an end," but when asked specifically if she wanted to hurt herself, Mrs. Pulcino denied any suicidal ideation.
>
> Mrs. Pulcino said her husband worried about her and often suggested she rest more, but was impatient with her chronic fatigue. When asked if she considered herself depressed, Mrs. Pulcino said, *yes*. She also wondered if there was something physically wrong that made her feel depressed.
>
> Dr. C. reiterated that none of the tests showed any significant physiological abnormalities, but he agreed that Mrs. Pulcino definitely felt ill and was depressed. He suggested that it would be valuable to have Mr. Pulcino come with her to the next visit. Dr. C. explained that Mr. Pulcino's input would help Dr. C. get a bigger picture of the problem and would be a chance for the three of them to work together on a treatment direction.

Involving the Partner

The patient's partner is an invaluable asset during assessment and treatment. A partner can provide information about depressive symptoms that the patient may not recognize. In cases where antidepressant medication is indicated, patients in a supportive, satisfactory marital relationship respond more favorably (10).

By seeing the couple together, the clinician can gain a better understanding of how their interactions may play a part in the patient's depression. Partners of depressed patients are often depressed themselves. It is important to assess whether or not the partner may be depressed, and, if so, to what degree the partner needs support. Even when partners do not report significant relational dissatisfaction they may still interact in ways that maintain the patient's depression.

The following questions to the partner can help the clinician gather more information and understand the interpersonal dimension of the patient's depression.

- How can you tell when your partner is depressed?
- What do you do when he or she is depressed? How does your partner respond?
- Can you describe times when your partner does not feel depressed?
- Have you yourself ever felt depressed?

- To both partners:

- How do you think your relationship has been affected by this problem?

After getting to know Mr. Pulcino, Dr. C. discussed Mrs. Pulcino's depression and her husband's perception of her illness:

At the conjoint interview, Dr. C. noticed immediately that Mrs. Pulcino was quieter and more withdrawn than in her individual visits. Mr. Pulcino watched her continuously and spoke to her in soothing tones. When she appeared unresponsive, Mr. Pulcino sat back, looked at Dr. C. and shrugged his shoulders.

Mr. Pulcino said his wife had been depressed for several months. He knew she was having a bad day if she was not dressed when he returned from morning chores for breakfast. They both reported that Mr. Pulcino tried to talk to his wife or hug her, but she would sometimes not respond and he would fall silent or leave suddenly for the barn. Mr. and Mrs. Pulcino thought their marriage was a good one, but they were both exhausted and edgy with each other because Mrs. Pulcino's depression was not lifting. The only time her depressive behavior seemed to decrease was when they watched TV together on Thursday nights. She might laugh then and Mr. Pulcino would feel better. When Dr. C. asked Mrs. Pulcino if she ever worried about her husband, she said she was concerned that he was becoming more moody. Mr. Pulcino agreed.

Mr. Pulcino's efforts to support his wife did not coincide with times when Mrs. Pulcino would accept his support. Mrs. Pulcino would consequently feel frustrated and then withdraw, whereas Mr. Pulcino would feel rejected and become more depressed. Mrs. Pulcino would then try to support her again and the cycle would continue. Dr. C. felt the Pulcino's had a strong marriage, but that they were stuck in a pattern that supported rather than alleviated Mrs. Pulcino's depression.

Suicide Assessment

All patients with depression should be carefully assessed for suicide risk. Suicide is the eighth leading cause of death in the United States, and most patients see their primary care clinician within 1 month of committing suicide. Major risk factors for suicide in depressed patients include being male, older, unemployed, unmarried or living alone, and substance abuse. The following series of questions (continued until the response is, *no*) are useful for suicide assessment:

- Have you thought that life is not worth living or that you wished you were dead? (passive ideation)
- Have you thought about hurting yourself?. . . killing yourself? (active ideation)
- Have you thought about the manner in which you might end your life? (plans)
- Do you possess what it would take (e.g., pills, firearms) to carry out your plan to end your life? (means)
- Do you intend to kill yourself with these means? (intent)

All patients with active suicidal thoughts should be referred to a mental health professionals, and those with plans need urgent evaluation. Those with the means and intent to commit suicide usually need immediate hospitalization.

Patients should initially be asked about suicidal ideation, when they are alone and may be more revealing about such thoughts; however, it can be very useful to involve partners and other family members in discussions about suicidal risk. Family members are often unaware of the suicide risk and, in cases of mild risk, can be helpful in monitoring the patient and his or her mood as well as removing dangerous items (e.g., pills and weapons) from the home. If family members become hypervigilant (e.g., not letting the patient out of their sight), however, or there is ongoing conflict, collaboration with a family therapist is indicated.

Life Stressors

Depressed persons report more stressful life events before the onset of depressive symptoms than nondepressed persons. These may include deaths, changes in work or financial status, the birth of a child, the departure of an offspring, geographical relocations, issues related to individual and family life cycles, and recent illnesses.

Some questions to guide the discussion of life stressors include:

What changes or stresses have occurred in your lives in the past year?
What impact have these changes had on you and your family?
Do you feel these changes play a part in your depression?

In the next segment, Dr. C. asked about suicidal risk, and the Pulcinos discuss the significant events that had recently occurred.

> Mrs Pulcino admitted that she had wished that she was not alive on several occasions over the past month, but never felt like hurting herself. She and her husband agreed that they should remove any medication from the bathroom cabinet that might be dangerous. During the last year Mr. Pulcino had taken a part-time job driving a delivery truck because of financial problems. To help out, Mrs. Pulcino had taken responsibility for keeping the books on the family business. It was then that she realized how serious their financial problems were. At the same time, Mrs. Pulcino's mother, who had lived down the road, moved to Florida after her retirement. This move had been particularly difficult for Mrs. Pulcino, who depended on her mother for support and childcare. As for the children, Emily, the oldest, had started kindergarten. Mr. and Mrs. Pulcino had not recognized how many stressful changes had occurred in the previous year. Mrs. Pulcino wondered if all the changes had been "too much" for her.
>
> With a clearer understanding of Mrs. Pulcino's symptoms and their relationship to her interpersonal context and life situation, Dr. C. began treatment with Mr. and Mrs. Pulcino.

Treatment of Depression in Primary Care

The choice of treatments of depression depends both upon the severity of the patient's symptoms, the patient's preference, and the clinician's skills (11). A treatment plan should be negotiated with the patient and his or her partner. Antidepressants and psychotherapy (cognitive-behavior or interpersonal) are equally effective for mild and moderate major depression. Patients with severe major depression or suicidal ideation should be referred to a psychiatrist for evaluation and medication. Minor depression (e.g., dysthymia or subthreshold depression) responds best to psychotherapy.

Depression is a chronic disease and should be managed using the principles of chronic disease management (12). This includes close collaboration with mental health professionals for medication management and/or psychotherapy and long-term follow up. Our discussion of treatment will focus on how to change individual and interpersonal behaviors that may perpetuate depression. We will conclude with guidelines for the use of antidepressant medication.

The Partner as a Collaborator in Treatment

By involving the partner, the clinician can help the couple interact in ways that may alleviate some of the patient's depressive symptoms. To that end it is important to gauge any overinvolvement or underinvolvement the partner may have with the patient's problem. Overinvolved partners take too much responsibility for the depressed person; thus, they inadvertently support the depressed person's feeling of helplessness. Underinvolved partners appear distant or even hostile toward the depressed person, who may then feel abandoned and hopeless (13).

The clinician can help the partner achieve a moderate level of involvement that is both supportive of the patient's needs and respectful of the patient's autonomy. For example, the partner who fixes all the meals for a depressed person may be encouraged by the clinician to prepare one meal per day while assisting the depressed person in preparing the others. On the other hand, to a partner who withdraws when the depressed person requests emotional support, the clinician may suggest he or she offer encouragement once per day before it is sought. In those ways the clinician can help bring balance to the partner's involvement around the patient's symptoms. A more balanced approach may also reduce pressure on the partner and benefit the couple's relationship as well. When relational discord makes it difficult for the couple to work together or is clearly a contributing factor in the patient's depression, the clinician should engage the couple in primary care couple counseling or negotiate a referral to a marital therapist (see Chaps. 14 and 25).

When involving the partner in treatment, it is important to:

1. Maintain an alliance with the patient and the partner.

A relationship already exists between the clinician and patient, so it is important to develop rapport with the partner, and try to maintain a balanced relationship with the couple.

2. Avoid blaming the partner for the patient's depression or making the partner responsible for alleviating the patient's depression.

The partner often feels overburdened by the patient's depression and may need to be relieved of excessive guilt or responsibility.

3. Focus on ways in which the partner can be a resource in treatment.

Emphasize the strengths in the relationship that may be utilized to help the patient, and ask the patient to tell his or her partner how he or she can be helpful.

4. Recognize and discuss the effect the patient's depression may have on the partner.

Partners of depressed people often experience depressive symptoms themselves.

5. Support the partner in looking after his or her own needs.

By addressing his or her own needs the partner may find additional strength and energy to help the patient.

Working with the Depressed Individual

How much primary care counseling the primary care clinician provides or whether the clinician refers the patient to a psychotherapist will depend upon the clinician's skills, interest, time availability, and the patient's preferences (see Chap. 25). There are some basic knowledge and skills, however, that all primary care clinicians should have when working with depressed patients.

Depressed people tend to feel powerless and angry about changing their situation. Because they often depend on others to meet many of their personal needs, depressed people are extremely sensitive to criticism and rejection. At times, their perception of whether or not others are critical or rejecting is distorted. Depressed persons have often experienced many losses and their grief is frequently unresolved. The pain of these negative experiences may only confirm their feelings of worthlessness. To protect themselves, depressed people may withdraw from what seems like a world that does not care, yet continue to hope that someone else will make things better. The further they withdraw, the more powerless they feel; the more powerless they feel, the more they count on others; the more they count on others, the more vulnerable they are to disappointment; the more disappointed they are, the more they withdraw; and so on.

Therapeutic approaches that are most effective with depressed patients are brief, goal-oriented, and focused on behavioral change. The central task of the clinician is to help the patient interrupt the downward spiral of depressive symptoms that results from feelings of powerlessness and dependency on others. Primary care counseling can aid the patient in identifying small, manageable tasks that will increase his or her sense of personal mastery and competence. Treatment strategies for working with the depressed individual follow:

1. Focus on changing behaviors.

An increase in meaningful activity has a positive effect on the patient's affect.

2. Go slowly.

Do not facilitate too much change too quickly when the patient's resources may be depleted.

3. Take small measurable steps.

Help the patient identify concrete, observable behavior that he or she can do (e.g., a patient who found it extremely difficult to leave the house started with a plan of going outside twice per week).

4. Utilize feedback from the patient's partner.

Involve the partner in observing positive changes in the patient and in giving the patient feedback on these changes.

These strategies are designed to increase the patient's sense of agency and self-determination. The resulting positive feedback can help the patient internalize those changes and begin to feel more self-confident.

Utilizing Antidepressant Medication

Most primary care clinicians have the skills to prescribe and monitor antidepressant medication for uncomplicated depression. Studies show that most primary care patients either do not take the prescribed medication or stop taking it within the first month or two. Ongoing psychoeducation about depression and antidepressant treatment has been shown to improve outcomes and should be provided by the primary care clinician (14). Patients should be seen within 2 weeks of starting antidepressants and followed regularly throughout treatment. At each visit the patient and his or her partner should be asked about side effects and compliance with medication and reminded that medication should be continued even when the patient is feeling better and is no longer depressed.

Medication is a family issue and should be treated as one. The effectiveness of antidepressants in major depression is well established, but it can be greatly influenced by relationship factors in the patient's life. For that reason, pharmacological treatment should be approached as a family issue and integrated into an overall treatment plan that includes ongoing counseling with the patient and partner. The involvement of significant others can improve compliance and provide the support the patient will need in the early stages of pharmacological treatment. By the same token, antidepressant medication can increase the patient's concentration, energy, and motivation to work on relationship issues. Combining medication and family counseling has a beneficial effect on both modalities.

When utilizing antidepressant medication as part of a comprehensive treatment plan, it is important to:

1. Present the option of using medication to the patient and partner together whenever possible.

This provides the clinician with the opportunity to educate the couple on the effects and side effects of antidepressant medication and to answer their questions.

2. Involve the patient and partner in a plan to monitor, decrease, and eventually discontinue the medication.

This may include planning a medication regimen together, monitoring signs of change, and continuing counseling during the transition from use to nonuse. The couples that work together around the use of medication can mirror and support other changes they are making in the relationship.

3. Look for signs of under or overinvolvement of the partner in the patient's treatment.

The underinvolved partner is unlikely to come to office visits and may have withdrawn emotionally from the patient. The overinvolved partner may have assumed or taken responsibility for the medication which may result in more passivity and depression in the patient or conflict in the relationship.

4. Request that the patient tell family members how they can be most helpful in assisting the patient's adherence to antidepressant medication.

Negotiating the amount and type of help that family members provide will help to prevent over or underinvolvement.

> After discussion with the couple, Dr. C. started Mrs. Pulcino on antidepressants and began seeing her every 2 weeks for brief primary care counseling and to monitor her medication. Mr. Pulcino agreed to attend these sessions as a resource to Dr. C. and as a support to his wife.
>
> During treatment Dr. C. helped the patient choose small, observable tasks to accomplish what both partners felt would help Mrs. Pulcino feel less depressed. For example, Mrs. Pulcino's first goal was to get up each day by 7:00 AM. Mr. Pulcino encouraged his wife and often reminded

her of this goal. When she did not get up, he would become critical and they would argue. Dr. C. helped Mr. Pulcino make changes in the way he offered support. Mr. Pulcino was encouraged by Dr. C. to give positive verbal feedback to Mrs. Pulcino on days she met her goal, but to say nothing when she did not. In discussing the issue, Mrs. Pulcino decided that getting up at 7:00 AM three times per week was a more reasonable goal.

Over the next few weeks Mrs. Pulcino was able to meet her new goal and the couple reported less conflict. Nevertheless, Mrs. Pulcino was still not sleeping well and had difficulty concentrating during the day. It was during this period that Mrs. Pulcino discussed feeling depressed at other times in her life, as had her mother. Mrs. Pulcino's father had died when she was 2 years old. She felt her mother was still sad about the loss. Mrs. Pulcino herself was tearful when discussing her father. Dr. C. discussed the use of antidepressant medication as a tool to help Mrs. Pulcino sleep better and regain some energy. He emphasized that the use of medication should be in conjunction with ongoing counseling to continue working on behavior changes and to monitor the effect of the medication.

Over the next 2 months Mrs. Pulcino began to sleep better and was able to accomplish her daily responsibilities, but the couple reported an increase in their arguing. Mrs. Pulcino felt her husband did not give her enough emotional support; and Mr. Pulcino said his wife demanded too much. Dr. C. suggested the Pulcinos see a marriage counselor to address these issues. He clarified that he would continue to see them together periodically to monitor the medication and would be in regular contact with their counselor.

The Pulcinos accepted the referral and saw a couples' therapist for a year during which time they were able to improve their relationship. Dr. C. proceeded cautiously with decreasing the medication and it was discontinued after 9 months.

The primary care clinician can effectively treat the depressed patient, especially if he or she has developed a network of professional resources with which to collaborate. Mobilizing the resources of the patient and family provides the foundation for comprehensive, integrated treatment. Focused primary care counseling and medication builds on this foundation to ensure successful treatment.

References

1. Katon W: The epidemiology of depression in medical care. *Int J Psychiatr Med* 1987;**17**:93–112.
2. Simon GE, VonKorff M: Recognition, management, and outcomes of depression in primary care. *Arch Fam Med* 1995;**4**:99–105.
3. Klinkman MS: Competing demands in psychosocial care. A model for the identification and treatment of depressive disorders in primary care. *Gen Hosp Psychiatr* 1997;**19**:98–111.

4. Whisman MA: The association between depression and marital dissatisfaction. In: Beach SR (Ed): *Marital and Family Processes in Depression* Washington DC: American Psychological Association, 2001.

5. Clarkin JF, Haas GL: Asssessment of affective disorders and their interpersonal contexts. In: Clarkin JF, Hass GL (Eds): *Affective Disorders and the Family*. New York: Guilford Press, 1988, pp. 29–50.

6. Joiner TE: Depression's vicious screen: Self-propagating and erosive processes in depression chronicity. *Clin Psychol. Sci Prac* 2000;**7**:203–218.

7. US Preventive Task Force (2002) Screening for depression. In: *Guide to Preventive Services Third ed*. International Publishing, 2002.

8. Whooley MA, Avins AL, Miranda J, & Browner WS: Case finding instruments for depression: two questions are as good as many. *J Gen Int Med* 1997; **12**:439–445.

9. Spitzer RL, Kroenke K, & Williams JBW: Validity and utility of a self-report version of PRIME-MD: the PHQ primary care study. *JAMA* 1999;**282**: 1737–1744.

10. Weissman MM, Prusoff BA, DiMascio A, Neu C, Gorklaney M, & Klerman GL: The efficacy of drugs and psychotherapy in the treatment of acute depressive episodes. *Am J Psychiatry* 1979;**136**:555–558.

11. Depression Guideline Panel: Depression in primary care. Vol, 2: treatment of Major Depression. Rockville MD: Agency for Health Care Policy and Research, US DHHS, 1993.

12. Dickinson WP: The management of depression as a chronic disease. In: DeGruy F, Dickinson P (eds): *20 Common Problems in Primary Care*. New York: McGraw Hill, 2002.

13. Coyne JC: Depression, biology, marriage and marital therapy. *Fam Proc* 1987; **13(4)**:393–407.

14. Katon W, von Korff M, Lin E, et al.: Collaborative management to achieve treatment guidelines: impact on depression in primary care. *JAMA* 1995; **273**:1026–1031.

Protocol: Assesment and Treatment of Depression in Primary Care

Screening for Depression

All patients should be screened:

- Over the past 2 weeks, have you felt down, depressed, or hopeless?
- Over the past 2 weeks, have you felt little interest or pleasure in doing things?

Questions to Ask If the Answers to Either of These Questions Is Positive

During the past 2 weeks, have you often been bothered by:

- Little interest or pleasure in doing things?
- Feeling down, depressed, or hopeless?
- Trouble falling/staying asleep, sleeping too much?
- Feeling tired or having little energy?
- Poor appetite or overeating?
- Feeling bad about yourself—or that you are a failure?
- Trouble concentrating on things (e.g., reading the newspaper)?
- Moving or speaking so slowly that other people could have noticed? Or being so fidgety or restless that you have been moving around more than usual?
- Thoughts that you would be better off dead or of hurting yourself?

A positive response to five or more of these questions is consistent with depression.

Questions to Explore the Family Context

To the Patient

- Who is most concerned about you?
- How do others respond to how you are feeling?
- What do others think is the cause of your depression?
- What do others suggest to remedy the situation?

To the Partner:

- How can you tell when your partner is depressed?
- What do you do when he or she is depressed? How does your partner respond?
- Can you describe times when your partner does not feel depressed?
- Have you yourself ever felt depressed?

To Both Partners:

- How do you think your relationship has been affected by this problem?

Assess for Suicide Risk

- Have you thought that life is not worth living or that you wished you were dead? (passive)
- Have you thought about hurting yourself?. . . killing yourself? (active)
- Have you thought about the manner in which you might end your life? (plans)
- Do you possess what it would take (e.g., pills, firearms) to carry out your plan to end your life? (means)

Treatment

- Negotiate whether to use medication, counseling, or both.
- Refer to a psychiatrist when severe or complicated depression or suicide risk.
- Consider referral to a psychotherapist for counseling.
- If there is marital distress or relationship difficulties, refer to a couple therapist.
- Involve partner in treatment
- See patient for regularly scheduled follow-up visits, even when patient is feeling better.

21
When Drinking or Drugs Is Part of the Problem: A Family Approach to the Detection and Management of Substance Use and Abuse

Although not always recognized as such, primary care clinicians see many patients with alcohol or substance abuse problems every day. Estimates are that one in five primary care patients seen in an average day have such problems (1, 2). These patients are often cleverly disguised, and most will leave the office with their secret safe; estimates are that only one in five is detected (3, 4). In addition, there may be family members of the patient being seen who have undetected alcohol or substance abuse problems. A family orientation improves a clinician's ability to detect alcohol and substance abuse problems in patients and their families by increasing the number of ways to access this information and improve reliability. Moreover, because virtually all treatments require some family involvement, family-oriented clinicians are in a good position to foster treatment success.

Considered by some the number one public health problem in this country, the effects of alcoholism and substance abuse for families and society stagger the mind. Substance use and abuse are chronic and serious biopsychosocial disorders that have repercussions across the entire biopsychosocial spectrum: from the physiologic effects of alcohol and drugs on organs and tissue, to the impact of the associated behaviors on family and society. Many well-known treatment approaches focus on the individual and consider the cellular and genetic aspects of the biopsychosocial spectrum. We will focus in this chapter on substance use and abuse as a disorder that involves and affects the family, and we describe the role of the family-oriented clinician in the detection, assessment and management of these problems. We will emphasize the importance of the family in all these aspects, while keeping both genetics and social context in mind.

Substance use in the form of tobacco dependence is a unique problem with profound consequences to the health of the individual, and in costs to society. The use of tobacco shares many principles of dependence with alcoholism and substance abuse, and strategies for behavior change have much in common. Even though some strategies for behavior change are borrowed from the tobacco dependence literature, (e.g., the five As: Ask, Assess, Advise, Assist, and Arrange), our primary focus for this chapter will be on other substance use and abuse.

Families and Substance Abuse

Since the 1970s, there is increased recognition of the role of the family in the understanding and treatment of alcoholism and substance abuse. For years, these problems were thought to be related primarily to genetics and/or individual psychopathology. There are clearly some genetic linkages, and individuals are responsible for their own behavior, but this is only part of the story. Norms for acceptable behavior with mind-altering substances are first encountered in families. Furthermore, conditions that exist in families may reinforce the maintenance of these behaviors. Once patterns of use are established, changing these patterns often involves and affects family members. Successful treatment will virtually always involve families in some fashion (5, 6). Primary care clinicians have some of the best opportunities for prevention, early detection, and assisting in the treatment of established substance abusers. A family approach to drug and alcohol problems is important for a number of reasons. Alcoholics and substance abusers live in families. The stereotype of the "skid row" alcoholic or drug addict who lives alone in the street represents a very small percentage of people who abuse alcohol or drugs (7, 8). Even addicted homeless people often have families who influence and are affected by their behavior. In addition, the impact of alcoholism and substance abuse on the patient and the family is determined more by the family environment (e.g., its rules, attitudes, and beliefs) than by the amount or pattern of alcohol or substance abuse (9).

Alcoholism and substance abuse runs in families. Patients who have two or more relatives with a history of alcohol abuse are at three times the normal risk of abusing alcohol themselves. Adoption and twin studies have demonstrated that both genetic and family environment increase this risk (9, 10). Some behaviorists view substance abuse as conditioned behavior that is reinforced by cues and contingencies within the family. Certain family rituals have been shown to protect against the transmission of alcoholism from one generation to the next (11). These findings emphasize the importance of obtaining a family history and identifying family members who are at risk.

A family approach allows earlier identification and treatment of alcohol or substance abuse problems. The earliest problems associated with alcohol and substance abuse are usually interpersonal, and they occur long before any medical complications. Alcohol and substance abuse problems often first present as marital disputes, parent–child conflicts, or work problems (9, 12). The clinician will identify underlying alcohol or substance abuse only by exploring these subjects (13). Family members are usually the first to recognize problems. They may alert the clinician to the problem and ask for help. For example, one common clinical presentation is a depressed woman with multiple somatic complaints and marital problems related to her husband's drinking. Caring for the entire family gives the family-oriented clinician the chance to intervene early, when treatment is easier and more effective.

Families are a major asset in the assessment and treatment of alcohol and substance abuse problems. Patients who abuse alcohol or drugs often deny having a problem. For example, alcoholics usually underreport how much they drink and the adverse effects of their drinking. Family members often provide a more accurate picture, although they sometimes also share in the denial. Acting alone, the clinician may have little ability to break down the denial, but allied with concerned family members, he or she can more effectively negotiate with the patient and begin treatment. Family treatment has been shown to be helpful both to initiate treatment and to increase the likelihood of success (14).

Families need treatment both to help cope with the effects of alcoholism and substance abuse on the family and to change family patterns that may have unwittingly contributed to the problem. Alcoholism and substance abuse are devastating illnesses that affect all members of the family. Marital conflict or divorce, child abuse or neglect, unemployment and poverty, along with numerous mental and physical health problems, are just a few of the possible consequences. Emotions like anger, blame, and guilt often run through these families and will persist even after abstinence, if the family does not receive treatment. A variety of family treatment modalities have been shown to reduce the emotional distress of family members (14).

In attempting to cope with the drinking or substance abuse, family members may inadvertently facilitate or enable it. This most commonly occurs when a spouse thinks he or she is protecting the abuser by keeping the substance use a secret or covering up the adverse consequences, such as missing work. Drinking or substance abuse can provide a function in some families in that it may be used as a solution to unresolved conflicts or unacceptable feelings. For example, anger or grief expressed while a person is drunk or high may be discounted because of the altered state. These families often display stereotypic patterns of interaction, which cycle between dry and wet phases (15, 16). Patients and families need help changing these dysfunctional patterns of interaction that can underpin addictive behavior. Family-based treatments are currently recognized as among the most effective approaches for adolescent drug abuse and have become increasingly effective for adult drug and alcohol abuse (17).

Clinician Barriers to Detection

There are many reasons that clinicians fail to recognize alcohol and substance abuse problems in their patients. There is a lack of education about alcohol and substance abuse. For example, only a small portion of medical school curriculum is devoted to the subject, and that is mostly lectures on medical complications. In one survey of practicing clinicians, only 27% reported that they felt competent to treat alcoholism (18).

1. The early signs of substance abuse are mostly psychosocial, not biomedical.

Substance abuse may masquerade as a physical problem. As a result, the biomedically focused clinician may be distracted by the presenting symptom(s) and be unaware of the problem.

Clinicians may have misconceptions about alcoholics and substance abusers based on prior professional and personal experience. Clinicians in training often care for skid row, end-stage alcoholics or substance abusers. These training contacts often generate feelings of aversion, hostility, and depression. Clinicians may also have had negative personal experiences with substance abuse and alcoholism in a friend or family member, which further colors their experience with patients. Clinicians may also be more likely to overlook substance abuse in patients of higher socioeconomic standing because they are most like themselves.

Pessimism about treatment may affect the clinician's inclination to screen for abuse. Many clinicians feel that substance abuse is not treatable and feel helpless when confronted with a patient who has these problems. Inadequate resources for treating substance abusers may add to this pessimism. As a result, clinicians may think that it is not worthwhile to screen for substance abuse.

2. Denial is perhaps the most significant clinician barrier to detection.

There may be a reluctance on the part of the clinician to impose his or her agenda or values on the patient who has come in for a different reason (4). Addressing issues of substance abuse often requires the clinician to change from a stance of caring and nurturance to one that is more challenging and confrontive. Many primary care clinicians are uncomfortable with this and prefer to avoid conflict. Denial may be further fueled by a desire to avoid an anticipated increase in time for the visit. As the clock ticks, the clinician may be more willing to ignore the issue in order to get to the next patient. Finally, the distinction between social drinking and alcohol abuse is not always clear. To diagnose alcohol or drug problems, the primary care clinician must address his or her own drinking and substance abuse, which can be threatening.

Sam Jones worked as a vice-president in a local construction firm, and had previously been seen for a variety of straightforward, mostly athletic-related, orthopedic problems. One week prior to the visit, Mr. Jones had been involved in a single-car motor vehicle accident that resulted in a visit to the local Emergency Department to repair a laceration. The Emergency Department did not obtain a blood alcohol level, but Mr. Jones confided to Dr. A. in a friend-to-friend fashion that he had "a few with the boys after work." Behind schedule, Dr. A. was happy to see a patient with such a time-limited problem like suture removal, and reassured that Mr. Jones was like himself, slapped him on the back on the way out the door, chiding him to drive more carefully.

The Five As: Ask, Assess, Advise, Assist, and Arrange

The presence, or serious potential, of adverse physical, family, social, occupational, or legal consequences best define alcohol and substance abuse. Dependence further includes the presence of withdrawal or tolerance. The practical definitions used by the past several editions of the *Diagnostics and Statistics Manual* (19) have been very helpful, from both clinical and research perspectives, by concretely labeling the disorders by their effects. Because of differing rates of metabolism, at-risk drinking, as defined by the National Institute on Alcohol Abuse and Alcoholism, changes depending on gender. For women, the limit is set at one drink per day or seven drinks per week; for men the quantity is double that (20). The acronym publicized by the U.S. Department of Health and Human Services (HSS) for its approach to tobacco dependence applies equally well to alcohol and substance abuse: Ask, Assess, Advise, Assist, Arrange.

Ask

Because of the high prevalence of alcohol and substance abuse, and their serious impact on health, all patients should be screened. Studies have shown that patients rarely bring up these problems spontaneously to their clinician (21). Unless the clinician specifically asks about drinking and drug use these people will remain anonymous (22). All patients should be asked:

1. "How much alcohol do you drink?" (Rather than, "Do you drink alcohol?")

It is helpful to get an average for the week so it includes weekends. Be sure of quantities without making assumptions. For example, one or two beers may be one or two of the 40-oz.-size beers.

2. "Have you experimented with drugs? Do you use any drugs?"

Drug use generally begins with experimentation.

3. "Have you ever had a problem with your health, your work, or your family because of drinking or drug use?"

This latter question has been shown to be particularly effective in identifying alcoholic patients (23).

When obtaining a family history, ask:

1. "Has anyone in your family ever had problems with alcohol or other substance abuse?"

Be as matter-of-fact as possible when inquiring about alcohol or substance use. Include these questions routinely with other medical background questions like previous surgeries and current medications. Show interest but not surprise about the amount or pattern of use during screening or assessment. Avoid derogatory terms unless the patient brings them up. Many patients will admit that they or their family members have had problems with alcohol or substance use, but have never considered it to be a disease. Be aware of the degree of defensiveness the patient exhibits in response to your questions. Remember the Shakespearean maxim, "Me thinks the lady doth protest too much."

There are a variety of quick screening and case identification tools that have been developed for use in the primary care setting to follow up suspicion of a problem. The most extensively studied instrument, the CAGE questionnaire (24), has been adapted to screen for substance abuse as well (25). Two or more positive responses are considered clinically significant.

C Have you ever felt you ought to Cut down on your drinking or drug use?
A Have people Annoyed you by criticizing your drinking or drug use?
G Have you ever felt bad or Guilty about your drinking or drug use?
E Have you ever had a drink or used drugs first thing in the morning to steady your nerves or get rid of a hangover (Eye-opener)?

> Mrs. Seacrest, a 44-year-old housewife and mother of three children, came to Dr. K. for her yearly Pap smear and check-up. She complained of feeling tired all of the time, and having difficulty sleeping. She attributed it to caring for three young children and an aging parent, but wondered whether she was beginning menopause. Further questions by Dr. K. revealed that Mrs. Seacrest was mildly depressed and that her husband was rarely at home, spending more and more time at work. As part of his routine interval history, Dr. K. asked about alcohol use. She replied that she usually had a drink before dinner while waiting for her husband to come home, and occasionally had a brandy to help her sleep. With more specific questions, she admitted to having one or two drinks regularly during most days and three or four each evening, but denied that it was causing any problems. At times she felt she ought to *cut down* on her drinking, and felt a little *guilty* about her drinking because she was very critical of her mother, who drank to excess. (Two affirmative answers to *CAGE* questions.)

A variety of other screening instruments have been shown to be useful in the primary care setting. The single question, "When was the last time you had more than five (for men, four for women) drinks on one occasion?" was found to have good sensitivity and specificity by Taj, Devera-Sales, and Vinson (26). The Short Michigan Alcoholism Screening Test (SMAST) (27) is another effective instrument that can be given to either a patient or significant other.

Assess

After asking all patients, a more thorough assessment needs to be done on all those who report significant drinking or substance abuse, give two *yes* answers to any of the CAGE questions, or present with a complaint related to alcohol or drug use. Whenever possible, involve family members as part of the assessment and before presenting the diagnosis of alcohol or substance abuse. Interviewing patients with family members present will usually provide more accurate information about the severity of the behavior and associated problems. Family members are the clinician's most important allies in the treatment process. They have often been concerned about the problem for years, but have not known how to intervene. When suspecting significant alcohol or substance abuse, ask the patient to return in 2–3 weeks with other family members to follow up on the presenting problem (see Chap. 7). With the patient and family members present, discuss the presenting problem and inquire about what seems to exacerbate the problem. If family members do not bring up the behavior, present it as a contributing factor and ask their opinion: "One of the things that I think is contributing to your husband's elevated blood pressure is his drinking. We know that alcohol raises blood pressure and can cause hypertension. What are your thoughts on this?"

> Dr. K. expressed concern about Mrs. Seacrest's chronic fatigue and said that he thought it might be due to an underlying depression made worse by her drinking. He asked her to return in 2 weeks to discuss the problem further and to review the results of the Pap smear and lab tests. He further requested that her husband accompany her to the next visit, as "he may help us understand what's contributing to your fatigue."

Assessment of the problem requires investigation into the quantity, time, and place of the behavior, along with identifying the patient's readiness for change.

1. Make a best effort to accurately assess the quantity of a substance ingested.

Quantify alcohol and substance abuse as precisely as possible. Denial and minimization are commonly encountered, and the clinician must pursue and probe for specific details. Obtain information about current usage, as well as larger trends over time. At some point, it may improve reliability either to ask family members in person or over the phone to corroborate details.

2. Ask about the time of ingestion.

Does the patient only drink on weekends? Does the patient only use cocaine after drinking? The clinician must be thorough and specific, and can end each phase of questioning with comments like, "Is there anything else I'm missing here? What are we leaving out?" to ensure completeness.

3. Assess the place and social setting for the behavior.

Does the patient drink at home, at bars, or both? Does the patient ingest substances alone, or with others? Many of these behaviors are context dependent, and an important part of treatment usually involves changing the patient's contact with the social context associated with the behavior.

4. Assess the patient's readiness for change.

Behavior change can be broken down into six different stages: precontemplation, contemplation, preparation, action, maintenance, and relapse (see Chap. 6). Successful treatment depends on an accurate assessment of the patient's current stage. Treatment often fails because the clinician fails to appreciate the step-wise nature of behavior change and tries to skip a step or two.

5. Record the patient's response in a prominent place in the medical chart.

A pertinent summary of alcohol and drug use should be located conveniently, as with such other basic medical information as allergies, previous surgeries, and current medications.

Advise

Once the clinician has made a thorough assessment, the next step is to advise the patient. Just like the assessment improves with family input, advice is more effective in a family context. Each patient's individual circumstances need to be accommodated, so advice can be specifically tailored for each patient. Personalized simple statements like, "I think you should quit or cut down for the following reasons . . . ," has been shown to be effective (28). In terms of advice giving, what applies to tobacco, applies equally well to alcohol and substance abuse. The U.S. Surgeon General recommends advice in the format of the five Rs: Relevance, Risks, Rewards, Roadblocks, and Repetition.

1. Relevance.

Link the risk-related behavior to current problems (i.e., medical, social, or legal) whenever possible. For example, drinking and its relation to ulcers or marital discord; substance abuse with its financial and legal ramifications.

2. Risks.

Beyond the current problem, describe other potential future problems with the risk-related behavior. Be broad and inclusive, but also be believable.

3. Rewards.

Help identify the unique personal and family rewards for behavior change. For example, decreasing alcohol use may lead to improved health as well because better social, financial, and/or legal circumstances are likely to ensue.

4. Roadblocks.

This portion of advice requires input from the patient, family, and clinician about particular challenges to success. Accurately anticipating these difficulties and strategizing together about ways to overcome them is critical to success.

In addition to the clinician's specific knowledge about the physical consequences of withdrawal, he or she can use his or her experience with other patients to help predict unanticipated challenges to behavior change.

5. Repetition.

The risk-related behavior should be prominently documented in the chart, and comments, however brief, directed toward facilitating behavior change should be made at every visit. Persistence pays off with these chronic problems.

> Johnnie Jordan, a 38-year-old Caucasian male, was admitted to rule out myocardial infarction secondary to cocaine ingestion. He had a long history of substance abuse, including tobacco dependence, alcohol abuse, and recently increasing cocaine dependence. He was admitted after 3 hours of crushing substernal chest pain with EKG changes consistent with ischemia. Over the course of his hospitalization, Dr. M. emphasized the connection between the chest pain and the cocaine use. Given his strong family history for coronary artery disease, Dr. M. pointed out that continued use of both tobacco and cocaine dramatically increased the likelihood that he would end up like his father (i.e., a "cardiac cripple"). The multiple rewards of improved sleep, smell, taste, and financial and legal situations were described. Marital reconciliation was also dependent on successful rehabilitation. Finding friends that did not smoke, drink, and use drugs was identified as a major roadblock to success. Direct referral to an intensive inpatient treatment program was arranged by hospital social work.

Assist

The kind of assistance indicated for patients with alcohol and drug problems depends on where they are on the readiness-to-change spectrum. For many, honest advice and education are all that can be realistically provided. When it is done in a family context, with family input and involvement, the family can reinforce the clinician's advice. The clinician and family need to appreciate their unique role in the patient's environment, and particularly need to understand the limits of their responsibility. It is the patient's responsibility to change his or her behavior.

The clinician may be able to push the patient, or sometimes just nudge, into the next phase of behavior change. For example, setting a quit date for patients in the preparation stage may move them into the action stage. The clinician may need to be patient, yet persistent, and work steadily over time, which is the advantage of primary care: Continuity of care allows the clinician to work steadily over longer periods of time.

Since the 1990s, increasing research has demonstrated the effectiveness of brief interventions (29). Brief interventions have been shown to be more effective than no intervention; they are often as effective as more extensive interventions; and they may provide a helpful base upon which further interventions can build. Fleming and his colleagues (29) demonstrated the effectiveness of a brief intervention consisting of two 15-minute visits 1 month apart and one nurse follow-up phone call. In these visits, patients were given "feedback about their current health behaviors, a review of the prevalence of problem drinking and adverse effects, a list of drinking cues, a drinking agreement, and drinking diary cards." This intervention was later shown to be cost-effective (i.e., the cost of the intervention was one fifth the ultimate cost of doing nothing) (30).

Pharmacotherapy is a concrete way in which the clinician can assist the patient. Medications for treating any underlying anxiety or depression will also be helpful in the treatment of alcoholism and substance abuse. Some research has shown that combining disulfiram with behavioral couples treatment improves outcome for patients with alcohol dependence (31).

Arrange

The final step in the pathway is to arrange follow up: Many patients with alcohol or drug problems will need some kind of referral. Patients with long-term addiction, severe problems, or who have previously failed primary care intervention or previous treatment are likely to need referral. The key to successful referral is to know community resources for substance abuse treatment and to establish a working relationship with a counselor. As with any therapy, the referral is more likely to succeed if the clinician can personally recommend an individual counselor and set up the appointment while the patient is still in the office. This counselor can also serve as a consultant to help the clinician with patients who refuse an evaluation. Establishing a personal relationship with a counselor permits a collaborative approach to treating the patient and family.

Once identified, substance abusing patients and their families should be followed closely, regardless of whether they go into treatment. If the patient or family refuses an evaluation, the clinician needs to work gradually with the patient, connecting the presenting problems and symptoms to abuse. If the patient enters a local inpatient treatment facility, a visit by the primary care clinician would help to support the program and the patient's progress. Regular appointments can be scheduled for the patient and family during and following outpatient treatment and aftercare. Close communication with the patient's counselor facilitates successful treatment.

The patient or counselor may occasionally ask the clinician to prescribe benzodiazepines or hospitalize a patient for detoxification. Detoxification with benzodiazepines should only be done in conjunction with a treatment program. The clinician should not prescribe such medication to patients who claim that they can quit on their own. On rare occasions, benzodiazepines can be prescribed as part of an outpatient-treatment program, but patients should be seen at least every other day to be sure they are not drinking or using drugs with the medication, and they should periodically be monitored with urine toxicology screens.

Substance abuse is a chronic, often lifelong disorder, and relapses are common. The patient, family, and clinician must recognize this so that they do not feel demoralized and helpless if the patient resumes the behavior. The clinician should try to see the patient and family as soon as the behavior is renewed. Family members can be instructed to come in for an appointment if the patient starts the abusive behavior again. During the visit, the clinician should support the patient and avoid criticism, and encourage the family to do the same. The clinician can congratulate the patient for abstaining as long as he or she did, and explain that relapse is common. The goal is to get the patient back into treatment as soon as possible. A counselor should be contacted while the patient and family are in the office and a follow-up appointment should be made as soon as possible.

Substance Abuse in the Family: When Family Members Present

Family members of substance abusers use the healthcare services more often than other patients (32). On routine visits, the clinician should screen for problems in the family as well as in the patient. Obtaining a genogram and asking about any family history often uncovers alcohol or substance abuse problems in the family. In addition, red flags may alert the clinician that a patient is experiencing a problem in the family. The most common associated problems include somatization, depression, and physical and sexual abuse.

When further history reveals that there is probable alcohol or substance abuse in another family member, the patient should be told the diagnosis and educated about its impact on the family. If the patient accepts that there is a problem in the family, he or she should be referred to Al-Anon (or Alateen for adolescents), or to a substance abuse counselor or Narcotics Anonymous. A variety of resources can help such patients understand what role they play in the pattern and how they must change to help the family member. Thus, the focus is on what the family member(s) can do.

If the patient does not accept that substance abuse in the family is a problem, the clinician should show how the presenting problem (i.e., depression, marital problems) is related. This may be a slow and gradual process. The clinician can refer the patient to a family therapist for the presenting problem, letting the therapist know that there is substance abuse in the family.

A family member will occasionally try to get the clinician to confront the substance abuser about their behavior. A family member may call the clinician and explain that the patient coming in for an appointment has a "drinking or drug problem." The implicit or explicit message is that the caller wants the clinician to confront the patient without revealing the source of the information. This effort to triangulate the clinician into a family conflict can occur with any problem, but it is particularly common in alcohol and drug abuse. In general, the clinician should avoid taking the "bait" and encourage the caller to accompany the patient to the appointment so that the concerns can be voiced directly.

> A telephone call:
>
> Mrs. K.: Dr. C., I just thought you should know before you see my husband next week that he's been drinking a lot lately and I think it's affecting his health. You see he's. . .
>
> Dr. C.: (interrupting) Mrs. K., these sound like important concerns about your husband's health. It sounds to me like you should come in with your husband to express those concerns directly to him in front of me.
>
> Mrs. K.: I can't do that. I just thought that as his doctor you could talk to him about his drinking.
>
> Dr. C.: I would have to tell him how I know about it. In situations like these I have definitely found its much more effective if you come in together.
>
> Mrs. K.: I'll have to think about it. You won't tell him that I called, will you?
>
> Dr. C.: Mrs. K., I will mention that you called, but that's all. If he called about you, I'd mention it to you. I hope to see you when he comes in next week. Good-bye now.

Conclusion

Substance use and abuse is a common, serious, and treatable chronic illness. Primary care clinicians need to be alert to the potential in all their patients. A family orientation gives the primary care clinician an advantage in the early diagnosis and treatment of these disorders. Access to the family increases early recognition and enables the clinician to utilize family members as allies in the treatment process. Family-oriented treatment is essential to change the context within which the problem arose, and to help patients and families establish and maintain new, healthier lifestyles.

References

1. American Society of Addiction Medicine: Public policy statement on screening for addiction in primary care settings. *J Addict Dis* 1998;**17**:124–127.
2. Fleming MF, Barry KL: Clinical overview of alcohol and drug disorders. In: Fleming MF, Barry KL (eds): *Addictive Disorders*: St. Louis: Mosby Yearbook, 1992, pp. 3–21.
3. Ashworth M, Gerada A: ABC of mental health. Addiction and dependence—II: Alcohol. *Br Med J* 1997;**315**:358–360.
4. Vinson DC, Elder N, Werner JJ, Vorel LA, & Nutting PA: Alcohol-related discussions in primary care. *JFP* 2000;**49**(1):28–33.
5. Edwards ME, Steinglass P: Family therapy treatment outcomes for alcoholism. *J Marital Fam Ther* 1995;**21**(4):475–509.
6. Liddle HA, Dakof, GA. Efficacy of family therapy for drug abuse: promising but not definitive. *J Marital Fam Ther* 1995;**21**(1):511–543.
7. Singer M: Family comes first: an examination of the social networks of skidrow ment. *Human Org* 1985;**44**:137–142.
8. Wolin SJ, Steinglass P: Interactional behavior in an alcoholic community. *Med Ann of DC* 1974;**43**:183–187.
9. Steinglass P, Bennett LA, Wolin SJ, & Reiss D. *The Alcoholic Family*. New York: Basic Books, 1987.
10. Goodwin DW. Alcoholism and heredity: a review and hypothesis. *Arch Gen Psychiatr* 1979;**36**:57–61.
11. Wolin SJ, Bennett LA, & Noonan DL: Family rituals and the recurrence of alcoholism over generations. *Am J Psychiatr* 1979;**136**:589–593.
12. Weinberg JR: Assessing drinking problems by history. *Postgrad Med J* 1976; **59**:87–90.
13. Doherty WJ, Baird MA: Treating chemical dependency in a family context. *Family Therapy and Family Medicine*. New York: Guilford Press, 1983.
14. Sprenkle D (ed): *Effectiveness Research in Marriage and Family Therapy*. Alexandria, VA: AAMFT, 2002.
15. Steinglass P. The alcoholic family at home: patterns of interaction in dry, wet and transitional stages of alcoholism. *Arch Gen Psychiatr* 1981;**38**:578–584.
16. Steinglass P, Davis DI, & Berensen D. Observations of conjointly hospitalized "alcoholic couples" during sobriety and intoxication: Implications for theory and therapy. *Fam Proc* 1977;**16**:1–16.
17. Rowe CL, Liddle HA: Substance Abuse. *J Marital Fam Ther* 2003;**29**(1):97–120.

18. Sadler D: Poll finds MD attitudes on alcohol abuse changing. *Am Med News* 1984;**27**:60.
19. American Psychiatric Association: *Diagnostic and Statistics Manual of Mental Disorders, fourth ed.* Washington DC: American Psychiatric Association, 1994, pp. 175–272.
20. National Institute on Alcohol Abuse and Alcoholism: *The Clinician's Guide to Helping Patients with Alcohol Problems.* Washington DC: U.S. Government Printing Office, 1995. NIH Publication no. 95-3769.
21. Ford DE, Kamerow DB, & Thompson JW: Who talks to clinicians about mental health and substance abuse problems. *J Gen Intern Med* 1988;**3**:363–369.
22. Woodall HE: Alcoholic remaining anonymous: resident diagnosis of alcoholism in a family practice center. *J Fam Prac* 1988;**26**:293–296.
23. Cyr MG, Wartman SA: The effectiveness of routine screening questions the detection of alcoholism. *JAMA* 1988;**259**:51–54.
24. Ewing JA: Detecting alcoholism: the CAGE questionnaire. *JAMA* 1984;**252**:1905–1907.
25. Brown Rl, Rounds LA: Conjoint screening questionnaires for alcohol and drug abuse: criterion validity in a primary care practice. *Wis Med J* 1995;**94**:135–140.
26. Taj N, Devera-Sales A, & Vinson DC: Screening for problem drinking: does a single question work? *J Fam Pract* 1998;**46**:328.
27. Selzer ML, Vinokur A, & Van Roooijen L: A self-administered Short Michigan Alcoholism Screening Test (SMAST). *J Stud Alcohol* 1975;**36**:117–126.
28. Bien TH, Miller WR, & Tonigan JS: Brief interventions for alcohol problems: a review. *Addiction* 1993;**88**:315–335.
29. Fleming MF, Barry Kl, Manwell LB, Johnson K, & London R. Brief physician advice for problem alcohol drinkers. A randomized controlled trial in community-based primary care practices. *JAMA* 1997;**277**:1039–1045.
30. Fleming MF, Mundt MP, French MT, Manwell LB, Stauffacher EA, & Barry KL: Benefit-cost analysis of brief physician advice with problem drinkers in primary care settings. *Med Care* 2000;**38**(1):7–18.
31. Rotunda R, O'Farrell TJ: Marital and family therapy of alcohol use disorders. Bridging the gap between research and practice. *Profession Psychol* 1997;**28**:246–252.
32. Liepman, M. Alcohol and drug abuse in the family. In: Christie-Seeley J (Ed.): *Working with the Family in Primary Care.* New York: Praeger, (in press).

Protocol: When Drinking or Drugs Is Part of the Problem:

A Family Approach to the Detection and Management of Substance Use and Abuse

Ask

C Have you ever felt you ought to *C*ut down on your drinking or drug use?
A Have people *A*nnoyed you by criticizing your drinking or drug use?
G Have you ever felt bad or *G*uilty about your drinking or drug use?
E Have you ever had a drink or used drugs first thing in the morning to steady your nerves or get rid of a hangover (*E*ye-opener)?

Assess

- Quantity of substance.
- Time of ingestion.
- Place or setting of abuse.
- Readiness for Change: Precontemplation, Contemplation, Preparation, Action, Maintenance, Relapse.

Advise

- Relevance: Link behavior to concrete social, occupational, or health consequences.
- Risks: Point out long-term adverse effects of current behavior.
- Rewards: Describe advantages of behavior change.
- Roadblocks: Anticipate hurdles to behavior change.
- Repetition: Persist in advice-giving as often as possible.

Assist

- Education: Provide information at the appropriate level.
- Brief Intervention: In addition to education, consider making a brief intervention (e.g., providing a list of drinking cues, a drinking agreement, and drinking diary cards).
- Consider pharmocotherapy: Treat depression and anxiety with psychotropic medications.

Arrange

- Close follow up: Provide frequent visits for patient and family.
- Referral: Make every effort to refer patients with long-term addiction, severe problems, or those who have failed primary care interventions or previous treatment.

22
Protecting the Family: Domestic Violence and the Primary Care Clinician

In Collaboration with Barbara Gawinski* and Nancy Ruddy[†]

When most clinicians first think of domestic violence, they think of partner abuse; however, the term *domestic violence* encompasses child abuse and neglect, partner abuse, and elder abuse. In this chapter, we will keep to this broader usage and discuss family violence in all its forms across all age groups. We propose that the clinician's main job is to recognize the signs of domestic violence and then use those resources that exist within the family and community to protect the individual and family. Abusive families lack the internal controls needed to create a safe environment. External controls by community agencies are consequently often required. The primary care clinician's role in treatment is to mobilize a safety network for the family to protect the individual and to initiate the work of change and healing that must occur in the family. With the help of the legal system, community agencies, and mental health professionals, the clinician can help set a process in motion that results in successful treatment for many of these families.

This chapter begins with a description of common elements to all three forms of domestic violence (i.e., child, partner, elder) while recognizing there are also important differences. The next sections in the chapter describe these more unique characteristics along with suggestions for screening, detection, and intervention. Because of the dearth of research, most of the material is based on expert opinion. For many clinicians, these issues bring up strong personal reactions, and the chapter concludes with our thoughts about continuity of care, when the perpetrator is your patient, and personal issues for the clinician.

* Barbara Gawinski, PhD, Associate Professor of Family Medicine, University of Rochester School of Medicine and Dentistry, Rochester, NY, USA.
[†] Nancy Ruddy, PhD, Associate Director of Behavioral Science, on the Faculty of the Hunterdon Family Practice Residency, Flemington, NJ, USA.

Domestic Violence: Common Elements

A complex combination of variables predisposes a family to domestic violence. An understanding of these factors can help a clinician recognize families that may be more vulnerable. At its core, domestic violence results from an abuse of power by the more powerful exerted on those with less power. A significant power differential may exist in any of a number of different dimensions: physical strength (men vs. women, adults vs. children or elders), physical capabilities (healthy vs. ill or pregnant), intellectual capacity (healthy vs. handicapped or delayed), competence with the prevailing language (natives vs. immigrants), professional status, social class, and financial resources, to name a few. In addition, certain family factors increase the risk of domestic violence: a history of violence or abuse across generations, substance abuse, blurred or confused generational boundaries, and family isolation (1–4). Making the problem even more complicated, barriers to detection and treatment, both in terms of the patient and in terms of the clinician, occur for all forms of domestic violence (5).

1. History of violence or abuse.

Domestic violence is twice as likely in families with a history of violence or abuse; however, most people who have a history of being abused do not become abusers, and often live their lives in fear of becoming abusers (1, 2).

2. Substance abuse.

Domestic violence is five times as likely in families where there is substance abuse. Domestic violence occurs both in times of intoxication and sobriety (3).

3. Blurred generational boundaries.

In families where child or elder abuse occurs, the boundary between the parent generation and the child generation is often unclear and at times nonexistent. Children may be seen as sources of reassurance about the parents' personal adequacy or self-esteem (4). When the child is unable to nurture the parent, the parent may feel rejected and may respond in a punitive manner. With elder abuse, the caretaking child may resent the change in roles, and the consequent reversal of dependency.

4. Family isolation.

These families, both as units and as their members individually, tend to be socially isolated. Social isolation fosters the belief that all the needs of family members must be met within the family. This belief increases the burden on already overburdened families, and also blocks members from reporting problems to those outside the family who may be able to help.

5. Patient barriers to detection and treatment.

Patients who are subjected to domestic violence may fear retaliation, either against themselves, their children, or their elders. They may feel ashamed of the situation, and think they should have done more to prevent it. They often perceive few personal and community resources, and may see clinicians as unhelpful. These people generally want to keep the family together, and *want the violence, not the relationships, to end*. They may fear that reporting the violence will destroy the relationships. In some circumstances, the violence may be culturally supported or proscribed by their religion, and reporting the violence may be perceived as violating those ties and beliefs.

6. Physician barriers to detection and treatment.

Clinicians may disregard clues as a result of: lack of training, overwhelming personal reactions, fear of offending, feeling powerless, or a desire to save time (5). Clinicians may want to avoid confronting perpetrators of violence due to their affection for, or their fear of, these people, or, in certain families, due to bias (e.g., in families of higher socioeconomic status).

Child Abuse and Neglect

Child abuse is the infliction of injury on a person less than 18 years of age by a parent, legally responsible guardian, or other adult. Physical abuse occurs when the child experiences an injury at the hand of the caregiver. *Child neglect* is defined as inadequate caregiving or parenting that has the potential for injury. This may include physical, emotional, educational, or medical neglect. These are legal definitions, not medical diagnoses; however, clinicians are legally compelled to file a report when acts of physical or sexual injury occur, or are suspected, or when children are exposed to substantial risk for any of these. According to the annual 50-state survey, in 1996, 1 million children in the United States were confirmed victims of child abuse and neglect, and 1185 children died from their injuries (6). These figures may reflect only a small percentage of the total amount of abuse that occurs but is never reported. For example, in one outpatient study 4.2% of mothers reported domestic violence, whereas physicians identified some type of abuse in less than 1% (7).

Identifying the Signs of Abuse

Clinicians may be the first to bring the problem of abuse to light. Identification depends on recognizing key signs of possible sexual and physical abuse. The signs of abuse will vary according to the age of the child (8, 9). Many of these symptoms are nonspecific to abuse; however, presentation of any combination of these symptoms should signal to the clinician the need to rule out abuse (see Table 22.1).

TABLE 22.1. Signs and symptoms of child abuse and neglect

5 years old and under	Preteen	Adolescents
Failure to thrive	Anxiety, fear, depression, insomnia	Psychosomatic complaints
Extreme clinging behavior		Changes in appetite or eating disorders
Sleep disturbances and night terrors	Sudden weight loss or gain	
	Encopresis and enuresis	Assumption of responsibilities in the house previously held by the mother
Hand marks, strap marks, pinch or bite marks	School failure or truancy	
Poorly explained sores or bruises in genital area, buttocks, or lower back	Knowledge of sexual behavior inappropriate to the child's age	Chronic depression and suicidality
Multiple bruises at different stages of healing	Preoccupation with or fear of sexual activity	Social isolation and running away
Burns (cigarette, scalding on hands and feet)	Inconsistent stories about bruises and sores in genital areas	Sexual promiscuity
Severe anxiety around physical examination		

Adolescent girls who are the victims of incest may have particularly complex family dynamics. They often exhibit extraordinary rebellious behavior, especially toward their mothers (10). They may be more forgiving of their father's abuse than of their mothers inability to protect them. Fathers in families with incest are often overly protective of their daughters. They may block their daughters from developing relationships outside the family, especially with males. Incest is frequently reported for the first time when the child enters adolescence and is prohibited by her father from developing peer relationships or boyfriends. The oldest daughter in families where incest occurs may be subtly encouraged to replace her mother as a parent and a spouse. These daughters function as parentified children, handling many of the maternal and domestic responsibilities in the household, while trying to meet the sexual and emotional needs of their fathers.

Some researchers believe that clinicians overlook sexual abuse of boys (8). While father–daughter incest is the most frequently reported form of abuse, 1 in 10 victims of sexual abuse will be male. Clinicians may apply many of the same identification criteria to both their female and male patients.

Physical abuse differs from sexual abuse in that the signs of physical abuse present both on the evidence of injury to the child as well as on the nature of the parent's presentation to the clinician. Parents of children who have been physically abused are often less distraught by their child's injuries than one would expect. Parental behaviors that may be evidence of child abuse include (11):

- unexplained delay in bringing the child for treatment
- implausible or contradictory explanation of the injury
- history of child having unusual injuries
- blunted emotional reaction to child's trauma

- parent blaming child for injury
- parent having history of previous abusive behavior

In factitious disorders (e.g., Munchausen by proxy), even though many of the preconditions are identical to physical abuse, the clinician will see just the opposite tone in parental behavior. Instead of being less distraught by the child's symptoms, the parent (almost always the mother) excessively worries about the child's condition, and will even create an illness or injury in order to justify concern. Although it is rare, the lethality of this disorder makes accurate diagnosis essential.

In the following case, the clinician's suspicion of child abuse is first raised by the nature of the child's behavioral symptoms.

> Mrs. Wooden brought Madeline, age 9, to see Dr. H. because she had been complaining of stomachaches at night and vaginal itchiness. Mrs. Wooden also took Dr. H. aside to say she was concerned about a report from the school that Madeline had written a note to a boy in her class asking if he wanted to "put his finger in her hole."
>
> Dr. H. asked Mrs. Wooden if she had noticed any other changes in Madeline's behavior. Mrs. Wooden reported that Madeline was often afraid to go to bed at night and wanted her mother to sleep with her. Madeline's teachers also reported that her grades were going down and that she seemed preoccupied and anxious. With this information in mind, Dr. H. proceeded with a complete physical of Madeline.

If there are signs of abuse that strengthen the clinician's suspicion, then he or she should proceed with further assessment and examination of the child. Based on the information gathered during this process, the clinician can make his or her decision about a treatment intervention.

Interviewing the Parent and Child

Interviewing cases of suspected child abuse and neglect requires sophisticated skills. Clinicians will vary on the point at which a referral is made, depending on their own competence, and availability of appropriate referral resources. For example, the way in which a primary care clinician in rural Montana proceeds may be quite different from a less-experienced clinician in a suburb near to a University Medical Center. In the following, we will describe what all clinicians should be able to do.

First, begin with the parent and the child together, and clarify that the goal is to understand thoroughly the concerns of the parent and the symptoms or injuries of the child. Gather a detailed history of the most recent symptomatology as well as previous incidents of a similar kind in the family. Explain that it may be necessary to talk with and examine the child alone.

When talking with the child it is important for the clinician to:

1. Slowly develop a relationship with the child.

Conversation should focus initially on less-threatening topics (e.g., friends, school, and the child's interests). A relaxed pace reduces the likelihood the child will become anxious.

2. Listen to what the child is willing to share.

It is important not to pressure the child for information about anything (e.g., the identity of a perpetrator).

3. Clarify the child's understanding of anatomy, and use the child's language when referring to parts of the body.
4. Do not assume the child is angry at the person who committed the abuse.

Abused children are often very attached to the abusive parent.

5. Encourage the child to share his or her feelings.

This may be the youngster's first opportunity to discuss a family problem.

6. Reassure the youngster that his or her safety is very important and that you are hopeful things will work out for the child and family.

> Dr. H. talked alone with 9-year-old Madeline, who he suspected had been sexually abused. Dr. H. found Madeline to be very talkative about her friends and her collection of dolls. Dr. H. explained that he was interested in Madeline's life and wanted to understand her situation. During their conversation Dr. H. learned that Mrs. Wooden often worked at night and Madeline's father would put her to bed. Madeline reluctantly shared that during the past several months he often stayed with her and touched her "privates." Sometimes he would ask her to hold his "thing" until "stuff" came out.

The interview provides the clinician with valuable information and also helps the child feel comfortable with the clinician before he or she proceeds with a physical examination. Some children may be less comfortable talking about events and may be more willing to draw a picture, and then perhaps describe what happened. Be sure to have paper, crayons, and pencils available.

Physical Examination and Laboratory Studies

The physical examination should be complete, from head to toe, in order to reduce the child's anxiety about examining any particular area of the body. A general exam can also be used to reassure the child that he or she is physically all right. Precise details of an appropriate examination can be found in a good text (e.g., 12, 13), but one should generally include:

1. A record of all bruises and burns according to size, shape, position, color, and age. Color photographs are required by law in many states. Every office should have a camera capable of instant pictures.
2. A careful description of genital anatomy.
3. A description of the child's affect during the exam, especially if there is out-of-proportion fear or ease with different parts of the exam.

Laboratory studies need to be done to confirm clinical impressions. These should be done carefully and with attention to their potential use in legal proceedings. Again, a complete list of all appropriate laboratory studies can be found in a good text (e.g., 11), but a short list might include:

1. A test for the presence of sperm in the vagina of females.
2. Tests for sexually transmitted disease in children of both sexes.
3. A pregnancy test for adolescent girls.
4. A skeletal survey of children under the age of 5 because clinical findings of fractures often disappear after 1 week.

Whenever possible the physical exam should be conducted with both a nurse and the parent present. The parent can provide valuable support for the child. Having the parent present also gives the clinician the opportunity to clarify what he or she will be doing and why.

> Dr. H. invited Mrs. Wooden and the nurse into the room for Madeline's physical. He explained to Mrs. Wooden and Madeline that a thorough physical was needed to help find out why Madeline was having stomach pain and vaginal itchiness. Noticing Madeline had brought a doll with her, Dr. H. examined her doll first to help Madeline understand what he would be doing. He then did a general screening physical of Madeline before examining her genital area and taking a culture from her vagina. His examination revealed some bruising around the vagina and evidence of an old hymenal tear.

It is very important that the clinician document his or her findings clearly and in detail; however, as many as 60% of children who have been sexually abused will have a normal physical examination (14). If the clinician's findings support his or her suspicion of abuse, the next step is to report the problem to a family member and to the appropriate child protective agency.

Reporting Suspected Child Abuse

All states require that clinicians and other professionals report *suspected* child abuse to the appropriate authorities, usually a local child protective agency or police. This step is often difficult for a clinician to take because he or she may not feel completely convinced that abuse has occurred. One study showed that physicians reported child abuse or neglect only 57% of the time they suspected it (15). Reporting one's suspicion is a legal responsibility and a critical step in providing for a child's safety as well as involving other professionals who can help strengthen the family's childrearing abilities. The clinician's job is to report allegations or suspicions, not to determine their validity.

The clinician should report suspicion of abuse when he or she suspects that

1. A family member has committed an act of sexual or physical abuse.

The clinician needs to decide whether or not to inform the parents of his or her intention to report suspected abuse. In most cases, the clinician should tell the parents first and then call Child Protective Services while the parents are in the office. The child's safety comes first, however, and disclosing the report to the parent(s) may put the child at increased risk. Unless there is a family member available who supports the child's story and can completely protect him or her, the child should not be allowed to return home until Child Protective has made a determination about the case. This plan reduces the risk of further abuse, punishment, kidnapping, or efforts to persuade the child to change his or her story. In extreme cases of physical abuse in which the injuries are severe, a child may need to be hospitalized to further assess his or her health, as well as to maintain the child in a safe environment.

> On the basis of Madeline's story and her physical exam, it seemed to Dr. H. that she had been sexually abused for at least 6 months by her father. Dr. H. told Mrs. Wooden that he was concerned that Madeline may have been sexually abused and that she was required by law to notify Child Protective Services. Dr. H. called Child Protective Services while Mrs. Wooden was still present. The protective worker said someone would come as soon as possible. Mrs. Wooden and Madeline waited 2 hours at Dr. H.'s office until the Child Protective worker arrived.

In these circumstances, it helps for the clinician to emphasize his or her legal responsibility to report any suspicion of abuse. Reporting is not intended as a personal judgment of the parents; rather, it is meant as a necessary step to clarify whether or not abuse has occurred. The clinician must keep in mind that he or she may be caring for this family for a long time and that extreme care must be taken to do this procedure correctly. We will discuss this further in the continuity of care section.

2. The parents have not provided for the child's safety and welfare in cases of extrafamilial abuse.

When the perpetrator is not a family member, the clinician should immediately report his or her suspicion to both parents. Guiding the parents to take action and report the incident to the police empowers the parents to care responsibly for the child. If the parents are unwilling, the clinician should let the parents know he or she will have to report them to the local Child Protective Agency for child neglect. The clinician should encourage the parents to support and reassure the child that they will protect him or her. In cases of sexual abuse the parents should emphasize that the child is not at fault.

> Mr. and Mrs. Lemanski, second-generation Polish-Americans, brought their son Jim, age 11, to Dr. X. because he was complaining of headaches and refusing to go to school. During the interview alone with Jim, Dr. X. learned that his gym teacher had been fondling Jim in the shower at school. Dr. X. had Jim's parents return to the exam room where he helped Jim share what had happened to him at school. Mr. and Mrs. Lemanski were shocked and hesitant to believe their son at first. With Dr. X.'s help Jim talked to his parents and they assured him they would protect him and that something would be done. Mr. and Mrs. Lemanski did not know what steps to take. Dr. X. instructed them to contact the police and to talk to school officials while he filed a report with child protective services. Dr. X. also recommended that the Lemanski's return in a few days to discuss the situation further.

In cases such as this the clinician should also encourage the family to see a mental health professional to help all the family members cope with the crisis. Including non-abused siblings in the therapy alleviates some of the confusion and symptomatic behavior they may be experiencing.

3. Involvement of Child Protective Services can provide parenting support and education.

In some cases the involvement of child protective services can help parents develop more effective parenting skills and prevent more serious harm to their children. For example, a clinician may suggest referral for preventive services to parents who use severe corporal punishment and may be at risk of seriously abusing their children.

> Dr. M. was concerned that 2-year-old Joey's bruises were inflicted by his mother. He noted how stressful it was to parent young children and asked Mrs. Campaneris how it was for her to be raising a 2-year-old. Mrs. Campaneris began to cry. She reported being tired all of the time and having little or no support. She and her husband had separated while she was pregnant with Joey. Mrs. Campaneris worried that she could hurt Joey. Dr. M. said Mrs. Campaneris deserved to have additional support and that Child Protective Services could be a resource to her. Mrs. Campaneris was fearful that Child Protective would remove Joey from the home. Dr. M. said he would call Child Protective while Mrs. Campaneris was in the office. Dr. M. learned that Child Protective often referred cases to a parent education program run by social services. The program provided home visits by a social worker as

well as a child care program. Child Protective would meet with Mrs. Campaneris to investigate the situation first and make a referral if it was warranted. Mrs. Campaneris was still anxious after the call, but was willing to go ahead with the plan. Dr. M. maintained contact with Mrs. Campaneris and Child Protective during the assessment. Mrs. Campaneris was referred to the parent education program.

Partner Abuse in Primary Care

Since the 1970s our understanding of the scope and ramifications of partner abuse has expanded enormously. Research indicates that this is not a rare problem, affecting somewhere between 20 and 35% of women over a lifetime (16, 17). The health risks are severe: Four women per day are killed by their partner (18, 19), and 10–25% of Emergency Department visits are due to domestic violence (20). In primary care, two studies have found lifetime prevalence of domestic violence of about 40% among primary care patients (21). Saunders and colleagues (22) found that women with a history of violent relationships visited their primary care physician more frequently than did women who had not been abused. Further, battered women may spend significantly more days in the hospital (23). In one study, the cost of healthcare for women who were victims of intimate partner violence was 92% more than a random sample of general female enrollees (24). The direct medical costs associated with partner abuse are estimated to be $1.8 billion per year (25).

Screening for partner abuse is also an important part of protecting children: Studies indicate that child abuse is about 15 times more likely in families in which there is partner abuse (26) and that about 70% of men who abuse their female partners also abuse their children (27). Stark and Flitcraft (28) found that almost two thirds of abused children were being parented by a battered woman. Even in the context of these high percentages, it is likely that much abuse goes undetected and unreported.

Many professional organizations have formally encouraged clinicians regularly to screen women for partner abuse [e.g., AMA Council on Scientific Affairs (29); American College of Obstetrician-Gynecologists (30, 31)]. The challenge for many primary care clinicians, however, is to screen in a timely and useful manner, and to respond when screening indicates that partner abuse is present. An understanding of the underlying dynamics in partner abuse helps frame the rationale for screening strategies and treatment recommendations. The Wheel of Power and Control [adapted from the Domestic Abuse Intervention Project, 1990 (32), and the New York State Office for the Prevention of Domestic Violence, 1993 (33)] succinctly summarizes these important dynamics (see Fig. 22.1):

Mrs. DeVries, a 28-year-old Serbian immigrant, came in to see Dr. V. ostensibly because of a cough. She was a stay-at-home mom with two

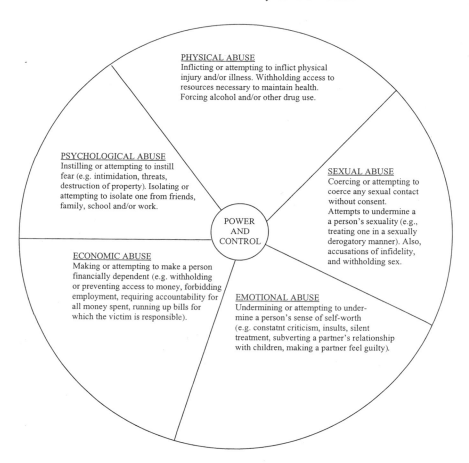

FIGURE 22.1. The wheel of power and control. (Adapted from references 32 and 33. Used with permission.)

preschool-age children. Her husband was a manual laborer who Dr. V. rarely saw. Mrs. DeVries was generally well, except for her difficulty with headaches, but she had always seemed a little depressed to Dr. V. While listening to her lungs, he noticed some bruising on her back that appeared to be in two different stages of evolution.

Dr V.: Ouch. I notice these bruises on your back. How did you get these?
Mrs. DeVries: I fell down the stairs. My husband tells me I have two left feet.
Dr. V.: It looks painful. When did you get them?

Most women do not present to their primary care clinician with abuse injuries (20, 34). It is critical that clinicians *ask about abuse*, as well as be aware of noninjury "red flags." The following are considered signs and symptoms of partner abuse worthy of follow up:

- Vague somatic complaints (e.g., headache, insomnia, hyperventilation, gastrointestinal problems, chest, back, or pelvic pain).
- Depression and anxiety.
- Injuries to head, neck, chest, breasts, and abdomen (especially breasts and abdomen during pregnancy).
- Contusions, lacerations, fractures, sprains, or burns.
- History inconsistent with presentation.
- Multiple injuries at various stages of healing.
- Use of minor tranquilizers or pain medications.

> After further questioning, it seemed clear to Dr. V. that there was more to this story than he was being told. The story did not match the injury and there was a subtle hesitancy in the way events were related.
>
> Dr. V.: I don't mean to pry, Mrs. DeVries, but I have an intuition there is more going on here. Are you okay? I'm sorry, but I really have to ask if you're getting pushed around at home?
>
> Further discussion revealed that indeed things were not going well at home. Increasing financial problems, marital conflict, and more drinking by her husband, combined with her two best friends moving away, all added up to more stress and more fights with her husband that had become increasingly physical. The increasing isolation and the lack of an income, however, made her feel both more vulnerable and powerless. Mrs. DeVries loved her husband and although frightened felt in no immediate danger and had no intention of moving out.

For general screening, Wasson and colleagues (35) found that a single-item screening question in the form of a word–picture chart that was added to a general health questionaire was very sensitive and specific for detecting partner abuse. Whether in the context of warning signs, or in regular screening (e.g., often accomplished at routine woman's health visits) it is helpful to follow these guidelines when screening for partner abuse:

- Ask questions in a nonjudgmental, nonthreatening manner.
- Ask about specific behaviors, rather than about "abuse" in general.
- For at least part of the visit, interview the woman alone, ensuring that her partner cannot overhear the conversation.
- Acknowledge the range of conflict and difficulties in relationships, and that partner abuse is not unusual.
- If there is known substance abuse in the home, specifically ask about how conflict is managed during substance use.

Many primary care clinicians find it helpful to have a structured interview to assist in approaching particularly difficult situations. One such pro-

TABLE 22.2. SAFE questions

Stress safety	Afraid/abused	Friends and family	Emergency plan
Tell me about the types of stress in your relationship? Do you feel safe in your relationship? Are there firearms in the home?	What happens when you and your partner disagree? Do you ever have yelling or screaming fights? Is there ever any pushing or shoving? Has your partner ever threatened or hit you?	Are your friends or family aware that you have been threatened or hurt? If not, do you think that you could tell them, and would they be able to give you support?	Do you feel you have a safe place to go in an emergency? If you feel you are in danger now, would you like help in locating a shelter, or developing an emergency plan?

tocol for domestic violence is the "SAFE questions" (Table 22.2, adapted from Ashur 1993, 36).

Many primary care clinicians are not sure how to proceed when a woman indicates she is experiencing partner violence. Some of the responses are relatively obvious: Treat any injuries, assess current safety, contact child protective agencies if children appear to be in danger, and document abuse. Some less obvious guidelines include: Avoid prescribing sedatives (they may cloud the patient's judgment), warn the patient of the potential lethality of partner abuse, and formulate a safety plan.

A safety plan should contain the following elements:

- A list of community resources for battered women (e.g., shelters, police, counseling centers, etc.).
- Agreed upon "safe houses." A good plan consist of three safe places (e.g., shelter, relative, or friend's home) and a means of getting to safety if needed.
- A stockpile of necessities in a safe place: clothes for patient and children, money, checking or savings account book, identification papers for patient and children, and comfort objects for children.

> In the end, Dr. V. felt reassured that for now the situation was unlikely to escalate significantly, but explicitly went through a safety plan with Mrs. DeVries and scheduled a follow-up visit in 1 week to reassess both her cough and the situation at home.

Throughout all interventions, it is imperative that clinicians stress their understanding of how difficult it can be to leave an abusive partner, and that they respect the woman's right to decide. Victims of partner violence often feel embarrassed about their inability to leave, and will avoid further discussion out of this embarrassment. In addition, many women in violent situations have accepted the violence as normal, still love their partner and do not want to leave, have few options because of their financial situation or child-care responsibilities, or believe the violence is their own fault. Pushing a woman to change her situation before she is ready can be counterproductive. Given that the violence occurs in the context of a controlling relationship, and that women often need to feel empowered before they are able to change their situation, a primary care clinician should strive to avoid being perceived as a controlling authority figure. Avoiding duplication of the power and control issues of the partner relationship in the clinician–patient relationship can be difficult. A long-term view of the problem (in the absence of immediate danger) is better, while noting increments of change toward empowerment and improved or changed home situation for the couple.

Clinicians often hear the distress in a couple's relationship, but physical violence has yet to occur, or the behavior is not defined as "abusive" by the couple. One partner is sometimes exerting an enormous amount of control over the other, and tensions frequently erupt. Arguments may have escalated to intimidation and destruction of property (e.g., punching walls, throwing things), but the patient denies that physical contact has occurred.

Situations in which physical violence has yet to occur are common, and these couples often resist referral. In terms of prevention research, the impact of intervening is unknown; however, it makes intuitive sense that the primary care clinician may successfully be able to intervene with some of these "previolent" couples. The primary care clinician can teach the couple basic anger management techniques (e.g., taking a "time out" from conflict, counting to 10, and explicitly listing the issues that lead to anger are time-honored strategies). Giving couples a venue to discuss their conflict and to problem solve together about avoiding future escalation can be a powerful message. Many couples respond to the clinician's strong statement that escalation is dangerous and must change; in fact, physical violence is against the law. Another good strategy is to agree at the outset that the couple will get outside assistance if they are not able to change the pattern with the clinician's suggestions. In these higher-risk couples, the clinician must assess for violence at each visit, and interview each person alone. If the dialogue appears to be increasing the frequency or intensity of the aggressive interactions, the individuals in the couple need to be referred.

Elder Abuse

As the population ages, increasing numbers of elderly are cared for by families. Many studies have noted the stress that caregivers face. This stress can sometimes escalate to mistreatment and violence toward the elderly (37). Mistreatment includes physical abuse and neglect, psychological abuse, financial exploitation, and violation of rights. It is estimated that more than 2 million older adults are mistreated each year in the United States (38).

Estimates suggest that only 1 in 14 elder abuse cases is reported to social service agencies (39, 40).

Screening for elder abuse is best accomplished by interviewing both the caregiver and the elder. A 1990 British study found that 45% of caregivers acknowledged engaging in abusive behavior, but few elders admitted to being a victim (40). Sixty-five percent of elder abuse is perpetrated by a spouse (about two thirds of whom are wives victimizing husbands), and about 23% of elder abuse is perpetrated by a caregiving child. Elder abuse may result primarily from the stress of the elder's needs. For example, elders with cognitive impairment or functional disability are at increased risk of abuse or neglect (38, 40); however, the behavior sometimes reflects long-standing patterns of behaviors or resentments.

In speaking with the caregiver, normalizing the stress of caring for someone is helpful. Pointing out how stress can sometimes result in resentment, anger, and frustration sets the stage for further discussion. Follow-up questions include asking about how caregivers handle difficult situations, and how they manage their anger and frustration. Just as with other types of abuse, asking if they ever feel they have, or fear they will, lose control when caring for the elder is crucial. In addition, because substance abuse is often part of the picture, all caregivers should be asked if they attempt to cope by using alcohol or drugs. The following are other "red flags" to watch for in caregivers:

- New self-neglect.
- Conflicting stories between caregiver and elder, or stories that change over time or do not match.
- Presentation.
- Mounting resentment.
- Caregiver excusing their own failure to provide appropriate care.
- Shifting blame for difficulties.
- Financial dependence on the elder.
- Aggressive/defensive behavior.

Uncovering abuse by interviewing the elder can be a challenge. Elders may be reluctant to disclose the abuse because they are afraid it will lead to institutionalization or retaliation by the abuser. Elders who suffer from mental incapacitation may not remember what has happened to them, or be confused by their situation. It does help to ask specific, behavioral questions about the caregiver's behavior while the caregiver is not in the room. Appropriate questions include:

- How do you and (name of caregiver) get along?
- Are they taking good care of you?
- Has anyone ever hurt you?
- Has anyone ever touched you without your consent?
- Has anyone scolded you?

- Has anyone taken things that belong to you without your consent?
- Has anyone forced you to sign papers, change finances, or the like, when you did not want to or did not understand?
- Has anyone made you feel afraid?
- Has anyone refused to care for you or help you when you really needed it?

If an elder or caregiver indicates that abuse is occurring, or that the caregiver is fearful of becoming abusive under stress, a primary care clinician has a number of options. In many states and localities, clinicians are mandated to report elder abuse to an agency specifically charged with investigating and managing elder-abuse cases. Check with your local office on aging to determine what actions are mandated. In addition, these offices can provide information about community resources that might relieve tensions. Some clinicians hospitalize a patient who they feel is at imminent risk, until another plan can be arranged. Provision of visiting nurse or other in-home supportive services can both clarify concerning situations, and offer respite for the caregiver. Clinicians can sometimes facilitate changes in the way the family as a whole is managing care for the elder. Assisting the family in obtaining regular respite care can provide the caregiver with periodic breaks and avoid a steady crescendo of stress. A family meeting that includes noncustodial relatives can result in reducing caregiving tensions by redistributing responsibilities or by just publicly acknowledging the work that is being done. Upon realizing that a change in living arrangements is imminent, elders may recant their story of abuse. The abuser may have used threats of institutionalization to intimidate the elder and prevent his or her disclosure of the abuse. Such retractions of stories should be viewed with caution, and the clinician may still want to take steps to reduce the level of stress on the caregiver or tensions in the home.

Continuity of Care

In virtually all cases of domestic violence, *maintaining contact with the family* is important, especially when reporting the problem to an outside agency has taken place. If the clinician has reported child abuse without notifying the parents beforehand, maintaining continuity may be particularly challenging. Most families initially react with intense anger, but they almost always remain in the clinician's practice and can benefit from his or her ongoing involvement. The clinician can provide important continuity of support for families who may be involved with a variety of legal, social service and therapeutic agencies, and professionals. Lawyers, therapists, social service workers, and judges may change frequently during the investigation and treatment of child abuse. The primary care clinician may be the one stable, ongoing contact with the family who can provide support and help the family work with these multiple systems.

To return to the Wooden case:

> Dr. H. contacted Mr. and Mrs. Wooden after Child Protective had seen them regarding possible sexual abuse of Madeline. Mr. Wooden was furious with Dr. H. and refused her offer to meet with them. Dr. H. called the Woodens again in 1 week. Madeline had been removed from the home and Mr. Wooden was scheduled to appear in both Criminal and Family Courts. The Woodens were very distraught and were now more open to meeting with Dr. H. Dr. H. met with the Woodens periodically over the next 3 years to provide support and help them understand and work with the judicial, social service, and therapeutic systems. Dr. H. talked with the Protective officer frequently, and also attended a meeting with the Wooden family and their family therapist. Madeline was eventually returned to her family and they continued in therapy for 1 year. Dr. H. maintained contact throughout the process and continued to provide medical care and support to the Wooden family.

Primary care clinicians can play a pivotal role in discovering, confronting, and perhaps preempting domestic violence in families. Recognizing the signs of abuse is the first step. By reporting one's suspicions to the appropriate authorities, the clinician activates community and legal systems that provide safety for the at-risk family member in a time of crisis. This step can also lead to involving resources that strengthen the whole family's ability to cope with stress in nonviolent ways. In this way, the clinician's actions protect individuals and the entire family.

When the Perpetrator Is Your Patient

Primary care clinicians who work with multiple members of the same family may confront situations in which the perpetrator of the violence is also their patient. This can be a particularly difficult situation. Disclosing one partner's story to the other is not appropriate. At the same time, it is difficult for a variety of reasons not to hear both sides, or attempt to intervene and change the perpetrator's behavior. The first priority is to maintain the safety of the victim. If a perpetrator believes that the victim has told the "secret" of the abuse, or is preparing to leave the relationship, it can increase risk greatly. The most dangerous time for the victim in a violent relationship is around the time of departure from the relationship (41). If patients expect to be asked about home life and stresses during primary care visits because the clinician has set this standard, it is relatively unlikely that such questions will make the perpetrator suspicious. On the other hand, if this line of questioning is not the norm, or if the clinician does not have an established relationship with the perpetrator, this topic should not be pursued. In addition, even if the clinician has a good relationship with the perpetrator, the frequency and intensity of the violence should be kept in mind. If the situation is particularly dangerous, the best course of action is to support the victim in finding safety.

When perpetrators respond to general questions about their home life or stresses in their lives by acknowledging the domestic violence, and take some responsibility for their behavior, they may be open to a referral to assist with anger management, ideally in a group for perpetrators of domestic violence. If the perpetrator acknowledges the violence but feels it is the partner's fault, or views it as normative, the perpetrator will be less amenable to referral, although it can be offered. The best course of action may be to support the victim in finding safety.

Personal Issues for the Clinician

The preceding portions of this chapter have detailed what the clinician must do when confronted with domestic violence. We have yet to touch on what is often the most challenging part of the job: what to do with one's own emotional response to domestic violence. Some have suggested that clinicians fail to detect domestic violence in large part because of their reluctance to address their own emotions. Just as there needs to be a specific set of guidelines for the clinician's behavior with patients in a domestic violence situation, there also needs to be specific guidelines for what the clinician does with his or her own feelings in response to these situations. Knowing what to do, both externally and internally, should reduce this avoidance, and help us to care better for our patients while we care better for ourselves.

Clinicians vary widely in their emotional response to situations of domestic violence. Some may feel fear; fear that is so compelling it is intimidating. Some may feel anger; anger that is so extreme it is rage. Some may feel a profound sadness, recognizing the tragedy of what will be a lifelong struggle. For all of us, we bring our own personal histories into the exam room and our emotional response is drawn from that deep well. For example, a clinician may have had personal experience with domestic violence and may experience all extremes of emotion. These might be manifest explicitly, or in an attempt to modulate their expression nothing might be said. On the other hand, another clinician might not have had any personal experience even remotely related, and even though he or she might be able to handle a purulent, draining abscess without blinking an eye, may experience extreme revulsion at the evidence for incest.

Because of this wide range of affective experience, and its deeply personal and unique nature, no set procedure for coping with each specific situation exists. Rather, a general set of guidelines can be offered:

1. Recognize your feelings.

This internal awareness may come about as a result of one's own therapy, or self-reflection, or come from feedback from supervisors, colleagues, friends, or family. A recognizable pattern can often make prediction easier. For example, a clinician may recognize that he or she initially always feels rage at an abusive spouse.

2. Focus on what is best for the patient when with the patient.

The patient is not the clinician's therapist, nor the perpetrator of domestic violence in the clinician's own life. Separate personal feelings from what is best for the patient. In addition, remember that silence may imply tacit approval. For the clinician to bring his or her own values into the exam room can be helpful, as long as what is in the patient's best interest is kept in mind.

3. Focus on self-care, when not with the patient; review every case.

No clinician is completely self-aware or able to take care of him- or herself alone. Domestic violence often generates some of the most intense affective responses the clinician will ever face, and every clinician needs a context for processing these feelings. A state bureaucracy is not an adequate forum for sharing these challenges. All clinicians deserve to have resources available to review each and every case: a partner, supervisor, mental health collaborator, or Balint-type group.

Domestic violence is the great psychosocial iceberg of our time. It takes an astute clinician to look below the surface for the hidden enormity of this problem. There are massive forces at work in a culture dense with violence (e.g., at the movies, on television, in the news), and the current is strong. In addition, the availability of firearms intensifies the consequences when violence does occur. The dedicated clinician must work both at the individual and family levels, and at the community and sociocultural levels to keep the vulnerable members of our society safe. Promoting an ethic of respect and co-humanity throughout his or her practice should be considered part of the job of every healthcare clinician.

References

1. Ross SM: Risk of physical abuse to children of spouse abusing parents. *Child Abuse Negl* 1996;**20**:589–598.
2. Burgess Rl, Garbarino J: Doing what comes naturally? An evolutionary perspective on child abuse. In: Finkelhor D, Gelles RJ, Hotaling GT, & Straus MA (eds): *The Dark Side of Families & Current Family Violence Research*. Beverly Hills: Sage Publications, 1983, pp. 88–101.
3. Kantor GK, Straus MA: Substance abuse as a precipitant of wife abuse victimizations. *Am J Drug Alcohol Abuse* 1989;**15**(2):173–189.
4. Kent JT, Blehar MG: Helping abused children and their families. In: *NIMH Science Monographs: Families Today: Volume II*. Washington, DC:

U.S. Department of Health, Education, and Welfare, 1982, pp. 607–630.

5. Sugg NK, Inui T: Primary care physicians' response to domestic violence: opening Pandora's box. *JAMA* 1992;**267**:3157–3160.

6. Wang CT, Daro D: *Current Trends in Child Abuse Reporting and Fatalities: The Results of the 1997 Annual Fifty State Survey*. Chicago: Center on Child Abuse Prevention Research, National Committee for Prevention of Child Abuse, 1997.

7. Kerker BD, Horwitz SM, Leventhal JM, Plichta S, & Leaf PJ: Identification of violence in the home: pediatric and parental reports *Arch Pediat Adolesc Med* 2000;**154**(5):457–462.

8. Finklehor D: *A Sourcebook on Child Sexual Abuse*. Beverly Hills: Sage, 1986.

9. Pressel DM: Evaluation of physical abuse in children. *Am Fam Physician* 2000;**61**(10):3057–3064.

10. Batten DA: Incest—a review of the literature. *Med Sci Law* 1983;**23**(40): 245–253.

11. Green AH: Current perspectives on child maltreatment. *Res Staff Physician* May 1979:150–163.

12. Giardino AP, Finkel MA, Giardino ER, Seidel T, & Ludwig S: *A Practical Guide to the Evaluation of Sexual Abuse in the Prepubertal Child*. Newbury Park, CA: Sage, 1992.

13. Giardino AP, Christian CW, & Giardino, ER: *A Practical Guide to the Evaluation of Child Physical Abuse and Neglect*. Thousand Oaks, CA: Sage, 1997.

14. Monteleone JA: *Child Maltreatment: A Clinical Guide and Reference*. St. Louis: GW Medical Publishing, 1998.

15. VanHaeringen AR, Dadds M, & Armstrong KL: The child abuse lottery—will the doctor suspect and report: physician attitudes towards and reporting of suspected child abuse and neglect. *Child Abuse Neglect* 1998;**22**(3):159–169.

16. Langan PA, Innes CA: *Preventing Domestic Violence Against Women*. Washington DC: US Department of Justice Statistics, 1982.

17. Straus M, Gelles R (Eds): *Physical Violence in American Families: Risk Factors and Adaptions to Violence in 8,145 Families*. New Brunswick, NJ: Transaction Publishers, 1990.

18. Browne A: *When Battered Women Kill*. New York: Macmillan, 1989.

19. Federal Bureau of Investigation: *U.S. Department of Justice Crime Reports: Crime in the U.S., 1985*. Washington DC: U.S. Department of Justice, 1986, pp. 9–12.

20. Campbell JC, Pliska MJ, Taylor W, & Sheridan D: Battered women's experiences in the emergency department. *J Emer Nurs* 1994;**20**:280–288.

21. Hamberger LK, Saunders DG, & Hovey M: Prevalence of domestic violence in community practice and rate of physician inquiry. *Fam Med* 1992;**24**:283–287.

22. Saunders DG, Hamberger K, & Hovey M: Indicators of woman abuse based on chart review at a family practice center. *Arch Fam Med* 1993;**2**:537–543.

23. Bergman B, Brismar B, & Nordin C: Utilization of medical care by abused women. *Br Med J* 1992;**305**:27–28.

24. Wisner C, Gilmer T, Saltzman L, & Zink T: Intimate partner violence against women: do victims cost health plans more? *J Fam Prac* 1999;**48**:439–443.

25. Miller TR, Cohen MA, & Rossman SB: Victim costs of violent crime and resulting injuries. *Health Aff* 1993;**12**:186.

26. Stacey W, Shupe A: *The Family Secret*. Boston: Beacon Press, 1983.
27. Bowker, Arbitrell, & McFerron: On the relationship between wife beating and child abuse. In: Yilo K, Bogard M (Eds): *Feminist Perspectives on Wife Abuse*. Beverly Hills: Sage, 1988.
28. Stark E, Flitcraft A: Personal power and institutional victimization: Treating the dual trauma of woman battering. In: Ochberg F (Ed): *Post-Traumatic Therapy and Victims of Violence*. New York: Brunner-Mazel, 1988.
29. Council on Scientific Affairs, American Medical Association: Violence against women: relevance for medical practitioners. *JAMA* 1992;**267**:3184–3189.
30. American College of Obstetricians and Gynecologists: *The Abused Woman* (Patient Education Pamphlet AP083). Washington DC, January 1989.
31. American College of Obstetricians and Gynecologists. *The Battered Woman*. (ACOG Technical Bulletin No. 124). Washington DC, January 1989.
32. Wheel of Power and Control, Domestic Abuse Intervention Project, 206 West Fourth Street, Duluth, MN, 1995.
33. Wheel of Power and Control, New York State Office for the Prevention of Domestic Violence, adapted from same developed by the Domestic Abuse Intervention Project, Duluth, MN, 1993.
34. Goldberg WG, Tomlanovich MC: Domestic violence, victims and emergency departments: New findings. *JAMA* 1984;**251**:3259–3264.
35. Wasson JH, Jette AM, Anderson J, Johnson DJ, Nelson EC, & Kilo CM: Routine, single-item screening to identify abusive relationships in women. *J Fam Prac* 2000;**49**(11);1017–1022.
36. Ashur MLC: Asking questions about domestic violence: SAFE questions. *JAMA* 1993;**269**(18):2367.
37. Costa AJ: Elder abuse. *Prim Care* 1993;**20**:375–389.
38. Swagerty D, Takahashi P, & Evans J: Elder mistreatment. *Am Fam Physician* 1999;**59**(10):2804–2808.
39. Hwalek MA, Sengstock MC: Assessing the probability of abuse of the elderly: towards development of a clinical screening instrument. *J Appl Gerontol* 1986; **5**:153–173.
40. Comijs HC, Pot AM, Smit JH, Bouter LM, & Jonker C: Elder abuse in the community: Prevalence and consequences. *J Am Geriatr Soc* 1998;**46**:885–888.
41. Sugg NK, Inui T: Primary care physicians' response to domestic violence. *JAMA* 1992;**267**:3157–3160.

National Domestic Violence Hotline: 800-799-SAFE

Protocol: Protecting the Family: Domestic Violence and the Primary Care Clinician

Domestic violence includes child abuse and neglect, partner abuse, and elder abuse. The clinician's main job is to recognize the signs of domestic violence and then utilize those resources that exist within the family and community to protect the individual and family. The safety of the vulnerable individual is the clinician's top priority.

Domestic Violence: Common Elements

- A history of violence or abuse.
- Substance abuse.
- Marital discord.
- Blurred generational boundaries.
- Family isolation.
- Patient barriers to detection and treatment include: fear of retaliation, shame, hopelessness, fear of the relationship ending. Patients generally want to keep the family together, and want the violence, not the relationship(s), to end.
- Clinician barriers to detection and treatment include: lack of training, wanting to avoid overwhelming personal reactions, fear of offending, fear of retaliation, sense of powerlessness, and desire to save time.

Child Abuse and Neglect

- Look for both direct and indirect signs and symptoms.
- Atypical parental behavior may provide clues to physical abuse.
- When interviewing suspected cases, start with parent and child together. When interviewing the child alone:
  - Slowly develop a relationship with the child.
  - Listen to what the child is willing to share.
  - Clarify the child's understanding of anatomy.
  - Do not assume the child is angry at the person who committed the abuse.
  - Encourage the child to share his or her feelings.
  - Reassure the child about his or her safety, and your hopefulness that things will work out for the child and family.
- Physical exams need to be thorough with all physical findings clearly documented. Photographs of abnormal physical findings are recommended.
- Laboratory studies can confirm clinical suspicions and may be used in a court of law.

Reporting Suspected Child Abuse

The clinician should report suspicion of abuse to local Child Protective Services when there is evidence that:

- A family member has committed an act of sexual or physical abuse.
- The parents have not provided for the child's safety and welfare in cases of extrafamilial abuse.

Involvement of Child Protective Services can provide parenting support and education. The clinician should almost always make a concerted effort to maintain contact with the family and provide continuity of support as the family works with various legal, social service and therapeutic agencies, and professionals.

Partner Abuse

Partner abuse is a way for one partner to gain power and control over the other partner. Most women do not present to their primary care clinician with injuries, rather, a multitude of indirect signs and symptoms will be present (e.g., headaches, abdominal or pelvic pain, anxiety, depression, or somatization).

The SAFE questions provide a structured format for addressing partner abuse:

- Stress/Safety.
- Afraid/Abused.
- Friends/Family.
- Emergency plan.

Elder Abuse

- Take time to interview elders alone.
- Few elders will admit to abuse due to their fear of retaliation, institutionalization, shame, or because of their cognitive impairment (e.g., dementia).
- Ask about caregiver stress, how they handle difficult situations, and if substance abuse plays a role in coping with stress; anticipate and acknowledge caregiver stress; recommend and facilitate respite care as indicated.
- Family meetings may be helpful to explicitly recognize the caregiver and possibly redistribute duties while nurturing healthy family coping and grieving, especially during transitions to different levels of care.

Personal Issues for the Clinician

- Recognize your feelings.
- Focus on what is best for the patient when you are with the patient.
- Focus on self-care when you are not with the patient.
- Review every case.

23
Family-Oriented Primary Care in the Real World: Practical Considerations for Comprehensive Care

Translating a family-oriented approach from theory into daily clinical practice presents a variety of broad pragmatic challenges. Such issues as, "How will I find the time? Who will pay for this approach? and How do I avoid getting caught in the middle?" need to be addressed. Questions about logistical details need to be answered (e.g., "How should I design my office brochure, the physical space, my records?"). In this chapter, we will provide very specific, family-oriented suggestions that take into account the reality of today's healthcare environment. Some of these ideas work best when starting a new practice, whereas others can be incorporated into existing practices.

A Family-Oriented Image

First impressions are important. Family-oriented clinicians can begin by proclaiming their family orientation with the word *family* in the name of the practice or group (e.g., Family Medicine Group, Family Health Associates, Family Practice Center, or Family Health Clinic). A practice logo that represents the family is another way to communicate a family orientation. Promotional material about the practice should emphasize its family orientation and services for families of all types.

The staff of the practice can further support and encourage a family-oriented approach. For example, staff members can attempt to get to know family members of patients, even if they are not members of the practice. When a patient calls, secretaries can communicate that family members are valued and included. Phone calls and visits by family members should be encouraged, and not viewed as intrusive. Family members in the waiting room can be invited into the examination room, if the patient so desires.

Enrollment of Patients and Families

A family orientation begins before the first visit (1). Whenever possible the entire family can be encouraged to register together with the same clinician at the orientation. Even when all members of the family do not have the same clinician, sufficient information about the entire family can be obtained at registration, or by mail, to construct a basic genogram. Self-administered genograms (2) and computerized genograms (3,4) can be completed at registration or before the first visit.

Family members can be encouraged to come in together for their first visit. For example, an older couple may make back-to-back appointments for complete physicals, or all the children in the family can be seen serially for well-child checks. This provides a time-efficient way to gather background health information about the family and to construct a routine genogram. This type of first visit gives the strong impression that the clinician is family oriented and will appreciate the entire family's participation in healthcare.

Despite a family invitation, the initial visit to the clinician often is by an individual patient. Even though not present, important information about other family members can be obtained by appropriate family-oriented questions (see chap. 4). "What kinds of illnesses run in your husband's/wife's side of the family? Is this his/her first marriage? What does he/she do for work?" It should not take long to obtaining an initial three-generation genogram. As such it provides an efficient representation of family, social, and genetic information. This initial "skeleton" template can be expanded at subsequent visits.

Physical Layout

Whenever possible, the physical layout of the medical office should be designed or adapted to accommodate families. Waiting rooms need to be large enough for several families and have reading material that is oriented to families. They should be accessible to the elderly and disabled and have separate play areas with toys for children. Pictures of families in the practice or babies delivered by the clinician can add a family touch to the waiting area or nurses' station. Exam rooms should ideally be large enough to seat at least two family members comfortably (approximately 100 square feet), and should be equipped with a third chair. Chairs can be readily moved from other exam rooms for additional family members. In addition, it is helpful to have at least one family conference or consultation room that can accommodate 8–10 people comfortably.

Range of Available Services

Whenever possible, a family-oriented medical practice should offer the services that a family most often needs. Pregnancy care, and the subsequent pediatric care, is an important part of family-oriented health care. Pregnancy and childbirth (see Chap. 10) is a crucial stage in the development of the family during which a family orientation and continuity of care is important. Clinicians that practice family-oriented maternity care have a more balanced mix of ages of patients, with more children in their practices than family clinicians that do not (5). High malpractice premiums are unfortunately forcing many family clinicians to stop practicing obstetrics (6). When a clinician does not do obstetrics, it is helpful to work closely with a family-oriented clinician that does provide maternity care to ensure as much continuity of care as possible. In some situations, a primary care clinician may participate in some of the prenatal care to maintain the continuity, even though he or she will not do the delivery.

Family-oriented practices can either directly provide or ensure easy access to other health-related services (e.g., social work or nutrition counseling) using health professionals that also value the inclusion of families and significant others. For example, dietitians need to consider that families usually share the same diet (7), that dietary interventions must consider the entire family, and that counseling the family about diet is more efficient and effective than counseling one individual. Whenever possible, a family therapist is part of the healthcare team (8), with an office in the same practice or building (see later for discussion of incorporating a family therapist into a medical practice and Chap. 25).

The family-oriented clinician needs to have a list of telephone and internet resources for services not provided in the practice. These resources commonly include other family-oriented mental health professionals, alcohol and drug services (including detoxification, inpatient and outpatient treatment facilities, AA, Al-Anon meetings, Adult Children of Alcoholics groups), self-help and support groups for chronic illness, bereavement, divorce, and advocacy organizations. Many communities maintain directories of these services.

A clinician can rent out space in the office, either when open or closed, to organizations that offer other related services to patients and families (e.g., Weight Watchers, Childhood Education Association, Alcoholics Anonymous, or other support groups). Patients and families may be more likely to attend a group that meets in their clinician's office. Larger multi-clinician practices may want to organize their own family-oriented groups focused on such specific areas as dealing with normative family development (e.g., prenatal and parenting classes), nonnormative family crises (e.g., divorce and separation), behavior problems like smoking and overeating, or chronic illness or chronic pain.

Incorporating a Family Therapist into a Medical Practice

Collaboration and referrals to family-oriented mental health professionals will be discussed in detail in Chapter 25. The most successful referrals occur when the family therapist practices under the same roof as the clinician. The clinician can personally introduce the patient or family to the therapist and, if necessary, can attend part or all of the first session. The therapist can easily meet with the clinician during a family conference or a regular office visit. Patients and families often prefer counseling sessions at the clinician's office, rather than going to a therapist's office or to a mental health center. Communication between therapist and clinician is improved: Each learns more about the other's work when they are practicing under the same roof.

There are several different models of collaborative family health care (8,9). In the most traditional model, the therapist has a private practice in the same building as the clinician. In a more collaborative model, the therapist may rent space within the clinicians office, but conduct a private practice that is financially independent of the clinician's practice. The therapist may do his or her own scheduling and billing, or he or she may contract with the clinician for secretarial and billing services. A therapist may be fully integrated into the medical practice as a partner or employee and treated as other healthcare clinicians in the practice. Services are billed by the practice, and the therapist is paid either on a straight salary or based upon a formula involving productivity or the overall profits of the practice. One unique model of collaborative practice is when a family clinician and family therapist see patients together as a team. Dym and Berman (10,11) have described the theoretical and practical aspects of this innovative approach. Regardless of the model used, the different theoretical orientation and style of practice between family-oriented medical practitioners and family therapists must be addressed directly (12).

When the therapist is seeing patients in a medical practice, a decision must be made whether the therapist's notes are included in the medical chart or are kept in a separate mental health chart, or if copies of the mental health notes are put in the medical chart. Close communication is integral to comprehensive care. The therapist can see what medical visits and problems have occurred since the last therapy session, and the clinician is kept up to date with the course of therapy. At the time of referral, the therapist should receive a referral note and should have access to the medical record containing the genogram and, if possible, the medical records of other family members. This method of communication encourages the integration of physical and mental health care. The clinician must be careful not to release the mental health notes to other clinicians or insurance companies, unless the patient specifically permits their release in addition to the medical records.

Record Keeping

Comprehensive family care includes family record keeping. In addition to the genogram, another tool in family-oriented care is the family chart or folder (13), in which the charts of all members of the family are filed together. *Family* is defined here for convenience as a group of persons sharing a common household. A relationship (not necessarily by blood or marriage) is implied (14). In addition to each family member's chart, the family folder includes a separate family card that goes in the front of the chart to be easily identified and accessible for each visit. On one side, there is space for the genogram with a brief list of standard symbols and a section for family history. Family problems or family assessments can be written on the back.

The advantages of a family chart are many. Information about the family, especially the genogram, can be obtained from different family members and is available for each family member's visit. Any family member can update the information at the time of visit. This important data does not need to be duplicated for each family member's chart. Without a family chart, the clinician may not otherwise know that two patients with different last names are closely related. It is particularly valuable to have a genogram readily available in the family chart when caring for remarried or blended families where relationships may be quite complex.

Having all the family members' charts in one family folder facilitates the detection of patterns of healthcare utilization, which may reflect family stress or dysfunction. Widmer (15) has shown that when one family member is depressed, other family members visit the doctor more frequently. These visits by different family members can be graphically illustrated by a family-care journal (16) in which dates and diagnoses (using a code such as ICD-9) for all family members is recorded graphically. Huygens (17) kept very meticulous and elegant journals or charts of familial patterns of illness for more than three decades in his practice in the Netherlands. In their classic study of family stress and illness, Meyer and Haggerty (18) used similar charts to demonstrate that streptococcal pharyngitis is often preceded by stressful family events.

Knowing about another family member's health problem at the time of a visit can be quite helpful. A family chart makes it easier to identify whether more than one family member has a cardiac risk factor (e.g., smoking or hypercholesterolemia). In such cases, an intervention aimed at the entire family may be more effective. Family charts also make family research easier to conduct. One can easily retrieve and compare information about the family. In time, however, family charts made of paper can become cumbersome because of their size. An electronic medical record solves this problem by providing instant access to all family members. In choosing an electronic medical record system, one should include consideration of how the system organizes family and household information. For example, a family record number located in the individual record could link the clinician to family-related information.

A family member often requests information about another family member's healthcare. For example, a mother at her yearly gynecological visit may inquire when her children should come in for their next visit or immunization. This information is readily available in the family chart. With family charts, however, the clinician must be particularly careful about confidentiality of information. The clinician should not provide information about an adult family member without that person's consent: A patient should not have access to the entire family chart without permission of the other members of the family.

Confidentiality

Confidentiality is a concern that often arises in family-oriented medical care (see Fig. 23.1).

> Chuck McNab, a 60-year-old African-American male, appeared for an appointment with Dr. D. He had been separated from his ailing wife, Martha, for more than 1 year. He was upset that his stepdaughter Cheryl had told him that his wife did not want him to visit her in the nursing home, and Cheryl would not tell him in which nursing home she was. Dr. D. knew the answer to Chuck's questions, but was reluctant to reveal this information to Chuck without his wife's permission. He also feared that telling Chuck might put him in a coalition with Chuck against his stepdaughter and possibly Martha, yet he thought Chuck should know where his wife was, so he was uncertain what to do.

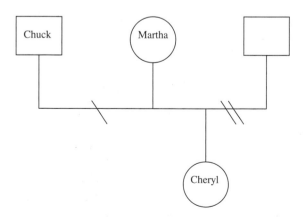

FIGURE 23.1. Confidentiality in a blended family.

In family-oriented primary care, it is important to determine the difference between a patient's request for legitimate confidentiality and colluding with a patient or family member about a secret that may fuel individual and family dysfunction.

Confidentiality is an essential ethical standard in medical practice, but secrets are destructive to healthy family functioning (19). To deal with this dilemma, the clinician should never provide information about an adult patient to another family member except when the patient has given explicit permission [or is in immediate danger to him- or herself (i.e., suicide) or others (i.e., homicide)] (20). Even with permission, this process is best accomplished with all relevant parties present. When the clinician suspects a secret that may be damaging to family relationships (e.g., an affair, or a serious or terminal diagnosis), the clinician can use his or her influence to advise the patient or family to disclose any important information; however, the clinician should not be the party to actually reveal the confidential information. One should consider referral to a psychotherapist to manage any serious fallout if the information is likely to be provocative.

> Dr. D. suggested to Chuck that he and his stepdaughter meet at the nursing home to discuss with Martha whether Chuck could visit his wife. Chuck agreed to abide by whatever decision Martha made about his visiting. Dr. D. called the daughter, who reluctantly agreed to tell Chuck which nursing home her mother was in, and to attend a family conference, as long as Chuck promised to respect Martha's wishes. Dr. D. met with the three of them at the nursing home. Martha said that she did not want her husband visiting often or for long periods of time, but told Chuck that he could visit every 2 weeks as long as Cheryl was not visiting. Chuck agreed to come every other Sunday afternoon for one half-hour. After several months of this schedule, Martha invited him to visit every Sunday for up to 1 hour.

By maintaining simultaneous strong alliances with each family member, the family-oriented clinician can be the most helpful to the patient and the family. In this case, Dr. D. avoided getting drawn into taking sides in the family feud and helped the McNabb family successfully deal with some of their conflicts.

There are situations where it may be unethical not to encourage the family to be involved in the management of a health problem (21). In certain circumstances, failure to inform or involve the family can result in serious harm to the patient or family members. When a patient is suicidal, family members should be informed and involved in treatment planning to help protect the patient's life, even if the patient does not want them told. The sexual partners of patients with AIDS or other serious sexually transmitted diseases should be informed of the risk, even when the patient refuses. Most state laws now permit or even mandate such disclosure. It is more common that there may be situations where the clinician should strongly urge the patient to involve or inform the family (e.g., when the diagnosis of a serious, fatal, or genetic disease is made, or when the patient decides to refuse treatment). In general, when the patient refuses or is reluctant to inform or involve the family in his or her healthcare, the clinician should inform the patient of the potential harm that may occur to the patient or the family if the family is not involved. The clinician must balance these risks with the patient's reluctance to involve the family.

Working with Other Professionals

Anytime more than two parties are involved with an issue, triangulation is a possibility (see Chap. 3). There is virtually always more than just the primary care clinician involved in today's healthcare, from physical therapists to case managers to any number of specialists. With each patient, the primary care clinician is at risk for triangulation in multiple ways, either with other members of the healthcare team or with the patient's family.

> Mrs. Smith, a 46-year-old Italian-American, presented several weeks ago to her primary care clinician, Dr. P., with a breast mass. Rapid work-up demonstrated carcinoma and Mrs. Smith met with Dr. S., the surgeon, and Dr. O., the oncologist. She and her husband were confused by what they perceived as conflicting messages from the two specialists. Dr. S. highlighted all the risks associated with surgery, including infection, bleeding, and death, and painted a rather pessimistic picture of her future. On the other hand, Dr. O. seemed to think that because of her age, general good health, and lack of co-morbidities, Mrs. Smith's prognosis was relatively good, and that if she needed chemotherapy, she would do well. Dr. P. reviewed the letters from the specialists, and concluded that there was agreement between the two, but guessed they had presented their views very differently, leading to the confusion. Dr. P. met with the Smiths and worked to elucidate the specialists' frames of reference so that their comments could be understood in the context of their respective professional disciplines—as a general rule, surgeons tend to emphasize risks, whereas oncologists tend to emphasize hope. In the end, this corroborated the Smiths' "gut feeling" and they were reassured that everyone agreed about the treatment and prognosis.

Key strategies to avoid triangulation are communicating clearly and avoiding taking sides, while maintaining patient advocacy. Encouraging direct communication between conflicting parties helps the clinician stay out of the middle. The primary care clinician may be tempted to overfunction for the patient and speak for them to specialists or other professionals in a well-intentioned effort to care for the patient; however, this robs the patients of their autonomy, fosters dependence, and often leads to impaired or inaccurate information exchange. The clinician can be helpful by offering to be present during a potentially difficult interchange.

Ms. Fernandez, a 28-year old Puerto Rican single mom, brought in her son, Jose, because of the school's concern that he had ADHD. Ms. Fernandez did not believe that he had ADHD and thought the school just wanted "to medicate everybody." Two of his teachers had done evaluations, but Jose had not yet met with the school psychologist. Dr. S. described the typical course of events in an ADHD evaluation (e.g., teacher input, testing done by the school psychologist classroom observation, etc.) and encouraged Ms. Fernandez to proceed because "some helpful information might be derived from the evaluation." Dr. S. offered her assistance in whatever way possible "to best serve Jose's interests," including being available either by phone or in person for school conferences.

Dr. S. avoided triangulation by providing education and facilitating direct interaction between Ms. Fernandez and the school.

Maintaining a position of patient advocacy and working to promote the patient's health is not equivalent to disregarding information from sources other than the patient. When there is conflict, the clinician may need to communicate directly with the other parties before making any judgment: There are always to sides to a conflict.

Mrs. Yarowsky contacted the family doctor on call. Dr. C. learned from Mrs. Yarowsky that she had recently had surgery done by her OB-Gyn (in a different office) for endometriosis, and had been given little pain medication postoperatively. Mrs. Yarowky lamented that her OB-Gyn doctor was callous and cold-hearted, and she desperately needed more pain medication. Dr. C. contacted the OB-Gyn, who reported that the patient had a history of prescription narcotics abuse, and had been given more than adequate supplies of pain medication. Following this second phone call, Dr. C. offered his sympathy to Mrs. Yarowsky, confronted her about the actual quantities of pain medication that had been prescribed, refused to call in a prescription for more pain medicine, and suggested that a visit to the office might be helpful in order to sort out issues around chronic pain and whether a referral to a pain treatment center was indicated. Dr. C. encouraged Mrs. Yarowsky to contact her OB-Gyn.

Conflicting interests between the individual patient and other family members presents another opportunity for triangulation. The clinician is often asked by the family or by other caregivers to decide what should be done in a situation where there is disagreement. In these circumstances, the clinician should avoid being drawn into the role of decision maker, unless the decision is clearly a medical one. The clinician should instead bring all relevant parties together and facilitate a process in which the group can discuss the problem (22). The best solution occurs when all parties can agree to support the outcome. If not, the patient retains the right to make his or her own decision, but does so fully informed as to what others are willing to do (23–25) (see Chap. 3 for more details on avoiding triangulation when there are conflicting interests).

Home Visits

Home visits or house calls augment family-oriented medical practice. They offer an opportunity to see the patient and family in their own natural setting and can provide valuable information about how the patient is functioning and how the family is adapting to the health problem. Siwek (26) has argued that house calls may be the best form of intervention during a family crisis. Home visits are particularly important for the frail elderly where a visit to the clinician's office during the winter may actually be dangerous. For homebound elderly, it can be helpful to arrange to meet other family members or the public health nurse at the home to get their assessments of how the patient is doing.

Home visits at the 2-week well-child visit can dramatically facilitate comprehensive family-oriented care. This can be a difficult time for the family to get to the office, and a home visit avoids exposing the newborn to infectious illnesses in the waiting room. A home visit is also the best way to assess how the family is adapting to the new baby (see Chaps. 10 and 11), how the feeding is going, and what kind of help and support the mother is receiving. Finally, making home visits is a very quick way to become known in a community. Word spreads through the neighborhood that the doctor is making a home visit, and one commonly has neighbors come by to meet this unusual doctor. For multiproblem or chaotic families, making a home visit sometimes may be the only way to assemble the entire family for a meeting. Such a home visit also may provide insights into the problems that the family is facing. Home visits are typically scheduled at the end of a session, and there are specific billing codes for these occasions.

Billing and Finances

A common concern about a family-oriented approach to medical care is that it takes too much time to implement and is not financially feasible. Involving the family in medical care takes some additional time up front, which pays itself back in the long run with reduced visits. Inviting the father to prenatal and well-child visits should not take additional time; having both parents present when discussing problems is usually the most efficient way to proceed. Involving the spouse of a patient with a chronic illness in his or her care similarly does not take additional time and can facilitate care and prevent later time-consuming phone calls.

Family conferences do take additional time, and that time should be billed at the same rate as other visits. Clinicians should not undervalue the worth of these family conferences or counseling by undercharging for them. The billing procedure needs to be flexible enough to take account of the family's income and insurance. In some cases the patient may be billed for an extended visit or consultation, or, if appropriate, for a counseling session. In other situations, different family members can be billed for portions of the session. Whatever method is used, it should be acceptable to the insurance company, and discussed and negotiated in advance with the family, so that the method of billing and payment is clear to everyone involved.

Termination of the Clinician–Patient Relationship

Despite everyone's best efforts, the relationship between clinician and patient occasionally does not work out. The clinician must make every effort to address the problems and to seek creative solutions. Even so, "irreconcilable differences" may exist. It is generally the patient who initiates a change and seeks out another clinician to provide care. When the patient initiates the termination, it is crucial to find out why. The change is often discovered when a written request for transfer of medical records arrives from another office. No clinician enjoys making contact with patients that reject or "fire" them, but calling the patient to obtain feedback can be enlightening to the clinician and therapeutic for the patient. It may also reduce the likelihood of a lawsuit. If the request for medical records comes from a law firm, contact should not be made with the patient. The rationale for the phone call should be honest and straightforward.

> Dr. T.: Hello, Mrs. Jones, this is Dr. T. I want to let you know that I received a request for transferring your medical records to Dr. A. We are in the process of doing that right now. In our practice, it is customary for us to call and find out if there were problems with how your healthcare was delivered so that we can try to do better with other patients.

People are usually quite pleased that the clinician took the time to call. Even though they may be hesitant in the beginning, they are eventually relieved and relish an opportunity to discuss the situation.

With some patients, clinicians may want to be cautious about allowing them to return to the practice, particularly if they left to doctor-shop or because the clinician set limits, perhaps on prescribing narcotics. Patients who leave the practice because they moved out of the area or because their insurance changed should, of course, be welcomed back if either of these situations change. All of these issues underscore the profound responsibilities of the clinician (and patient, and family) to attend to the relationship issues that promote health partnerships.

On the rare occasion when a clinician initiates the termination, it is the clinician's responsibility to outline the impasse. The patient rarely denies the problem once it is pointed out and the termination is usually mutually agreed upon. It is customary for the clinician to provide emergency care for 30 days after formal receipt of a termination letter; otherwise, the termination is considered abandonment of a patient. It is important to avoid blaming the patient, and instead to ascribe the need for termination in terms of lack of fit between patient and clinician. Care must be taken to insure that the patient has other available resources for obtaining healthcare (i.e., a clinician-initiated termination may not be possible in some remote areas.) Even though it is rare for a clinician to discharge a patient from his or her practice, it is a possibility that when recognized may help both parties attend to improving the relationship. Instead of feeling trapped and forced to care for all patients, the clinician may feel freer to talk explicitly with patients about the strengths and problems in their professional relationship. A patient who realizes that he or she may be discharged from the practice may work harder to maintain responsible and mature relationships with his or her healthcare providers.

Conclusion

In the end, the practice of family-oriented primary care is time-efficient, cost-effective, and, perhaps most importantly, care-effective. At first glance, it may seem like gathering a genogram, for example, takes "extra" time, but this is time well spent. It is often time that must be spent in order to make a proper diagnosis and arrange appropriate treatment. This chapter has described some methods and strategies for streamlining these processes. Arranging an office system that facilitates the practice of family-oriented primary care minimizes the up-front time while maximizing patient care. Finally, a family-oriented approach allows us to know our patients as people. With today's focus on speed and the bottom line, there is no substitute for the satisfaction derived from this human connection.

References

1. Christie-Seeley J: Establishing a family orientation. In: Christie-Seeley J (Ed): *Working with Families in Primary Care.* New York: Praeger Press, 1983.
2. Rogers JC, Cohn P: Impact of a screening family genogram on first encounters in primary care. *Fam Prac* 1987;**4**:291–301.
3. Ebell MH, Heaton CJ: Development and evaluation of a computer genogram. *J Fam Prac* 1988;**27**:536–537.
4. Gerson R, McGoldrick M: The computerized genogram. *Primary Care* 1985; **12**:535–545.
5. Mehl LE, Bruce C, & Renner JH: Importance of obstetrics in a comprehensive family practice. *J Fam Prac* 1976;**3**:385–389.

6. Weiss BD: The effect of malpractice insurance costs on family physicians' hospital practices. *J Fam Prac* 1986;**23**:55–58.

7. Eastwood MA, Brydon WG, Smith DM, & Smith JH: A study of diet, serum lipids, and fecal constituents in spouses. *Am J Clin Nutr* 1982;**36**:290–293.

8. Glenn M: *Collaborative Health Care: A Family-Oriented Model*. New York: Praeger, 1987.

9. Seaburn D, Lorenz A, Gunn W, Gawinski B, & Mauksch L: *Models of Collaboration: A Guide for Mental Health Professionals Working with Health Care Practitioners*. New York: Basic, 1996.

10. Dym B, Berman S: Family systems medicine: family therapy's next frontier? *Fam Ther Network* 1985;**9**:20.

11. Dym B, Berman S: The primary health care team: family physician and family therapist in joint practice. *Fam Syst Med* 1986;**4**:9–21.

12. McDaniel S, Campbell T: Physician and family therapists: the risks of collaboration. *Fam Syst Med* 1986;**4**:1–4.

13. Froom J, Culpepper L, Kirkwood RC, Boisseau V, & Mangone D: An integrated medical record and data system for primary care. Part 4: family information. *J Fam Prac* 1977;**5**:265–270.

14. A Glossary for Primary Care. Report of the North American Primary Care Research Group (NAPCGR). Presented at the Annual Meeting of NAPCRG, Williamsburg, VA, March 1977.

15. Widmer RB, Cadoret RJ: Depression in family practice: changes in patterns of patient visits and complaints during subsequent developing depression. *J Fam Prac* 1979;**9**:1017–1021.

16. Froom J: An integrated system for the recording and retrieved of medical data in a primary care setting. Part 4: family folders. *J Fam Prac* 1974;**1**:49–51.

17. Huygens FJA: *Family Medicine. The Medical Life History of Families*. New York: Brunner-Mazel, 1978.

18. Meyer RJ, Haggerty RJ: Streptococcal infections in families: factors altering individual susceptibility. *Pediatrics* 1962;**29**:539–549.

19. Karpel M, Strauss E: *Family Secrets. Family Evaluation*. New York: Gardener Press, 1983.

20. Christiansson CE: Ethical issues in family-centered primary care. *Counsel Values* 1985;**30**:62–73.

21. Boszormenyi-Nagy I: Ethics of human relationships and the treatment contract. In Lennard HL, Lennard SC (Eds): *Ethics of Health Care*. New York: Gondolier, 1979.

22. Sherlock R, Dingus CM: *Families and the Gravely Ill: Roles, Rules, and Rights*. New York: Greenwood Press, 1988.

23. Brody H: Ethics in family medicine: patient autonomy and the family unit. *J Fam Prac* 1983;**17**:973–975.

24. Sider R, Clements C: Family or individual therapy: the ethics of modality choice, *Am J Psychiatr* 1983;**139**:1455.

25. Williamson P, McCormick T, & Taylor T: Who is the patient? A family case study of a recurrent dilemma in family practice. *J Fam Prac* 1983;**17**:1039–1043.

26. Siwek J: House calls: current status and rationale. *Am Fam Physician* 1985;**31**(4):169–174.

Protocol: How to Set Up a Family-Oriented Practice

Use a Family-Oriented Image

- The practice name should contain the word *family*.
- Staff should support and encourage a family-oriented approach.

Provide a Range of Available Services

- The practice should offer pregnancy and pediatric services when possible.
- Social work and nutritional services should be offered.
- A family therapist should be part of the practice or available for close collaboration.
- A comprehensive list of other family-oriented resources in the community should be available to the clinician, patients, and families.

Enroll Patients with Their Families

- The entire family should be enrolled together with an initial joint visit whenever possible.
- A genogram should be obtained on all families at the time of their first visit.

Use a Family-Oriented Medical Record

- The charts of all members of the household ideally should be filed together or electronically linked.
- There should be easy access to family information.

Plan the Physical Layout to Support a Family Orientation

- The waiting room should be able to accommodate families with all age members, including small children and disabled elderly.
- Examination rooms should be large enough to accommodate families.

Implement Flexible Scheduling

- Patient scheduling should be flexible enough to meet the needs of the families and allow longer appointments for family counseling.

Use Home Visits

- Home visits should be a regular part of the practice.
- When possible; homebound elderly, terminally ill, and postpartum patients should be seen in the home.

Bill for Family-Oriented Services

- Family conferences and counseling should be billed appropriately.
- The waiting room should be able to accommodate families with all age members, including small children and disabled elderly.

24
Acute Hospital Care: Letting the Family In

George Mayer, a 67-year-old German-American male, did not look well when he arrived at the emergency room (ER). Clutching his chest, he was pale, anxious, and sweating. "The pain in my chest started several hours ago and just won't go away," he told the nurse as she attached him to a cardiac monitor. "I thought it was just indigestion, but maybe it's my heart." The nurse hooked up the oxygen, adeptly inserted an intravenous catheter and called for the clinician.

George's wife, Sarah, accompanied her husband to the ER and remained by his stretcher trying to reassure him that everything would be okay. The nurse asked her to leave and wait in the ER waiting room while her husband was being evaluated. As she left the room, her husband slumped over, the cardiac monitor showed ventricular tachycardia, and the nurse shouted "Code Blue." Cardiopulmonary resuscitation was begun as Sarah was escorted to the waiting room. George responded to intravenous lidocaine and electric cardioversion, and he regained consciousness as his rhythm became regular again. His EKG showed he had suffered a large anterior wall myocardial infarction (MI). He was sedated and transferred to the Intensive Care Unit (ICU).

Sarah remained in the waiting room throughout this time. Each time she went to the emergency desk to get information, she was told her husband was being evaluated, and the doctor would be out shortly to talk with her. After an hour, the ER physician appeared and spoke with her. He explained that her husband had suffered a serious heart attack, that his heart had briefly stopped, but they had been able to restart it. He was now stable and on his way to the ICU. He directed her to the ICU waiting area and said that she could see her husband as soon as he was stable.

Admission to an acute-care hospital is usually a crisis for patients and their families. It may occur because of an acute illness (e.g., pneumonia, myocardial infarction, or a newly diagnosed cancer) or because of an exacerbation of a chronic illness (e.g., asthma, congestive heart failure, or renal failure). It is a time when families usually pull together: Family members come from out of town, old conflicts are put aside, and the family tries to do whatever they can to help. Family support is particularly important during such a crisis, but hospital procedures unfortunately often result in families being cut off from their hospitalized member and from his or her medical care. When a patient is admitted to the hospital, the family literally hands the care of the patient to the hospital. The hospital staff takes over, and provides everything from meals and personal care to intensive medical procedures and surgery. Families are only allowed to visit during restricted visiting hours, usually during the afternoon and evening hours. These visits may even be viewed as interference or a nuisance by the hospital staff.

Families often encounter difficulty getting information about the health condition and medical care of the patient. Clinicians may be hard to contact, and nurses may be unfamiliar with the details of care or reluctant to share them with the family. This communication problem is compounded when there are multiple medical specialists involved, some of whom have different recommendations for the patient. Families are rarely consulted about treatment plans and typically participate little in the care of the patient, except when the patient is unable to make decisions about care. By contrast, after leaving the hospital, most of a patient's healthcare is provided by family members. The family then reassumes their roles as the primary healthcare givers. Lack of coordination of care during the transition, from home to hospital and back again, results in poorer care of the patient, and the family suffers as well.

A family-oriented healthcare system cares for the patient in a way that encourages families to actively assist in hospital care and prepares families to care for the patient in the home. To implement this, a team approach involving the clinician, other healthcare professionals, the hospital and all its services, staff, and the family is necessary. As part of the team, the clinician needs to have knowledge and understanding of the family, the hospital, and insurance reimbursement, and be able to work as a negotiator between multiple systems. Most community clinicians communicate regularly with the families of their hospitalized patients and acknowledge the importance of their support to the patient. This chapter will provide a framework for thinking about this family orientation and extending it in new ways.

The Changing Hospital Environment

Gone are the days when a clinician could electively admit a patient to the hospital for the evaluation of a worrisome symptom and discharge the patient, when the clinician, patient, and family thought the patient was ready. Economic pressures at national, state, and local levels are restricting the use of hospitalization to briefer periods of time and for only the most serious medical problems. Hospitalization rates and lengths of stay in the hospital have dropped dramatically. Patients in the hospital now are sicker, and they require more intensive and higher technological care. Hospital staffs are providing more services with fewer personnel, and they are busier than ever before. Nurses and clinicians complain that they have less time for the "caring" part of their work (e.g., talking to and consoling ill patients and their families).

Many patients, especially the elderly, are being discharged from the hospital before they are able to function independently. With less time for adequate discharge planning, patients are sent home when they no longer need acute hospital care, although they may not quite be ready to return home or adequate services may not have been set up completely. Patients are sicker and have more healthcare needs than before. Community and home services still lag behind the need for such services. Most insurers reimburse for acute medical and nursing care, but they may provide little support for rehabilitative or custodial care.

Modern medicine, with all its financial limits, makes the role of the family even more important in the care of patients in the hospital. To ease the transitions in and out of the hospital, outpatient services need to be coordinated closely with in-hospital care. Families are an integral part of the healthcare system and need to be involved at the time of hospital admission, throughout the hospitalization, and after discharge. Adequate services in the community also need to be available and affordable to patients and their families so that families can get the help they need to care adequately for their sick members.

Involving Parents in the Care of the Hospitalized Child

Pediatrics led the way in family involvement in hospital care. Until the 1950s, hospitalized children were isolated from their parents, and parents were discouraged from visiting. Because the children cried after their parents visited, it was believed that seeing their parents was emotionally upsetting and therefore unhealthy for the children! As a result of studies by Robertson (1) and others (2), the adverse effect of the child's separation from his or her parents was recognized, and dramatic changes have occurred in hospital policies concerning the involvement of parents in the care of their children. In most hospitals today, parents may stay with their child continuously throughout the hospitalization (3). Cots or beds are provided for parents to sleep with the child. Parents may accompany their child for tests. Some hospitals even allow a parent to accompany a child into the operating room while anesthesia is being induced and into the recovery room to be present when the child awakens. All these policies have helped to make the hospital visit a less-traumatic experience for the child and parents. The child is less anxious when accompanied by the parent, and parents feel they can help and care for their child.

Adult healthcare has not yet caught up with pediatrics in this domain. Children are not the only ones who need their families at their bedside in the hospital. Family members are still considered "visitors" in most hospitals, and families' access to patients continues to be restricted. Entire hospitals, not just the pediatrics or obstetric wards, need to become more family friendly and welcoming so that families can be used as a resource in the care of patients, rather than seen as a nuisance that interferes with appropriate care. To accomplish this will involve changes in hospital policies and the attitudes and behavior of all healthcare professionals (4). As advocates for patients and their families, primary care clinicians should lead the way in this movement by modeling appropriate behavior for hospital staff and using their influence to change hospital policies.

A landmark study by the Institute of Medicine on the quality of care recommended that healthcare institutions "accommodate families and friends on whom patients may rely, involving them as appropriate in decision making, supporting them as caregivers, making them welcome and comfortable in the care delivery setting, and recognizing their needs and contributions" (p. 50) (5). The Joint Commission on Accreditation of Healthcare Organizations (JCAHO) strongly encourages hospitals and long-term care facilities to involve families to ensure patient safety and quality care (6).

The Institute for Family-Centered Care (www.familycenteredcare.org) is one of the leaders in promoting family-centered care in all healthcare settings. They publish guidelines and checklists to help hospitals become more family-centered (7). These recommendations range from environmental design to policies and practices. The Institute encourages open or flexible visiting hours for families, family advisory panels, family resources rooms, and active involvement by families in all aspects of hospital care.

Family-Oriented Hospital Care

The primary goal of family-oriented hospital care is to address the needs of the patient and the family and to utilize the family's resources in the care of the patient throughout the hospitalization. Working with the family can directly benefit the patient in several ways:

1. Families can assist in the medical evaluation of the patient.

As in most medical situations, family members are usually excellent observers and can provide additional valuable information about the patient at the time of admission and throughout the hospitalization. The acutely ill patient is often less able to give a reliable report of the illness. Interviewing family members may be especially useful in the hospital setting for several reasons.

a. A family member may give critical historical information about the illness that the patient may have forgotten or neglected.

For example, a middle-aged man was admitted with severe abdominal pain and diarrhea. During an interview with the family, his son recalled a camping trip with his father to the Adirondacks a month earlier. Giardia cysts were found on microscopic examination of the patient's stool.

b. The family may recognize a pattern that the patient does not.

A young woman was admitted to the hospital with another exacerbation of her asthma. Her husband commented to her clinician that her wheezing became much worse whenever the heat was on in their house. Upon checking the furnace, a mold was found growing on the filter.

c. The patient may minimize symptoms.

The wife of a cardiac patient contradicted her husband's claim that he was having very little chest pain. She explained to his clinician that he went through three bottles of nitroglycerin tablets each week. On cardiac catherization, he had severe triple-vessel coronary artery disease.

d. The patient may completely deny symptoms or behaviors.

A 60-year-old woman was admitted with unexplained ataxia. On the second hospital day, when the patient developed a tremor and hallucinations, her son admitted that the patient had been a heavy drinker for many years, something unknown to her primary care clinician. She was diagnosed as having alcoholic cerebellar degeneration.

e. The patient may be unaware of some symptoms.

An 80-year-old man was seen in the ER after an apparent blackout spell at home. After interviewing the patient's wife, the clinician learned that the patient had fallen and struck his head 3 days previously, and that morning he had had a grand mal seizure, not syncope. A CT scan revealed a subdural hematoma.

The family provided essential information in each of these cases, which led to the diagnosis. Even during hospitalization, family members can provide important information about the patient, information of which the hospital staff may be unaware. For example, a 78-year-old man was having episodes of unexplained confusion for several days after a hip replacement. His wife, who had been at his bedside each day, said that she thought he became confused shortly after receiving one of his medications. She reported that a similar reaction had occurred several years previously after surgery on his prostate. The offending medication was stopped and the confusion was resolved.

2. Reducing the family's anxiety will reduce the patient's anxiety and speed recovery.

Children are strongly influenced by their parents' perception of health problems and medical procedures. Pediatricians have long recognized that a child's fear of doctors or immunizations often reflects parental fears transmitted (usually unconsciously) to the child. Dealing with the parent's anxiety can be more effective than trying to allay the fears of the child directly. Studies have shown that adults are similarly influenced by perceptions of those closest to them, especially family members (8, 9). Some surgeons realize the importance of speaking with the spouse or adult child of a patient about a planned operation. Family members who have doubts or concerns about the surgeon or the operation will often communicate these to the patient either directly (e.g., "I don't think you should have this operation, Mom") or indirectly (e.g., "This is a pretty small hospital to be doing this kind of surgery. I wonder how many of these procedures they've done?"). Keeping the family informed and addressing their emotional needs will help them to be more supportive and confident with the patient.

3. Involving family members in the hospital will help them to assume the appropriate healthcare responsibilities after discharge.

With shorter hospital stays, patients are returning home with greater nursing and healthcare needs. Although some of these are met by home health services, family members provide most. If family members are not involved in the care of the patient while in the hospital, they are unlikely to be prepared physically or emotionally to care for the patient when he or she returns home. Family members who develop the skills and confidence to provide for the patient while still in the hospital will provide better care at home and hasten recovery.

> Although she was 86 years old, Mrs. Phemore, a Portuguese immigrant, had never been hospitalized until she fell and broke her hip. On admission she was very agitated and mildly confused. She initially refused to consider surgery, saying that she would rather die at home than in the hospital. The orthopedic surgeon met with the patient and the daughter and son-in-law with whom she lived, and explained the procedure, its risks and benefits, and how it would speed her recovery to return home. The patient's daughter and son-in-law told Mrs. Phemore that they wanted her to return home as soon as she was able, and the operation would help her do this. She consented to the surgery, which was uneventful. Mrs. Phemore's daughter participated in her mother's physical therapy and learned the exercises and how to help her walk. With the help of the hospital social worker, the daughter set up home services that included Meals on Wheels, physical therapy and public health nurse visits to supervise her rehabilitation. Mrs. Phemore was discharged back to her home 2 weeks after admission.

Surveys of the families of acutely ill or dying patients have identified what families want most during hospitalization (10). In order of priority, these include:

- To be with the ill person.
- To be helpful to the ill person.
- To be assured of the comfort of the ill person.
- To be kept informed of the medical status of the ill person.
- To be able to share their emotions.
- To receive acceptance and support from the hospital staff.

The family-oriented clinician can assist family members in getting these needs met, and the clinician is directly responsible for some (e.g., keeping the family informed of the patient's medical status and maintaining the maximal comfort of the patient). For others, the clinician must work with the hospital staff to provide emotional support to families, encourage them to share their feelings, and find ways that they can be helpful to the patient. Finally, clinicians can influence hospitals to become more family oriented with unlimited visiting hours for close family members and for family participation in patient care.

The rest of this chapter will present specific suggestions for implementing a family-oriented approach to hospital care that meet the needs of patients and their families.

Hospital Family Conferences

Family conferences are an efficient and effective way to deal with family and patient anxiety that occurs around a hospitalization. It is helpful to have contact with the family as soon after hospital admission as possible. The family has often brought the patient to the hospital and desires more information about the patient. (Because the basic skills of convening and conducting a family conference are covered in Chaps. 5 and 7, this section will cover aspects of the family conference that are particular to the hospital setting.)

Family meetings during hospitalization are often impromptu and informal. They may be as simple as talking to a spouse in the emergency room to obtain more history, or as complex as meeting with an extended family of a dying patient about limiting treatment or whether to resuscitate (DNR). Several principles are useful:

1. Involve the patient in family meetings whenever possible.

Healthcare clinicians and family members often exclude the patient from these family meetings because they feel that the patient is either too sick to participate or will become emotionally upset. Some families have a rule not to discuss health problems directly with an ill family member. Although a patient may sometimes be too ill to participate or may be undergoing a procedure, the patient can in most cases listen and often actively participate. Involving the patient in the family conference can be helpful because it:

a. Is time efficient. The clinician can give medical information to the patient and family at the same time and does not have to repeat it.
b. Allows the patient to comment on and correct important medical information.
c. Encourages the family to discuss the illness and hospitalization together, and to share information and emotional reactions.
d. Helps to keep the family focused on the immediate and specific issues faced by the patient and the family.
e. Prevents secrets from developing (e.g., when the clinician gives the family a prognosis and the patient is not told, or vice versa).
f. Allows the clinician to see how the family interacts with the patient (e.g., blaming, overprotective, etc.).

It is occasionally necessary to meet briefly with the patient or family alone after a family meeting that includes the patient. The family may not be willing to share information or feelings with the patient present, despite the clinician's urging. For example, Mrs. Bramer was admitted with "falling spells." After a meeting with the patient and the family, Mr. Bramer pulled her doctor aside and explained that she "drank a lot." In such cases, the clinician should be clear about not keeping secrets, and should address these issues directly with the patient and the family together. Dr. C. met again with the family and the patient and asked the family to share this information with the patient. He thanked her family for being so concerned about her health that they would tell him about the drinking and he emphasized that this information was very important in understanding her health problems and treating her successfully in the hospital.

2. Find the best place to meet with the family.

It is often difficult to find a quiet, private place to meet with patients and their families. Patients may be bedbound and unable to travel to a family conference room. The best place to meet with the family is often at the patient's bedside, whether the patient is in the emergency room (ER), the intensive care unit (ICU), or a private room. This may require assembling enough chairs for everyone, or remain standing in the ER or ICU. If the patient is in a semi-private room and the roommate is ambulatory, the roommate can be asked to leave the room during the conference; otherwise, use the curtain to separate the room to provide some privacy. Failure to attend to this basic, but often overlooked, need for a quiet and private place to meet with families can sabotage the clinician's best efforts.

3. Invite participation, either directly or indirectly, of relevant staff in the family conference.

If the hospital has a primary-nurse system, in which one nurse is responsible for developing and coordinating a nursing care plan, the primary nurse is a key person to get involved with the family. Nurses, not physicians, provide most of the care for patients in the hospital, and they have the most contact with families. Social workers often know the most about insurance reimbursement for services and placement possibilities. Physical therapists know the most about the patient's physical limitations.

4. Obtain a skeletal genogram to identify important family members and their relationship to the patient.

This common outpatient tool can be especially valuable to inpatient care. Constructing a basic genogram of the patient's immediate family usually takes only a minute or two, and it may become invaluable during later contacts with the family. It should be placed in the chart to help other care clinicians (e.g., nurses, residents, dietician, physical therapist) orient themselves to the family, and it can be developed further during the hospitalization. For many families, the primary care clinician will already have a genogram that can be shared with the rest of the healthcare team (see Chap. 3).

5. Review events leading up to the hospitalization, acknowledging the helpful information provided by the family, and then state the current assessment and treatment plan for the patient.

Reviewing the history gives the patient and family the opportunity to correct any misinformation or confusion about the events prior to admission, and reassures the family that you have a clear understanding of the situation. Pertinent test results should be explained, and a simple, clear assessment of the illness should be presented. The treatment plan, the prognosis, and the anticipated length of stay in the hospital should be discussed. The patient and family members are encouraged to ask questions and express their concerns. Depending upon the complexities of the problem, family conferences can last from a few minutes to 1 hour. When decisions regarding such options as surgery or whether to resuscitate must be made by the patient and family, extra time is necessary to be sure that all family members understand the issues involved (see Chap. 16 for a discussion of DNR conferences). If the illness is of sudden onset or the diagnosis is grave, the patient and family are often in a state of shock or disbelief and may not remember or seem to understand what is told to them. Explanations must be kept quite simple and nontechnical, and they should be repeated several times over the ensuing days.

6. Be prepared to respond to strong affect from family members.

The hospitalization of a loved one is often a frightening experience for family members. Providing accurate and timely information about the patient is an effective way to help reduce family members' anxiety; however, some family members may respond with overwhelming anxiety or anger. The clinician should be prepared to address these feelings in family members. If key family members do not visit the patient in the hospital, it may indicate that they are responding to their fear by withdrawing from the patient.

7. Clarify the channels of communication between you, the family, and the hospital staff.

Families are reassured when they have a reliable way of contacting either the clinician or the hospital during the day or night. With unstable patients, the clinician may want to call the family at certain times during the day or when there is any change in the patient's status. Giving the family a way to reach the primary clinician for urgent questions is very reassuring to the family and is rarely abused.

> Shortly after George Mayer was transferred to the ICU, his family clinician, Dr. T., arrived at the hospital. After examining George, reviewing his test results, and discussing the case with the senior resident in the ICU, Dr. T. and his primary nurse spoke with George's wife, Sarah, in George's room. Although George was mildly sedated, he was well-oriented and could participate in the meeting. While reviewing the events leading up to the hospitalization, Sarah added that her husband had been having chest pain for several weeks prior to this episode, which was something George had not mentioned.
>
> Dr. T. explained the heart attack, the cardiac arrest, and the resuscitation to George and Sarah. He said that George's cardiac rhythm was now stable and he was through the riskiest part of a heart attack. "You will be in the intensive care unit for about 3 days while your heart begins to heal," he explained. "After you are transferred to a regular floor, we will develop a plan to get you on your feet and home." George's nurse demonstrated how the cardiac monitor and other equipment worked, and gave Sarah the ICU telephone number to call at any time. Sarah was allowed to sit with her husband in the ICU for an hour while he slept. She was comforted to see how much care he was receiving and how well he slept. She felt that simply holding his hand was helping him during this critical period.

Although it is best for the clinician, nurse, or social worker to give information directly to as many family members as possible, this is not always possible. It is helpful to have the family choose one member who will be responsible for communicating with the healthcare clinicians and passing on information to the family. This person can be so designated on the genogram. This approach helps to prevent getting phone calls and messages from numerous family members requesting the same information. If the family has difficulty choosing one spokesperson, or if the clinician still gets calls from several family members, it may be a sign of a distressed or dysfunctional family and may warrant reassembling the family to explore the situation. There will occasionally be a family member who lives out of town but plays a particularly important role in the family (e.g., someone in a health profession). It may be necessary to speak with these family members directly to be sure they understand what is happening and that they support the treatment plan.

While George Mayer was still in the ICU, Sarah asked Dr. T. whether George should be considered for coronary artery bypass surgery (CABG). She explained that her daughter was a surgical resident in a distant hospital and had raised this question to her. Dr. T. explained why George was not being considered for CABG surgery at that time, but agreed to call her daughter and discuss this question directly with her. After calling the daughter and discussing her father's care with her, the daughter was reassured by Dr. T.'s competence and supported his plans to the rest of the family.

Family Involvement During Hospitalization

The family-oriented clinician can help the family to be actively involved in the hospital care in a number of ways.

1. Maintain regular contact with the family.

One way to do this is to inform the family when you plan to visit the patient and encourage them to be present at that time. An update on test results and further plans can be given to the patient and family at the same time. On the other hand, a regularly scheduled phone call can be arranged.

2. Encourage family members to be present and supportive of the patient however they can.

All departments in the hospital should have the most liberal visiting policies possible for family members. Close family members should be allowed unrestricted visiting hours as long as they do not disrupt essential hospital care or disturb the patient. Even in the ICU, where routine policies allow visiting for 10 minutes out of each hour, policies should be developed that allow for a spouse, child, or parent to stay with the patient for longer periods of time. Some ICUs even provide cots or beds for family members to spend the night in the patient's room (6). Small children free of communicable disease should be allowed and encouraged to visit a parent in the hospital. When visiting policies are more restrictive, the clinician can assist the family in requesting extended visiting hours.

> An elderly Hispanic woman with Alzheimer's disease became quite agitated during the first few nights in the hospital. Despite attempts to restrain and medicate her, she screamed throughout the night and crawled out of bed on several occasions. Finally, the patient's daughter spent the night with her mother sleeping on a cot provided by the staff. When her mother awoke during the night her daughter would reassure her, coax her back to bed, and sing her a song to help her sleep. Sleep medication and restraint were stopped and the woman's day–night reversal improved. After 2 nights, the hospital staff tape-recorded the daughter's voice and her singing, and played it to the woman at night to help her sleep.

Participating in the hospital care of a family member can be stressful. If children or others are at home, the family member may feel pulled between responsibility to the hospitalized patient and those at home. Routine family care is disrupted. Family members may have to take time off from work to be in the hospital, with resulting loss of income and financial stress. At times, it is important to encourage a family member to attend to their own needs: to go home, get adequate sleep, take care of their own health problems, or care for others in the family.

3. Find ways in which the family can participate in the care of the patient.

Hospital policies should promote and encourage participation. Some elderly patients require help to feed themselves, which is a time-consuming task for the nursing staff, but one that family members may enjoy. If visiting hours start in the afternoon, family members cannot help at breakfast or lunch. In addition to helping with hospital meals, family members can bring in appropriate foods for the patient. Home-cooked foods are generally more appetizing and likely to be eaten, and family members who learn from the dietician what foods are allowed in the diet and how to prepare them will be more likely to incorporate them into the diet at home.

Family members can also help with other aspects of care of the patient. During physical or occupational therapy, family members can learn what activities the patient participates in and which exercises the patient should do after discharge. When dressing changes or other simple procedures will continue after discharge, a member of the family can work along side the nurse and learn the procedure in the hospital.

The kinds of procedures and care the family can participate in will depend upon the desires of the patient and the interests and capabilities of the family. In one randomized clinical trial, women participated in their husbands' post-MI exercise stress test. The women who actually walked on the treadmill were more confident of their husbands' physical and cardiac capacity and less fearful of another MI than were women who did not participate or who simply observed the test (11).

Participating in some aspects of care, however, may be too stressful for families and have an adverse effect. Another study of high-risk cardiac patients and their families found that family members who learned cardiopulmonary resuscitation (CPR) were more anxious about the patient's health than were those who did not, and the patients in these families were also more anxious and had poorer adjustment to their illness (12). The investigators suggested that the CPR sessions had a "rehearsal component" that made the normal and healthy repression of thoughts of sudden death more difficult to maintain. In addition, family members reported feeling responsible for keeping the patient alive, and in some cases feared leaving the patient lest he have a cardiac arrest while alone. In general, it appears that family involvement is most beneficial for procedures and treatments that emphasize the patient's recovery and wellness, rather than potential adverse outcomes.

Several hospitals have developed innovative programs, which involve family members in every aspect of hospital care (13). Patients are admitted with their spouse or other relative and stay in apartment-style rooms. The family members are taught to perform many of the tasks traditionally performed by the nursing staff. These units are very popular with patients and their families. Patients report reduced anxiety, and family members feel more competent to handle medical problems when the patient returns home. In addition, these units require fewer nurses (an important advantage during the current nursing shortage) and cost approximately half as much to run as traditional hospital units.

Family members can help with personal care (e.g., bathing) even in the ICU, as well as with the emotional support that is important to a patient's recovery. Such simple measures as holding the patient's hand can have a powerfully reassuring effect on both the patient and the family, and help to humanize this frightening and highly technical environment. Cardiologist James Lynch (14) has documented the importance of human touch in the ICU (i.e., how it can reduce the resting heart rate and improve or abolish some arrhythmias).

Involving the family in a patient's care helps to meet the needs of both the patient and the family. It provides the patient with additional care and family support to reduce anxiety and speed recovery. It permits the family to be with the patient and to feel that they are being helpful to him or her. It also provides the clinician with the necessary information and resources to treat the patient successfully.

> George Mayer was transferred to a regular medical floor and began cardiac rehabilitation 3 days after his heart attack. He and his wife attended several cardiac teaching classes together in the hospital. They learned about the role of diet and exercise in cardiac rehabilitation and met with the dietician to review their diet. Together they negotiated which high-cholesterol foods would be eliminated from both of their diets, and which only George would avoid (i.e., Sarah did not want to give up ice cream). Sarah purchased the American Heart Association cookbook and brought a couple of home-cooked meals to George in the hospital. George underwent a limited stress test on his seventh hospital day that revealed no ischemia or arrhythmia. Sarah accompanied him to the exercise lab. After watching George on the treadmill, Sarah was invited by the cardiologist to try the treadmill out to experience what her husband had endured. She was amazed at how strenuous the exercise was and felt reassured that George could safely tolerate it.

Working with a Hospitalist

The rise of the "hospitalist movement" since the 1990s poses special challenges to family-oriented hospital care (15). Primary care clinicians who decide not to provide inpatient care often refer their patients to hospitalists, who provide and supervise all hospital care for their patients. Studies suggest that adult care by hospitalists is associated with shorter hospital stays and perhaps better medical outcomes (16). Continuity of care is usually broken with hospitalist care, however, and hospitalists rarely have long-term relationships with patients and their families.

Primary care clinicians who do not provide inpatient care must carefully chose hospitalists who are family-oriented and communicate effectively with patients, families, and the referring clinicians. Most of the principles of collaboration and referral to mental health professionals, which will be outlined in Chapter 25, apply to working with hospitalists. Regular and sometimes daily communication with the hospitalist about patients in the hospital is essential. Liberal use of faxes or e-mails from the hospitalist to the primary care clinician is an efficient way to stay informed. Family members often trust the primary care clinician and may call about a patient in hospital, even when he or she is not directly caring for the patient. He or she may need to explain the reason for using a hospitalist and how he or she will stay informed about the patient's hospital course. The primary care clinician who uses a hospitalist may chose to make (and bill for) a social visit to a patient and family in the hospital to help maintain continuity. This is particularly important if the patient is critically ill or decisions about placement or end-of-life care must be made.

Discharge Planning

With shorter hospital stays and patients being discharged with greater medical needs, planning for home care by the family has become an increasingly important aspect of hospital care.

1. Discuss discharge plans with the family early and on a regular basis.

This may be as simple as telling the patient and family how many additional days the patient is likely to be in the hospital, or as complex as discussing nursing home placement. Discuss discharge as early as possible. Patients or families are unfortunately often given less than 24 hours notice that the patient will be discharged.

2. Ask the social worker or public health nurse to contact the family in a timely fashion to determine their postdischarge needs.

This can be useful even when there are no obvious home-care needs. A social worker or public health nurse is usually better able to assess home-care needs and is more aware of resources in the community. For instance, the patient may benefit from a hospital bed or commode, or he or she might be able to take advantage of a community service (e.g., Friendly Visitors, Meals on Wheels) or group (e.g., Multiple Sclerosis Association). In addition, these professionals can help the family determine what they can afford and what services their insurance will cover.

3. Discharge the patient when both the patient and the family are ready.

Sending a patient home when there are insufficient services or the family is unprepared to care for the patient is inappropriate medical care. If discharge planning is started early, an adequate plan can be set up prior to the time the patient no longer needs acute hospital care.

4. Consider a family conference prior to discharge.

Try to get all the members of patient's household to be present, but encourage as many other family members as possible to attend. Invite the hospital staff that have been involved with the patient's care or helped with discharge planning, which usually includes the primary nurse and the social worker or public health nurse, but may also involve other consulting clinicians, physical, occupational, or speech therapists, or the dietician.

a. Update the current medical status of the patient (i.e., diagnosis, treatment received, and prognosis). Have the other staff report on their areas of involvement.
b. Outline the treatment plan (including medications), the needs of the patient at home, and services to be provided.
c. Elicit the patient's and family's understanding, questions and reactions to the patient's discharge, and the discharge plan. Anticipate difficulties by asking how they think the plan will work, and what problems are likely to arise.
d. Encourage the patient and family to negotiate the roles and responsibilities they will assume in the patient's care (see Chap. 18 on chronic illness for details of this negotiation).

5. Arrange a follow-up appointment with the patient and family.

Depending upon the nature and severity of the problems, this may occur in the office or the home 1–6 weeks after discharge. Patients and their families should be encouraged to call sooner if problems arise.

> The day before George's discharge from the hospital, Dr. T. met with the couple, their daughter who had flown in from out of town, George's primary nurse, the cardiac nurse educator, and the dietician. George's medical condition, diet, medication, and exercise program were all reviewed with the family. George and his wife were referred to a cardiac rehabilitation program at the local YMCA. The family was encouraged to share their feelings and concerns about George and his health. Sarah was most concerned that George would push himself too hard and not

tell anyone if he was having any chest pain. Dr. T. helped the couple negotiate how they would handle these issues. George agreed to tell his wife if he was having chest pain. Sarah agreed that he would be responsible for his level of activity, but that she would give him one reminder if she felt he was overdoing it.

Dr. T. briefly met with the couple alone to discuss guidelines for sexual activity. He took a brief sexual history and explained that based upon George's stress test and his level of activity, they could safely return to their normal sex life. He said that they may experience some anxiety or even some sexual difficulties in the beginning, and that this was normal. He scheduled them for a follow-up visit in the office for 1 month. If all was going well at that time, he told George that he would gradually be able to return to work after that.

Family-oriented care in the hospital offers special opportunities and challenges for the primary care clinician. They can provide invaluable information in an assessment of a problem. Their input is critical to the long-term success of any treatment plan. In addition, because families are often in a state of crisis, they can greatly benefit from regular communication and support from the clinician. During the hospitalization, they have the opportunity to learn more about their family member's illness and how to assist in their loved one's care.

References

1. Robertson J, Robertson J: Young children on brief separation. *Psychoanalyt Study Child* 1971;**26**:264–315.
2. MacCarthy D, Lindsay M, & Morris I: Children in hospital with mothers. *Lancet* 1962;**i**:603–608.
3. Institute for Family-Centered Care: *Hospitals Moving Forward with Family-Centered Care*. Bethesda, MD; IFCC, 2000.
4. Institute for Family-Centered Care: *Changing the Concept of Families as Visitors: Supporting Family Presence and Participation*. Bethesda, MD; IFCC, 2003.
5. Committee on Quality Health Care in America, Institute of Medicine: *Crossing the Quality Chasm: A New Health System for the 21st Century*. Washington DC: National Academic Press, 2001.
6. Committee on Quality Health Care in America, Institute of Medicine: *Changing the Concept of Families as Visitors in Hospitals. Advances in Family-Centered Care* 2002;**8**(1):1–6.
7. Institute for Family-Centered Care: *Self-Assessment Tools for Evaluating Family-Centered Care Practices*. Bethesda MD: IFCC, 2001.
8. Chatham M: The effect of family involvement on patients' manifestations of postcardiotomy psychosis. *Heart Lung* 1978;**7**:995–999.
9. Schwartz L, Brenner Z: Critical care unit transfer: reducing patient stress through nursing interventions. *Heart Lung* 1979;**8**:540–546.
10. Daley L: The perceived immediate needs of families with relatives in the intensive care unit setting. *Heart Lung* 1984;**7**:231–237.

11. Taylor CB, Bandura A, Ewart CK, Miller NH, & DeBusk RF: Exercise testing to enhance wives' confidence in their husbands' cardiac capability soon after clinically uncomplicated acute myocardial infarction. *Am J Cardiol* 1985;**55**: 635–638.

12. Dracup K, Guzy PM, Taylor SE, & Barry J: Cardiopulmonary resuscitation (CPR) training: Consequences for family members of high-risk cardiac patients. *Arch Intern Med* 1986;**146**:1757–1761.

13. Berg B: A touch of home in hospital care. *New York Times Magazine*, 1983; No. 27:90–98.

14. Lynch JJ: *The Broken Heart: The Medical Consequences of Loneliness.* New York: Basic Books, 1977.

15. Wachter RM, Goldman L: The hospitalist movement 5 years later. *JAMA* 2002;**287**:487–494.

16. Wachter RM, Goldman L: The who, what, when, where, whom, and how of hospitalist care. *Ann Intern Med* 2002;**137**:930–931.

Protocol: Checklist for Family Involvement During Hospitalization

[ ] Contact the family as soon as possible, at least within the first 24 hours of hospitalization.
[ ] Establish a method for the family to communicate with the treatment team.
[ ] Make regular contact with family members during hospitalization.
[ ] Encourage the family to support and assist the patient in the following ways:
    ( ) Visit as much as possible.
    ( ) Help with meals and bathing, or other grooming needs.
    ( ) Assist with dressing changes and other medical treatments.
    ( ) Participate in physical, occupational, and speech therapy.
    ( ) Learn about any special dietary needs and bring in home-cooked meals.
    ( ) Accompany the patient to medical tests and procedures.
    ( ) Stay overnight when appropriate.
    ( ) Attend educational courses and instruction on the patient's illness.
    ( ) Obtain books and other written material about the illness.
[ ] Discuss discharge planning with the patient and family, as early as possible and on a regular basis.
[ ] In anticipation of discharge, encourage the family to:
    ( ) Meet early with social worker to determine needs at home.
    ( ) Learn from the patient's nurse about medication to be taken after discharge.
    ( ) Obtain dietary instructions from the nutritionist.
    ( ) Learn about postdischarge treatments and therapies.
[ ] Meet with the family prior to discharge to be certain they have the necessary information and are prepared for home care.
[ ] Schedule a follow-up appointment for the patient and family.

25
Working Together: Collaboration and Referral to Family-Oriented Mental Health Professionals

Successful behavioral health referral is an art form. It requires understanding the patient's motivation to change, ensuring a sense of safety during a vulnerable time, combating the stigma of psychotherapy, fostering hope that the venture can be successful, and promoting confidence in the therapist. The primary care clinician can sanction and bless the psychotherapy in ways that enhance the likelihood, and success, of treatment, but that is just the beginning.

Collaboration between medical and behavioral health professionals is characterized by a common mission and a synergism of professional expertise. Numerous books (1–9), articles and research, and demonstration projects have defined and expanded collaborative care. There are various ways to collaborate with behavioral health clinicians, from referral with limited ongoing contact between professionals, to incorporating a family-oriented therapist in a primary care practice (see Chap. 23). Coordination of care is easier when clinicians have more contact with one another, whatever the practice arrangement (3,5). Seaburn and colleagues (5) have identified a spectrum of collaborative models that reflects the range of communication among clinicians:

Parallel delivery occurs when each clinician is aware of the other, but has clearly defined and nonoverlapping roles and responsibilities. For example, a pediatrician works with the child and her parents to manage her mild intermittent level of asthma, whereas the family psychologist helps the family with school adjustment issues.

Informal consultation is the common "hallway consult" (10) in which either the primary care or mental-health clinician briefly consults with the other colleague about a clinical question or specific case. The consultant does not have contact with the family, and the consultee chooses whether to incorporate the suggestions into any care plan. Informal consultation is facilitated by geographical proximity of the clinicians, or by an established relationship in which brief telephone or e-mail consultations are included.

Formal consultation involves direct contact between the family and the consultant, who makes recommendations to the primary clinician or to the patient and family. This model is common among primary care clinicians who request psychiatric consultation or assessment about an ongoing and complicated family.

Co-provision of care occurs when both behavioral health and primary care clinicians have ongoing relationships with the patient, and when they have similar treatment goals. For example, a woman who repeatedly visits her physician with worries about cancer occurring in various organ systems can benefit from a referral to a medical family therapist, while continuing to see the physician regularly. Case scenarios like these require careful communication among the clinicians to maintain consistency about clinician messages. In a co-provision of care model, conjoint sessions allow both clinicians to meet with the patient and family to insure that a joint plan and message is utilized.

All of these levels include some degree of collaboration, but the fourth level (i.e., co-provision) is the model often described in the literature about collaborative care. In this form, collaborative care is more than *cooperation* among healthcare professionals (11). Colleagues can cooperate and have "parallel arrangements" without consulting with one another. Pediatrician Ellen Perrin (12) noted how collaboration is also more than *help*. A professional can help another colleague, but have little say or power about implementation of a plan. Collaborative partners strive to have relatively equal status and power, but different skills and knowledge.

This model of integrated family healthcare provided by professionals who complement and support one another is increasingly a reality rather than a goal. Research on patient preferences (13,14) demonstrates that patients prefer collaborative models of care when loved ones need assistance; however, satisfaction with care is only a part of effectiveness. In randomized controlled studies, collaborative care has demonstrated better outcomes for such issues as depression, somatization, support for caregivers, and some health behavior changes (15–19). Research has also documented that collaborative care can be integrated cost-effectively into health delivery systems. Large scale studies of Medicaid patients in Hawaii (20) and of BlueCross BlueShield claims data (21) have documented decreases in medical use following collaborative psychotherapeutic interventions. Other emerging research has begun to document cost effectiveness of collaborative care (22,23) for other clinical populations.

The professional journal, *Families, Systems and Health* (www.fsh.org) (24), published since 1983, provides a vehicle for advancing collaborative research and clinical models. An interdisciplinary organization, The Collaborative Family Healthcare Association (www.cfhcc.org) has emerged to promote this vision of healthcare, and to facilitate communication among clinicians, researchers and policy makers. Interest in collaborative care is both a North American interest, and a reflection of the work of clinicians throughout the world (8,25–27). This interest is also not confined to primary care. Enhancing integrated care systems among multiple clinicians, families, and patients is required within settings as diverse as oncology and cardiac units, child and geriatric settings, and transplantation and rehabilitation centers. This chapter will make practical suggestions for building collaborative models in which primary care clinicians can work with mental health professionals to maximize outcome for the patient and the providers.

How to Find a Good Family-Oriented Psychotherapist

Primary care clinicians do not need to be convinced of the value of trusted behavioral health specialists. A number of possible arrangements encourage these relationships. Chapter 23 described how practice arrangements might include on-site therapists, either on a fee-for-service basis, or as a practice employee. It should be noted that some insurance plans make collaboration difficult because they require referral to the behavioral health service plan carve-out. In those situations, the primary care clinician generally has little choice about the referral, although it may sometimes be possible for the physician to make the case for an out-of-network referral. Other insurance plans include panels of participating behavioral health providers. Collaboration will be most possible for these patients, and for those who have choice about their psychotherapist. This makes knowledge of available psychotherapy resources very important.

For individual concerns, most practicing primary care clinicians have identified psychiatric emergency and other mental health resources. It is also important to identify family-oriented resources and psychotherapists. The challenge of finding compatible family-oriented colleagues may be more difficult than identifying other kinds of specialists. Clinicians often base their referral practices on direct experience of working, for example, with a cardiologist or a surgeon in the hospital. Referrals to psychotherapists are more similar to referrals to dermatologists or physical therapists, in which referral is based on reputation. Repeat referrals occur because of positive feedback from the patient and a sense of compatible mission. Providers new to a community have several options to identify competent family-oriented therapists.

1. Ask respected colleagues who they use and why.

Behavioral health clinicians often have unique areas of interest or expertise, so it is useful to ask the colleague about the therapist's range of services and style of practice.

2. Use professional directories and state licensing boards to identify family-oriented mental health professionals in your community.

Psychotherapists hold a bewildering array of professional degrees and theoretical orientations. Psychiatrists, family therapists, psychologists, social workers, nurse practitioners, and licensed mental health counselors are the most common mental health professions. Most of these professions have state licensing or certification processes, with available lists. Therapists who are part of insurance panels or approved listings generally have positive reputations. National organizations often have referral capabilities, especially the American Family Therapy Academy, The American Association for Marriage and Family Therapy, and the Collaborative Family Healthcare Association (see list of web addresses at the end of this chapter).

3. Ask the patients.

Some patients in any primary care practice are or have been in psychotherapy. Ask about therapy experiences, and ask patients who they have seen, whether they are satisfied, and why. If a patient is currently in therapy, discuss whether it could be helpful for you to contact the therapist to facilitate coordinated care.

4. Arrange a face-to-face meeting with the therapist to discuss his or her orientation to evaluation and treatment.

A lunch or a meeting at either professional's office provides first-hand information about how the therapist interacts, as well as his or her theoretical orientation, beliefs about treatment, experience with the medical system, and whether your working styles will be compatible. A phone call may substitute, but a face-to-face meeting is preferred.

Avoiding Potential Problems in Collaboration

Even though much has been written and studied about building successful collaborative relationships with behavioral health professionals, misunderstandings still can block effective patient care (28). These difficulties are rooted in differences in training and differences in professional goals and roles. These differences need to be acknowledged and understood for effective collaboration to result. Table 25.1 identifies some of the common differences in working styles and goals between primary care and behavioral health professionals.

The following example illustrates extreme ways that professional differences can plague collaboration and referral. In a sense, it is a lesson about how to prevent collaboration and bring out defensiveness and professional arrogance in colleagues. In the example, a stereotyped primary care physician calls a stereotyped mental health professional to make a referral.

> Dr. P.: Hello, this is Dr. Psycho.
> Dr. M.: Hi, Sue? This is Dr. Medic at the Family Medicine Center. I have this patient I'd like you to see, but I just have a minute to tell you about her as I'm already 45 minutes behind in my appointments. She's a 16-year-old primigravida at 34 weeks gestation, complicated by some intrauterine growth retardation and mild preeclampsia.

TABLE 25.1. Differences in the cultures of primary care and behavioral health professionals

	Primary care Clinicians	Behavioral Health Clinicians
Language or	Medical	Humanistic, psychoanalytic,
Traditional paradigm	Biomedical	systemic
New paradigm	Biopsychosocial	Cognitive-behavioral, psychodynamic
		Family systems
Professional style	Action-oriented, advice-giving	Process-oriented, avoids advice
	M.D. takes initiative	Patient takes initiative
Treatment orientation	Fix-it	Facilitate
Standard session time	10–15 minutes	45–50 minutes
Demand for services	Around the clock	Scheduled sessions (except emergencies)
Use of medications	Frequent	Infrequent
Use of individual and family history	Basic	Extensive
At risk for	Somatic fixation	Psychosocial fixation

The problem is that this lady just won't come in for her prenatal visits or any of the tests she needs. I've tried everything to get her in. She's really impossible! I keep telling her that the baby is going to die if she doesn't do what I tell her. Can you see her? Maybe you can convince her that she's got to come in for these appointments.

Dr. P. (talks slowly and calmly): Well, Dr. Medic, I can hear you're really upset. What do you think is going on? Could she be depressed?

Dr. M.: I don't know, that's your department. She doesn't look very happy, but who would in her situation? Say, if you want to put her on an antidepressant, let me know so I can be sure it's a safe one for pregnancy.

Dr. P.: Seems like you're jumping to medications rather quickly, Dr. Medic. I feel I need to know something about the patient, you know, her history and her family, before we rush into pharma-cotherapy. What do you know about her family?

Dr. M.: I don't have time for that stuff. It's hard enough dealing with all her medical problems. All I know is that I've seen her boyfriend and I'm sure he's on drugs. I've checked the lady for AIDS and she's okay so far, but she's not cooperating with me.

Dr. P.: Boy, sounds like this case is really getting to you. You're pretty angry at her, you know.

Dr. M. (getting increasingly frustrated): I am not the patient here. Will you see this patient or not? Just convince her to come back for her tests.

Dr. P.: Calm down, Dr. Medic. I'm going to need some time to do a complete evaluation on this patient. I've got an opening in 2 weeks.

Dr. M.: Two weeks—she'll have a dead baby by then! Besides she probably won't show up. I'm calling now to get an appointment for her, which I'll give to her social worker so I can be sure she'll get there.

Dr. P.: That's being too directive. We need to use her ability to secure an appointment and get to my office as a measure of her motivation for change. I can't badger her to come. That's her decision.

Dr. M.: Look, I don't have time for this. Forget about seeing the patient. I'll just call Child Protective. They'll do something about this.

Dr. P.: I'm sorry, Dr. Medic. I'm trying to be helpful to you. I have to tell you I'm concerned you're falling back on strong-arm tactics instead of demonstrating the caring and sensitivity that's supposed to be part of being a health professional.

Dr. M.: Big help. Thanks a lot.

Dr. P.: Good-bye.

This extreme example illustrates the many ways primary care and behavioral health professionals can misunderstand and miscommunicate with each other. Each professional has unique job demands, a preferred style of working, and differing expectations of each other. There is room for the full spectrum of biopsychosocial care. Recognizing ways to appreciate differences, negotiate working styles, and coordinate care helps us move toward a vision of seamless healthcare for patients and families.

What Triggers a Referral to a Therapist

Primary care includes education, support, and some counseling for psychosocial problems. Chapter 1 described the levels of clinician involvement with families, in which Level 3 includes emotional support for families, Level 4 is family assessment and primary care counseling, and Level 5 requires either specialty training or referral to a mental health clinician. Table 25.2 distinguishes problems that might be appropriate for primary care counseling, and those that indicate a referral. In addition to these problems, which may be treated with short-term counseling, other problems (e.g., somatization and substance abuse) often require a period of primary care counseling to mobilize the patient and family for a specialist referral. The decision to refer to a behavioral health specialist is influenced by the kind of problem or patient, and the comfort and training of the clinician.

Patient Factors That Trigger a Referral

Severity of the Problem

By definition, problems in this category require time, specialized training, and an intensity of treatment not practical in a primary care setting. These are complicated, serious, and sometimes frightening psychosocial problems. These situations often result in relatively easy referrals, particularly if there is a crisis. A family of a patient experiencing an acute psychotic break or suicidal episode, a patient who has been recently raped, or a couple

TABLE 25.2. When to treat and when to refer problems seen in primary care

Problems Commonly Seen in Primary Care (Level 4)
adjustment to the diagnosis of a new illness
adjustment to a new developmental stage or change
individual, marital, or family crises of limited severity and duration
mild depressive or anxiety reactions
uncomplicated grief reactions
behavior problems

Problems Commonly Referred to a Mental Health Specialist (Level 5)
suicidal or homicidal ideation, intent, or behavior
psychotic behavior
recent sexual abuse (e.g., incest or rape), or a history of abuse that continues to influence
    the patient's feelings or behavior
recent physical abuse (e.g., child, spouse, or elder), or a history of abuse that continues to
    influence the patient's feelings or behavior
substance abuse (e.g., alcohol or drugs)
somatic fixation
most marital or sexual problems (e.g., especially those involving affairs, separation, or
    divorce, or active consideration of any of these)
multiproblem, complex family situations (e.g., two pathognomonic signs are families in
    which it is difficult to determine a genogram, or the "thick chart")
problems resistant to change in primary care counseling

considering divorce may all be sufficiently anxious and motivated that they will typically agree (or even request) to see a mental health specialist.

With long-standing problems, patients and families are less anxious, more familiar with their difficulties, and more resistant to a referral to a mental health colleague. Problems in this category may include substance abuse, a history of sexual or physical abuse, somatization, and some multiproblem family situations. The families may require more support and reassurance from their primary care clinician, or the situation may have to escalate into crisis before the patient or family will successfully connect with a behavioral health specialist (see Chaps. 19, 21, and 22 for suggestions about referral for somatization, substance abuse, and physical or sexual abuse).

Chronicity of the Problem

If either the provider or the patient has been concerned about a psychosocial problem for greater than 6 months, it is generally useful to consider evaluation or referral. For example, a patient reports that she and her husband had been working with the school for the past year to try to help their son with his behavior problems, but the same problems emerged in September with a new teacher. As another example, a physician may contract for six monthly primary care counseling sessions with a couple experiencing adjustment problems in their first year of marriage. At the end of that time, both the provider and the couple agree that some moderate improvement has occurred, but that problems still exist. A further example might be a woman who drinks two beers every day, but denies a drinking problem. Her family is very concerned, and she agrees to prove to them that she can abstain from any alcohol. At the end of the agreed-upon 6-month period, the patient and family report that she reduced her drinking, but that she was unable to abstain altogether. All of these situations call for referral based on chronicity of the problem.

Patient Request

A patient or family may directly request a referral to a mental health specialist. A primary care clinician who is interested in providing primary care counseling can inform patients of that alternative, but should not make them feel uncomfortable if they prefer a different provider. Some patients and families prefer the privacy of counseling with someone other than their regular primary care provider.

Clinician Factors That Trigger Referral

Constraints on the Clinician's Time or Interest

Most clinicians who incorporate primary care counseling limit their practice to an afternoon per week or to one or two daily appointments. Other physicians prefer to do less counseling, and have a lower threshold for referring their patients and collaborating with mental health specialists.

Limits of a Clinician's Training

Physicians differ in their training experiences in assessing and treating psychosocial problems. Some obtain specialized training in marital and family problems, alcohol counseling, or hypnosis. Others have basic training in the management of psychiatric disorders. The trigger for referral may occur with the sense that, "I'm in over my head," or, "This is out of my league." As in other areas of primary care, the provider's training should determine his or her threshold for referral.

Recognition of a Need for Further Assessment

Even with specialized training, a clinician may recognize that something in the history is missing, or that the information just does not "add up". A referral for further evaluation is always appropriate in these cases.

Stagnation or Failure of Primary Care Counseling

It is always useful to contract for a specific number of sessions for primary care counseling (e.g., somewhere between three and six). This contract serves to increase the patient's or family's motivation, and targets a time to evaluate whether the goals are being reached. Referral should usually occur at the contract's end, if either the health professional or the patient is dissatisfied with the treatment. It may be tempting to negotiate a new contract, but we should be careful that this does not perpetuate the lack of change.

Personal Issues

Personal issues can make it difficult to work effectively with a particular patient, family, or problem. A clinician who is very stressed in his or her own life may have little energy for patients' problems. At those times, it is important to protect ourselves and use our referral network. Problems that "hit close to home" (e.g., alcoholism for a clinician from an alcoholic family, or marital problems for a physician separating from a spouse), may require early referral. Other signs may signal potential countertransference problems (e.g., the feeling that "this patient is driving me crazy" or a sense of dread when a particular name appears on the day's roster of patients). At a minimum, a consultation in these situations might be useful to ensure that the primary care provider is able to separate his or her personal issues from those of the patient. The consultation might then result in either a referral to the consultant or in new ideas about how to handle the case. The positive side of identification is that the clinician may have a high investment in helping the patient and the patient may feel understood (29). The negative tendency is to lose a clear view of the patient's problem because of the clinician's own difficulties (see Chap. 26 for further discussion of clinician's own family issues and how they influence practice).

How to Make a Successful Referral

A successful referral begins with a successful contact between the primary care clinician and the mental health specialist.

> Mental Health Specialist: Hello, this is Dr. Frank.
> Primary Care Physician: Hello, Dr. Frank, this is Dr. Ho at the Primary Care Unit. I have a patient over here that I'm scheduled to see again tomorrow and I'd like some help with her. She is a 35-year-old married woman with three children who has become pregnant again. She is unsure about carrying the pregnancy, and I think it is very risky. Her husband does not want more children and favors an abortion. I have tried to talk to this patient, but she says unless the pregnancy is life-threatening she doesn't think she wants an abortion. I can't tell her she'll die, but another pregnancy does jeopardize this woman's health. I wonder if it would be possible for you to see her and provide another perspective.
> Therapist: That sounds like a very interesting and difficult situation, Dr. Ho. Could you tell me about the medical implications of this woman carrying another child?
> Physician: I wish I knew for sure. In her last pregnancy, she had severe toxemia and bad gestational diabetes. I warned her against getting

pregnant again. She states the timing is bad, in the best of circumstances, and is not morally opposed to abortion, but says she herself would rather not go that route. I suppose we could manage it if she does decide to carry the pregnancy, but it is risky.

Therapist: I would be happy to meet with this woman and her husband to discuss their decision. At least if the two of them could agree one way or the other, we could be assured this woman would have some family support whatever they decided. I would see my role as protecting this woman's right to make a final decision on this, but I would try to help her remain open to her husband's input and to understand the medical implications of both decisions clearly. Please have the patient call me after your appointment tomorrow. Then, if I or either member of the couple has any further medical questions, we will call you, as that's your area; otherwise, I'll try to see the couple before your next scheduled appointment with them, and get back to you immediately. Would you rather I drop you a note, or give you a call?

Physician: It would be great if you could call right after the session so I know where things stand. You can even leave a message on my private line. Then please drop me a short note for the chart.

Therapist: Fine, and if they wish to pursue this beyond one session, I'll let you know. I do understand there is time pressure here if the possibility of abortion is to be a real option, so I'll get right on it. Thank you for your call.

Physician: I'll look forward to hearing from you. Good-bye.

Having clarified the request to the specialist, secured his or her agreement to see the patient, and gotten the specialist's input on making the referral, the next step is to present the referral in a way that makes sense to the patient.

Dr. Ho: Hello, Mrs. Fortune. I'm sorry to see your husband was unable to join us today.

Mrs. Fortune: He had to work. He said to tell you maybe he could come next time.

Dr. Ho: I know from our last conversation that you have a lot of mixed feelings about your current pregnancy. How are you feeling about it now?

Mrs. Fortune: About the same. My husband and I have been round and round about it. We've even had a few arguments. I just don't know what to do. Now his mother is getting involved, telling me I have to get an abortion. I'm really angry that he even told her.

Dr. Ho: Sounds like it's hard to figure out exactly how you feel with so many people around you having strong opinions.

Mrs. Fortune: Yeah, that's right.

Dr. Ho: I wonder if you and your husband have ever considered seeing a counselor?

Mrs. Fortune: No, we've never had a big problem.

> Dr. Ho: You certainly don't have to have a big problem to be helped by seeing a good counselor. You and your husband have a lot of good history. This decision, though, is a real tough one; I think the two of you could make good use of seeing a counselor colleague of mine for a consultation. She has seen other patients in similar circumstances and has sometimes been able to help them sort out what they really want to do. She will not make the decision for you, but she may help you and your husband see the situation a little more clearly so you can support each other whichever way you decide. Without trying to pressure you, there are some time constraints about your decision. I'd really encourage you to talk with Dr. Frank. I think you'll like her.
>
> Mrs. Fortune: Isn't this something we could just talk out on our own?
>
> Dr. Ho: That's certainly a possibility; however, I know you're having a rough time and I think it's a difficult enough situation that it might be useful to accept some special support and expertise.
>
> Mrs. Fortune: Well, maybe you're right. I haven't been sleeping well, I've been so worried.
>
> Dr. Ho: Please give Dr. Frank a call today for an appointment. She'll be expecting to hear from you. And be sure to make it for a time when your husband can go as well. Do you think that will be a problem?
>
> Mrs. Fortune: He may not like the idea initially, but he has been very upset about this whole thing.
>
> Dr. Ho: How about if I give him a call and tell him why I think it might be a good idea? That way if he has questions I could answer them.
>
> Mrs. Fortune: Okay, you could reach him at home late this afternoon.

This example illustrates the importance of the primary care physician, the specialist, and the patient having clear communications around the time of the referral. This clarity helps to avoid such problems as the primary care physician feeling that the specialist did not focus on the referral request, the specialist not communicating with the primary physician after the consultation, or the patient feeling abandoned by the primary care physician.

Guidelines for Making a Successful Referral

Attention to the process of making a referral can greatly impact the primary care clinician's satisfaction with the referral. Clinicians are more likely to get the assistance they want from a referral when they are clear about how and why they want to collaborate. Setting up careful referrals requires attention to communication with the therapist, and with the family.

Enhancing Collaboration with the Therapist

1. Clarify the consultation or referral question in your own mind.

If it is not clear, let the specialist know that you are not sure. A discussion could help clarify the referral question.

2. Refer to someone you know and trust whenever possible.

Suggest a meeting if the person is unknown.

3. Consult with the intended therapist as early as possible to share ideas and strategy, even prior to the time of presenting the referral to the patient.

With the patient's permission, send any records that may facilitate treatment.

4. Make explicit what kind of communication you want from the therapist.

Discussion should cover:

a. Specific preferences for communication. Some providers wish to be called after the first session or two, then receive a report for the chart at the beginning and end of treatment. Discuss whether private phone messages can be used.
b. Frequency of contact. Be specific about how frequently you want to communicate. At a minimum, request reports at the beginning and end of therapy, and calls about any crisis that might influence ongoing medical care.
c. How much information is desired. Be specific if you wish a brief, one-paragraph report, or if you want a lengthier description of the case that might clarify some patient and family dynamics, and impact care.

5. Identify your preferences for collaborative style.

It is reasonable to ask therapists to:

Provide timely feedback.
Provide a succinct and useful evaluation and treatment plan.
Support your relationship with your patients.
Communicate directly about any problems, especially with patient complaints.
Welcome communication with you.
Inform you of the ending and outcome of treatment.

6. Clarify your own availability with regard to the case.

"I am very busy right now in my practice. This is the second time this adolescent has run away. I would like you to see this family and take charge of these issues. I would see myself as providing support and back-up for your treatment, as you work to help this family establish a different way of relating."

7. Negotiate and clarify what you and the patient will address, what the therapist will cover, and how you will work together.

Patients often bring the same issue to their primary physician that they bring to their therapist, in part to see if they both say the same thing. The potential for clinician splitting and miscommunication is lessened if collaborators identify which issues will be addressed in therapy (e.g., a recent affair), which issues will be dealt with in primary care (e.g., the medical aspects of the wife's sexual dysfunction), and what topics will be handled by both (e.g., both professionals will support the couple's strong parenting skills in the face of their current marital stress). Being explicit about the treatment plan allows the medical provider to redirect, for example, the wife who is looking for support after her husband's affair (e.g., "That sounds painful. I think you need to discuss these issues further in your therapy"). It also allows the therapist to appropriately return medical issues to the physician (e.g., "You have many concerns about your poor lubrication and your lack of interest in sex. You need to make an appointment with your physician and describe these concerns. Then we can continue to work on other factors that may be inhibiting your desire for your husband").

Enhancing Collaboration with Patients and Families

Describe the Referral in Ways that Maximize the Patient's Motivation

1. Use the patient's language and beliefs about the problem to describe the referral.

For example, "You are very worried about whether to carry this pregnancy. I am also concerned about you. I think you and your husband deserve to discuss this with someone who has special expertise in this area."

2. Refer for "evaluation," "consultation," or "counseling."

Avoid referring for "family therapy," unless the patient or family specifically requests it. Some patients think therapy is only for people who have severe troubles, or feel blamed for their problem.

3. Refer to the specialist as a "counselor" or an "expert" who "helps patients with problems such as yours."

It is often most helpful to use a generic description of the mental health specialist, rather than such specific labels as "family therapist," or even "psychiatrist" or "psychologist." Specific labels can be confusing. It is most significant for patients to feel that you have confidence in the specialist.

4. Elicit family support for the referral.

If necessary, conduct a brief family meeting to discuss the problem. If the family is resistant or refuses to attend the family conference, inform the psychotherapist and let that person manage who will or will not be a part of the treatment.

5. Have the patient call the therapist for an appointment before he or she leaves your office.

6. Avoid a battle if a patient strongly resists a referral.

This can often result in patient's becoming entrenched in their refusal. Some difficult referrals take 1–2 years to accomplish. State that you believe this could be helpful, but that it is the patient's decision. Ask the patient to consider a future referral if they do not improve over a specific time period. A referral may be more likely if a crisis occurs.

7. Support treatment with the behavioral health specialist.

If a patient complains about the specialist, encourage them to talk directly with the therapist. If the complaints continue, ask whether it might be helpful if you communicated with the therapist (see Chaps. 3 and 26 for discussion of ways to avoid triangulation).

Communicate Regularly with the Therapist

1. Let the patient know you and the therapist are a team and that you communicate regularly.

Ask patients to complete release of information forms to facilitate communication between you and the therapist. Reassure the patient that if he or she wishes to keep some information confidential, the wish will be respected.

2. Follow up with the Patient after Making the Referral.

Set up an appointment with the patient soon after the counseling begins to support treatment and reassure the patient of your interest. An appointment with the patient soon after counseling ends can similarly show interest and help perpetuate the changes that have occurred.

Collaborative arrangements between medical and behavioral health professionals result in high-quality, cost-effective patient care, as well as support for the clinicians. Consultation from or referral to a behavioral health specialist is a powerful primary care intervention. Even if the referral is refused, the discussion demonstrates the clinician's interest, and it may encourage the patient and family to view their problem differently, or motivate them to make changes. When the referral is successful, the patient and family are the beneficiaries of coordinated care that addresses the full range of their health and illness.

Useful Web Sites: Collaboration Between Therapists and Primary Care Clinicians

Collaborative Family Healthcare Association, www.cfhcc.org
Interdisciplinary organization of physicians, therapists, nurses, and health policy analysts committed to models of collaborative care. Includes membership lists as well as training and educational resources.

American Family Therapy Academy, www.afta.org
Organization of senior family-oriented behavioral health clinicians from multiple disciplines. Includes membership list, conference opportunities, and resources.

American Association for Marriage and Family Therapy, www.aamft.org
The national association for marriage and family therapists. Includes a therapist referral process, educational resources, and state and national conferences.

Cummings Foundation, www.thecummingsfoundation.com
A private foundation dedicated to excellence in behavioral healthcare, particularly systems of care in which behavioral care is integrated into primary healthcare.

Integrated Primary Care, www.integratedprimarycare.com
An independent web site that identifies resources about models of healthcare that integrate medical and psychosocial providers.

The Counselling in Primary Care Trust, www.cpct.co.uk
A private foundation that works to establish behavioral health counseling services in general practice settings throughout the United Kingdom.

References

1. Doherty WJ & Baird MA: *Family Therapy and Family Medicine*. New York: Guilford Press, 1983.
2. Wynne L, McDaniel SH, & Weber T: *Systems Consultation: A New Perspective for Family Therapy*. New York: Guilford Press, 1986.
3. Glenn M: *Collaborative Health Care: A Family-Oriented Model*. New York: Praeger, 1987.
4. McDaniel SH, Doherty WJ, & Hepworth J: *Medical Family Therapy: A Biopsychosocial Approach to Families with Health Problems*. New York: Basic Books, 1992.
5. Seaburn DB, Lorenz AD, Gunn WB, Gawinski BA, & Mauksch LB: *Models of Collaboration: A Guide for Mental Health Professionals Working with Health Care Practitioners*. New York: Basic Books, 1996.

6. Blount A (Ed): *Integrated Primary Care: The Future of Medical and Mental Health Collaboration*. New York: WW Norton, 1998.

7. Cummings NA, Cummings JL, & Johnson JJ (Eds): *Behavioral Health in Primary Care: A Guide for Clinical Integration*. New York: Psychosocial Press, 1998.

8. Bor R, Miller R, Latz M, & Salt H: *Counselling in Health Care Settings*. London: Cassell, 1998.

9. Patterson J, Peek CJ, Heinrich RL, Bischoff RJ, & Scherger J: *Mental Health Professionals in Medical Settings: A Primer*. New York: WW Norton, 2002.

10. Hepworth J, Jackson M: Health care for families: models of collaboration between family therapists and family physicians. *Fam Relations* 1985;**34**: 123–127.

11. McDaniel S & Hepworth J: Family psychology in primary care: managing issues of power and dependency through collaboration. In: Frank R, McDaniel SH, Bray J, & Heldring M (Eds): *Primary Care Psychology*. Washington DC: American Psychological Association Publications, 2002.

12. Perrin E: The promise of collaborative care. *Devel Behav Pediatr* 1999;**20**:57–62.

13. Katon W: Collaborative care: patient satisfaction, outcomes and medical cost-offset. *Fam Syst Med* 1995;**13**:351–365.

14. Mauksch LB, Tucker SM, Katon WJ, Russo J, Cameron J, Walker E, et al.: Mental illness, functional impairment, and patient preferences for collaborative care in an uninsured, primary care population. *J Fam Prac* 2001;**50**:41–47.

15. Katon W, Von Korff M, Lin E, Walker E, Simon GE, Bush T, et al.: Collaborative management to achieve treatment guidelines: Impact on depression in primary care. *JAMA* 1995;**273**:1026–1031.

16. Mittelman MS, Ferris SH, Shulman E, Steinberg G, & Levin B: A family intervention to delay nursing home placement of patients with Alzheimer disease: a randomized controlled trial. *JAMA* 1996;**76**:1725–1731.

17. Morisky DE, Levine DM, Green LW, Shapiro S, Russell RP, & Smith CR: Five-year blood pressure control and mortality following health education for hypertensive patients. *Am J Publ Health* 1983;**73**:153–162.

18. Smith GR, Rost K, & Kashner TM: A trial of the effect of a standardized psychiatric consultation on health outcomes and costs in somatizing patients. *Arch Gen Psychiatr* 1995;**52**:238–243.

19. British Family Heart Study: A randomised controlled trial evaluating cardio-vascular screening and intervention in general practice: principal results of British Family Health Study. *Br Med J* 1994;**308**:313–320.

20. Pallack MS, Cummings NA, Dorken H, & Henke CJ: Medical costs, Medicaid, and managed mental health treatment; The Hawaii study. *Man Care Q* 1994;**2**: 64–70.

21. Mumford E, Schlesinger HJ, Glass GV, et al.: A new look at evidence about the reduced cost of medical utilization following mental health treatment. *Am J Psychiatr* 1984;**141**:1145–1158.

22. Von Korff J, Katon W, Bush T, et al.: Treatment costs, cost-offset, and cost-effectiveness of collaborative management of depression. *Psychosomatic Med* 1998;**60**:143–149.

23. Olfson M, Sing M, & Schlesinger HJ: Mental health/medical care cost offsets: opportunities for managed care. *Health Affairs* 1999;**18**:79–90.

24. Bloch D: Family systems medicine: the field and the journal. *Fam Syst Med* 1983; **1**:3–11.
25. Navon S: The non-illness intervention model: psychotherapy for physically ill patients and their families. *Am J Fam Ther* 1999;**27**(3):251–270.
26. Petersen I: Comprehensive integrated primary mental health care for South Africa. Pipedream or possibility? *Soc Sci Med* 2000;**51**(3):321–334.
27. Jenkins CJ: Promoting and measuring behavioral health service in family medical practices in the United Kingdom. *Fam Syst Health* 2002;**20**:399–413.
28. McDaniel SH & Campbell T: Physicians and family therapists: the risks of collaboration. *Fam Syst Med* 1985;**4**(1):4–8.
29. McDaniel SH, Doherty WJ, & Hepworth J: *The Shared Experience of Illness: Stories of Patients, Families, and Their Therapists*. New York: Basic Books, 1997.

Protocol: the Dos and Don'ts of Referral to Behavioral Health Specialists

With a Behavioral Health Specialist, Do

- Clarify the consultation or referral question.
- Whenever possible, refer to someone you know and trust.
- Consult with the intended therapist as early as possible.
- Make explicit the kind of communication you want from the therapist.
- Indicate your preferences for collaborative style.
- Negotiate and clarify what you and the patient will address, what the therapist will cover, and how you will work together.

With Patients and Families, Do

- Describe the referral in ways that maximize the patient's motivation.
- Use the patient's language.
- Refer for "evaluation," "consultation," or "counseling."
- Refer to the specialist as a "counselor" or an "expert on helping people with problems such as yours."
- Elicit family support for the referral.
- Have the patient call the therapist for an appointment before he or she leaves your office.
- Support treatment with the behavioral health specialist.
- Communicate regularly with the therapist.
- Let the patient know you and the therapist are a team.
- Follow up with the patient after making the referral.

With Referrals to Behavioral Health Specialists, Don't

- Assume the behavioral health specialist has a similar working style as a primary care physician: Work to get to know the differences between yourself and a therapist you respect.
- Wait until the last minute to refer a difficult patient or family.
- Use medical or psychiatric diagnoses with patients when making a referral.
- Refer to a "family therapist" for "family therapy." Many patients hear these labels as conferring blame or inadequacy.
- Battle with patients when they resist a referral.
- Allow patients to pit you against a therapist.
- Continue to refer to a therapist who does not provide adequate feedback or effective treatment.

26
Managing Personal and Professional Boundaries: How the Clinician's Experience Can Be a Resource in Patient Care

Family-oriented primary care begins at home. Empathy and sensitivity are resources that are largely developed in the clinician's own personal and family life. A clinician's appreciation of the richness of emotional life, the complexity of human problems, and the humility inherent in human suffering forms the foundation for empathy and for a successful clinician–patient relationship. A practitioner may be drawn initially to primary care because his or her upbringing has resulted in a highly developed sense of responsibility and altruism. Many primary care clinicians played a caretaking role that was highly valued in their original families and led to a commitment to serve others with a sensitivity to illness and loss.

This early family training can be useful to the clinician interested in the art of medicine. Caretaking roles can contribute to the growth of individuals as excellent, caring health professionals. These same dynamics make it very important for clinicians to establish clear boundaries between work and family life in order to offset a tendency to get overinvolved with patients, patients' families, and work issues in general. This can be particularly challenging in rural settings, where the clinician interacts with patients in a variety of settings and multiple relationships are inevitable. Anxiety can result in a desire to control people or situations, which leads to overinvolvement (1). In social settings, communicating clearly that medical concerns are discussed in the office or in a professional phone call can be useful. A clear sense of boundaries between the personal and the professional can prevent this problem and support the healthy dynamics that led an individual to choose a career in primary care medicine.

This chapter will discuss several aspects of managing personal and professional boundaries, including mindfulness in practice, recognizing when one's family of origin or current family issues are influencing a patient encounter in a positive way, and when to refer a patient to a colleague because of the potential negative effects of the clinician's personal issues. We will also discuss the importance of role clarity when one's own family member is ill, and provide some warning signals for problems in this area.

Mindfulness in Practice

The first step to understanding boundary issues in practice is being a reflective practitioner (2), aware of oneself and one's own personal and interpersonal issues. *Mindfulness* refers to a nonanxious, reflective approach that includes attentive observation, critical curiosity, "beginner's mind," and presence (3–5). Methods to promote mindful practice include a commitment to observe one's own process, ask open, reflective questions that invite curiosity, think out loud during an interview, and invite feedback. A mindful approach to a patient or family interview is anchored by the clinician's awareness of his or her own past and current personal and family issues (see Fig. 26.1).

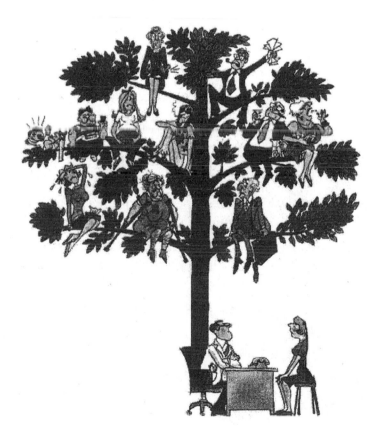

FIGURE 26.1. The clinician's family tree. (*Source*: Crouch M, Roberts L., 1987. *The Family in Medical Practice.* New York: Springer Verlag.)

Clinicians' Family of Origin Issues

A clinician's past and current personal issues can be either a major resource or a profound hindrance in the clinician–patient relationship (6). Styles of caretaking and authority as well as tolerance for affect are all learned in our families of origin. Many clinicians are able to use their past experiences to enhance their empathy and their credibility with patients; however, current problems or unresolved struggles from the past can cloud or distort our perceptions of patients and their families. Using personal issues as a resource depends on being able to recognize these issues when they occur in our work. When the clinician recognizes that a patient or family is stimulating an important personal issue, the clinician then has the opportunity to decide whether to treat, collaborate with a colleague, or refer.

> Dr. Brown came from a family of Irish-American high achievers and heavy drinkers (see Fig. 26.2). When her parents divorced during her adolescence, she began attending Alateen while her mother attended Al-Anon. After his second marriage, her father finally entered alcohol treatment and began attending AA regularly. Alcoholism had caused Dr. Brown much pain in the past and became an area of interest to her as a clinician. She read articles and sought supervision during residency for patient problems that involved alcoholism. Drawing on her experience with her own family, supervision helped her recognize that alcoholic patients and their families were the only people who could decide to change the problem. Dr. Brown saw her role as assessing the problem, and providing advice and support. By using her personal experience and professional training to great advantage, she became known for her skill in evaluating alcoholic families and frequently getting them into treatment. She felt great pride and satisfaction in helping these patients and became a referral source for colleagues who recognized that they did not have the same skills.
>
> By contrast, Dr. Lane always had difficulty with her alcoholic patients. Her father, from a large Italian-American family, was also a drinker (see Fig. 26.3). She suspected that his drinking contributed to the loud

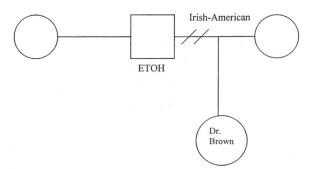

FIGURE 26.2. A physician who uses her past as a resource to help patients.

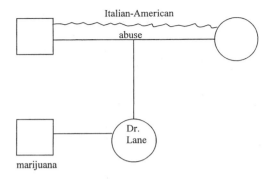

Figure 26.3. A physician with unresolved personal issues.

arguments and occasional physical fighting that still characterized her parents' marriage. Her father denied he was a "problem drinker" because he said he drank half as much as did his own father, who "did have a problem." Dr. Lane drank very little herself, as did her husband, but her husband smoked marijuana on a daily basis because, "It helps me relax." Dr. Lane found herself very interested in getting her alcoholic patients into treatment, but felt she was never successful. She told her colleagues: "Alcoholics never change. There's no point in wasting your breath trying to convince them."

In the first example, Dr. Brown was able to recognize and understand alcoholism clearly. She knew what she could contribute as a clinician and what the patient and family would have to go through themselves. She also had respect for the difficulty of the process. All these factors helped to make her comfortable working with alcoholic patients, whether they were actively drinking or working to stay sober. Dr. Lane, on the other hand, was not clear how substance abuse had affected her own life. This same confusion occurred when trying to evaluate patients about whether they had a problem with drinking. As her personal experience remained unchanged, she eventually became pessimistic about the potential for change for her patients. For personal issues to be a resource, it is critical that the clinician be able to recognize when an issue can be used to enhance professional skills (as with Dr. Brown) and when it is unresolved (as with Dr. Lane). We all have issues in the latter category, and when patient problems overlap with them it is important to either refer, collaborate, or seek consultation. We do not do ourselves, or our patients, a service by treating these problems in isolation when our own unresolved personal experiences are a factor in their care.

A clinician may be able to understand a particular problem in depth because of personal experience; on the other hand, the clinician may not perceive a patient accurately because that patient reminds him or her of the clinician's own family member. Recognizing countertransference in primary care, when a patient or family triggers a personal issue, is not always easy and requires sensitivity and experience. Each professional will have a set of idiosyncratic signals, often such strong affect as anger or sadness, that alert him or her to a personally relevant dynamic occurring during an interview. The following are *signals* that a patient or family may be activating a personal issue for the clinician:

1. Overinvolvement with a particular patient or family.
   - Routinely having longer than usual visits with the patient.
   - Allowing this patient or family easier access than is typical for you (e.g., allowing them to call you at home or interrupt you with another patient).
   - Your own family members complaining about this patient's behavior because it is invading family life.
2. Underinvolvement with a particular patient or family.
   - Expanding the time between patient visits because you would rather not see a patient.
   - Not returning a patient or family member's phone call.
   - Routinely asking your secretary or nurse practitioner to "take care of the problem."
   - Feeling reluctant to see a patient when you see his or her name on the schedule.
3. Undue pessimism that people can change a particular problem behavior.
4. Insistence that a patient must change a particular problem behavior.
5. Prescribing the same treatment, or "educating" a patient over and over again, despite the fact that it is not working.
6. Confusion about why your treatment is not working with this particular patient when it typically works with others.
7. Boredom, anger, or sadness with a patient or family that is out of proportion to the patient's problem.

In the next examples, Dr. Holmes is able to recognize and utilize the signals that he is overreacting to the family, whereas the second clinician, Ms. Smith, does not attend to these signals and loses her patient.

> Dr. Holmes, a middle-aged English-American physician, felt particularly badly about having to tell a long-time patient that he had terminal cancer. Just after finishing with this patient and his family, he noticed that Mrs. Gerber, an older French-American woman, was next on his schedule. His eye twitched, and he wondered if he was getting a headache. Mrs. Gerber was a demanding patient who made Dr. Holmes feel as if he never gave her enough. "I wonder what her complaint will be today," he thought. Sure enough, Mrs. Gerber looked irritated when he walked in the room. "What took you so long?" she asked. Dr. Holmes found himself wanting to say, "I had someone with

a *real* illness to deal with". Instead, he said, "I'm sorry. We get backed up here from time to time. What can I do for you today?"

After the session, while reflecting on his day, Dr. Holmes wondered why Mrs. Gerber got to him so much. While discussing it with his partner, he realized Mrs. Gerber made him feel the way he used to with his mother: No matter what he did, he felt that he could not please her, and perhaps for the same reason—as an adult Dr. Holmes had come to realize that his mother had a long-standing underlying depression. He began to wonder about Mrs. Gerber's psychosocial situation, how much support she had, and whether she might be clinically depressed. He decided to do a more in-depth evaluation of her mental status and her affect, and to try to involve her family and friends in the evaluation to test her support network. After the conversation with his colleague, Dr. Holmes realized he was actually looking forward to the next session with Mrs. Gerber because he was curious to find out what was driving her unhappiness.

Ms. Smith, an African-American woman, had the reputation of being a caring, effective clinician. She was responsible and responsive, although she did not have many friends. Ms. Smith did a lot of counseling in her practice. Even though she did not enjoy it much, she felt it was part of her job as a nurse practitioner, and she also was convinced that few patients would accept a referral to a mental health specialist. Today, she had to see Mrs. Griot, a Canadian patient in the ICU who had come very close to overdosing on the antidepressant Ms. Smith had prescribed for her. The overdose surprised Ms. Smith. She had been doing individual counseling with this young housewife for 4 months and described the patient in her chart as "bright and sensible." At the hospital, Mrs. Griot told her that she had another argument with her husband, became frustrated, and "wanted a way out." Ms. Smith decided this woman was more impulsive than she had realized, and bluntly told her in the hospital that she needed to see a psychiatrist. The patient was offended by Ms. Smith's abruptness. She decided Ms. Smith did not truly understand how miserable she felt, and she switched to another primary care clinician.

Without realizing it, Ms. Smith was repeating a pattern established in her own family of origin (see Fig. 26.4). When she was 10, her own mother had committed suicide after several counseling sessions with her internist. The family had handled this death by trying to "move on." Ms. Smith's father remarried quickly and her mother was rarely discussed in family gatherings. Ms. Smith worked hard to take care of her brother and sister. She felt she had adapted to this tragedy as well as possible, but in fact she had little support and had spoken to virtually no one about the loneliness and confusion that plagued her memories of her mother. Ms. Smith instead poured herself into her work and was vulnerable to taking on too much counseling, too much responsibility with patients, and not recognizing patients at high risk for major depression or suicide.

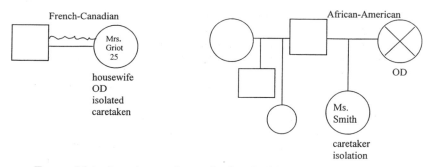

FIGURE 26.4. A patient and a professional with mirroring personal issues.

Most professionals find that utilizing personal issues as a resource requires trusted colleagues with whom to discuss challenging cases. Balint groups (7), and their latter-day offshoots that add a family perspective (8, 9), allow clinicians to explore their own personal issues vis-à-vis clinical cases. Some of these groups use both the patient's and the clinician's genogram as tools to discover any similarities that may be meaningful in the doctor–patient relationship. Several family-oriented primary care clinicians have recommended that clinicians use a transgenerational approach (10) to work on their own family of origin issues as a method of becoming more effective professionally (11–13).

The Clinician's Current Family Issues

Issues in the clinician's current family life can also be either a resource or a problem for patient care.

> Dr. Orion's lively, Ukranian parents visited her for the first time in her new home soon after the arrival of her first child. Because Dr. Orion practiced obstetrics, she was prepared for the joy, the physical pain, and the fatigue that accompanied having a child. She was not prepared, however, for what happened when her parents visited. Her parents were clearly delighted at the arrival of their first grandchild; however, her mother could not stop telling her what to do with the baby. No matter what Dr. Orion did with her baby, her mother had a better way to do it.
>
> After breathing a sigh of relief at her parents' departure, Dr. Orion returned to patient care and found herself interested in how new parents negotiated the change in their relationship with their own parents. She collaborated with a family therapist on a study of the relationship between new parents, grandparents, and infant morbidity. She also developed clinical guidelines for patients to obtain support and guidance from their own parents, either before or soon after the delivery of their first child. Dr. Orion tested the guidelines by applying them to

her relationship with her own parents and recognizing them in their new role as grandparents.

Where Dr. Orion was able to use her own experience to be helpful to her patients, Dr. Waters found himself discontent and overwhelmed with patients whose problems resembled his own.

> Dr. Waters, a young English-American man, felt drained and tired at the end of each workday. He realized that ever since he and his partner had been discussing separation, his tolerance for hearing about patients' relationship problems was very low. One female patient with whom he had previously enjoyed working now seemed demanding and needy. An immigrant from Taiwan, she complained that her husband did not listen to her and cared more about work than he did about her, complaints amazingly close to those of Dr. Waters' own partner, Jeff. Dr. Waters continued to see this patient, although he spaced her appointments out as much as she would tolerate.

All personal experiences have the potential to enrich our professional lives; however, private stresses and struggles that are occuring in the moment, thus by definition are unresolved, run the biggest risk of leading to difficulties in the doctor–patient relationship. A trusted colleague or a Balint-type group can be very helpful in sorting out these issues. It is important to us and to our patients that we give ourselves permission to collaborate or to refer when patients' problems hit "too close to home."

Studies have shown clinicians to have particular difficulty with depression and substance abuse (14–16). In addition, they are susceptible to having problems in their own marriages related to workaholism, or what Gerber calls being "married to their careers" (17). Several strategies are important to *help the clinician deal with current family problems*:

- Develop a willingness to seek help oneself when it is needed.
- Develop a lifestyle that provides a balance between work and personal life.
- Establish appropriate boundaries between work and home life so that some time is protected for personal and family needs to be met without the intrusion of patients.
- Develop clarity about when one is in a professional role, with the challenges and rewards of being a professional, and when one is in a family role, with the challenges and rewards of being a family member.

Role Clarity: To Be or Not to Be Your Own Family's Clinician

A natural facet of being a family member is caring about the health and well-being of loved ones. This function is somewhat complicated when one or more family members is a health professional. When and how much to use one's professional expertise with family members can be a challenging issue. Many families consciously or unconsciously train their children to be caretakers of some kind. It is quite natural then, when one becomes a healthcare professional, to feel some conflict about how much to advocate, translate, and take care of one's own family's medical concerns. If the clinician refuses to use his or her special expertise with family members, the patient/family member may feel uncared for or abandoned and the clinician may feel badly about not being "helpful" in an area where he or she does have some special skill.

Being clear about whether one is functioning as a professional or as a family member is essential to resolving this dilemma. These roles can merge and be very difficult to separate when a loved one is seriously ill and involved in the complex healthcare system (18). With serious illness, it is generally difficult to develop the neutrality and distance necessary to make clear diagnoses and to implement potentially difficult treatment plans if one is a family member of the patient. It is also difficult to allow oneself to advocate for and to care deeply about a family member if one is responsible for his or her medical care.

One solution is to develop a relationship with a respected primary care clinician who is outside the family. Turning to this person frees the clinician to enjoy the family member role, yet have confidence that the patient is receiving quality medical care. Some clinicians refer all health problems for family members because of the recognition that one's judgment may be skewed and any complication would be a nightmare; however, many other clinicians offer family members advice about minor health problems (e.g., otitis media, conjunctivitis, or urinary tract infections). These clinicians draw the line with any problem that could potentially carry a serious diagnosis, or when treatment could have a bad outcome. Clear boundaries are useful whenever a family member is ill; consulting with a colleague and having clear guidelines can allow one to be a strong advocate for a loved one's care without taking over as the responsible clinician.

Without a clear distinction between the roles of healthcare professional and family member, it is easy for the clinician to become either overinvolved or underinvolved in the family member's medical care. Some clinicians may characteristically overfunction in their professional role; therefore, they tend to become overinvolved in the medical care of family members. In this situation, it is easy to avoid important emotional issues by intellectualizing or medicalizing about a loved one's condition. Others may underfunction and not provide concern or support unless a family member has a "truly serious" illness. Either problem is dangerous because it results in the underfunctioning of a clinician as a family member. Every clinician needs to examine his or her style, philosophy, and practice setting, and consciously set boundaries with regard to dealing with family medical issues. The specifics of these boundaries will vary from individual to individual. Some practice settings with few clinicians (e.g., those in rural settings) make setting boundaries more challenging, but they are all the more important. The following are general *warning signs of overinvolvement* with your own family's medical concerns, signs of slipping into the difficult role of being your own family's clinician:

1. When you counsel or advise family members about some serious health issue without referring them to their clinician.
   - When you repeatedly give advice about a family member's significant health concern and learn that the relative does not go to his or her clinician about the problem.
   - When you repeatedly try to get a family member to adopt a more healthy lifestyle and change such behaviors as diet, smoking, and exercise.
2. When you, and only you, take care of family health matters.
   - When you are the only person who speaks to your ill family member's specialist.
   - When you are the person who coordinates the care of the family member among the specialists (rather than the primary care clinician).
3. When you, rather than an independent clinician, evaluate a family member's serious illness.
   - When you do a physical exam of a family member.
   - When you order tests for a family member.
   - When you write a referral letter to have a family member evaluated further.
4. When you treat a family member for an illness for which most people see a clinician.
   - When you write a prescription for medication for a family member.
   - When you assist in the surgery of a family member (deliver a baby, run a code, etc.). (19)

The following is an example of a clinician who became overinvolved in her grandmother's medical care.

> Dr. Rudder, an African-American woman, was raised by her grandmother after her mother died at a very early age. Her grandmother was very proud of "her granddaughter, the doctor." Soon after Dr. Rudder set up a practice as a primary care clinician in a distant urban setting, her grandmother had a stroke in her rural hometown.
>
> Dr. Rudder rushed to the hometown hospital to see her grandmother and found her in the care of an older clinician who she was unsure was medically "up to date." Dr. Rudder was quite upset about her grandmother's illness and the thought that she might die, but she had difficulty focusing on these feelings. Instead, she found herself making demands of the floor nurses as if she were the attending, and strongly suggesting alternative treatment plans to her grandmother's clinician.

> Dr. Rudder knew there was much she wanted to say to her grandmother: how she appreciated all her sacrifice in raising her; how she admired her stubborn strong will; how she loved her. She found herself instead obsessed with her grandmother's medical care. Frustrated that perhaps it was not the best, Dr. Rudder suggested to her grandmother that she change physicians to one of her colleagues in residency who had opened a practice not too far away. To Dr. Rudder's disappointment and irritation, her grandmother made it clear that she had a long-term relationship with her physician, that she had complete confidence in him, and that she had no desire to change physicians at this point in time.
>
> During the hospitalization, Dr. Rudder functioned as the primary family link to her grandmother's physician. Other family members pumped her for information and relied on her to relay any questions to her grandmother's doctor. Dr. Rudder felt trapped, unsatisfied with her role, worried about her grandmother, and exhausted. Her grandmother died 1 week after being hospitalized.

Dr. Rudder unfortunately confused her role as clinician with her role as family member. Her medical knowledge interfered with her being able to deal successfully with the important emotional issues that confronted her with the illness and impending death of her grandmother. Her lack of confidence in her grandmother's doctor made it that much more difficult for her to leave her medical care in his hands. As a result, she was unable to maintain a clear boundary around her most important role in this situation—that of granddaughter.

Although some clinicians tend to become overinvolved in family member's health issues, others respond to the same stress by becoming underinvolved. The following are *warning signs of underinvolvement* with your own family's medical concerns (i.e., signals that the rest of the family may read as a lack of caring):

1. When you do not want to hear anything about a family member's symptoms.
2. When you never comment on or discuss the medical issues of a family member.
3. When you do not provide support or sympathy for the everyday symptoms, or aches and pains, of family members.
4. When you avoid contact or conversation with the ill family member.

The following is an example of a clinician who was underinvolved in his children's lives.

> Dr. Santiago had a style his patients likened to Marcus Welby. He was always available to them, morning, noon, and night. They worshiped him, and even stopped his children on the street to tell them what a wonderful man he was. His family was organized around supporting

Dr. Santiago's dedication to his job. His wife ran the household and raised the children. His children were used to the fact that he rarely came to their baseball games or school plays. They also knew that unless they had some dire illness or injury, their father was unlikely to show much concern. "He sees so much serious illness, he knows this is not a problem," their mother would tell them. His children unfortunately grew up not realizing either their father's loneliness or the depth of feeling he had for them.

Under- or overinvolvement in family member's medical concerns can lead to personal pain and interpersonal difficulty. Conscious decisions about boundaries between work and family life make a balanced lifestyle more likely.

Conclusion

The dictum, "Physician, heal thyself," may be one of the most powerful therapeutic agents for any clinician's patients. Clinicians' unresolved past or current personal problems play a role in their attitude and impression of patients, either wittingly or unwittingly. In an essay that called for clinicians to examine their personal and societal stands regarding the family, Stephens said: "Let us boldly become more "pro family," perhaps attending first to ourselves in our own family roles" (20) The secret to successful caretaking may be the recognition that we cannot change another's behavior; rather, we can only change our own. Even though we are responsible for professional medical care (e.g., the diagnosis and treatment), the patient remains in charge of his or her own health (e.g., reporting symptoms, collaborating in the history and exam, and final decision making regarding treatment). Patient care can benefit from clinicians establishing these boundaries and focusing on changing our own behavior when needed.

References

1. Guggenbuhl-Craig A: *Power in the Helping Professions.* Irving, TX: Spring Publications, 1979.
2. Schon DA: *The Reflective Practitioner: How Professionals Think in Action* New York: Basic Books, 1983.
3. Epstein RM: Mindful practice. *JAMA* 1999;**282**:833–839.
4. Epstein RM: Mindful practice in action. (1): technical competence, evidence-based medicine and relationship-centered care, *Fam Syst Health* (In Press), 2002a.
5. Epstein RM: Mindful practice in action. (2): cultivated habits of mind, *Fam Syst Health* (In Press), 2002b.

6. McDaniel SH, Hepworth J, & Doherty WJ: *The Shared Experience of Illness: Stories of Patients, Families, and their Therapists*. New York: Basic Books, 1997.

7. Balint M: *The Doctor, His Patient, and the Illness*. New York: International Press, 1957.

8. McDaniel S, Bank J, Campbell T, Mancini J, & Shore, B: Using a group as a consultant in Wynne L, McDaniel S, & Weber T (Eds). *Systems Consultation: A New Perspective for Family Therapy*. New York: Guilford Publications, 1986.

9. Botelho R, McDaniel S, & Jones JE: A family systems approach to a Balint-style group: an innovative CME demonstration project for primary care physicians. 1988 (Submitted for publication).

10. Bowen M: Toward the differentiation of self in one's family of origin. In *Family Therapy in Clinical Practice*. New York: Jason Aronson, 1978.

11. Christie-Seely J, Fernandez R, Pardis G, Talbot Y, & Turcotte R: The physician's family, in Christie-Seely J (Ed). *Working with the Family in Primary Care*. New York: Praeger, 1983.

12. Crouch M: Working with one's own family issues: a path for professional development, in Crouch M, Roberts L (Eds). *The Family in Medical Practice*. New York: Springer-Verlag, 1986.

13. Mengel M: Physician ineffectiveness due to family-of-origin issues. *Fam Syst Med* 1987;**5**(2):176–190.

14. Juntunen J, Asp S, Olkinuora N, Aarimaa N, Strid L, & Kauttu K: Doctors' drinking habits and consumption of alcohol. *Br Med J* 1988;**297**:951–954.

15. McCue JD: The effects of stress on physicians and their medical practice. *N Engl J Med* 1982;**306**:458–463.

16. Vaillant GF, Sobowale AB, & McArthur C: Some psychological vulnerabilities of physicians. *New Engl J Med* 1972;**272**:372–375.

17. Gerber L: *Married to Their Careers*. New York: Tavistock Publications, 1983.

18. Klein BS: *Slow Dance: A Story of Stroke, Love, and Disability*. Toronto: Random House, 1997.

19. LaPuma J, Priest ER: Is there a doctor in the house? An analysis of the practice of physicians treating their own families, *JAMA* 1992;**267**:1810–1812.

20. Stephens G: On being "pro family" in family practice. *J Am Board Fam Prac* 1988;**1**(1):66–68.

Protocol: How to Manage Personal and Professional Boundaries as a Healthcare Professional

Patient Care

Signals that a patient or family may be activating a personal issue for the physician:

1. Overinvolvement with a patient or family.
2. Underinvolvement with a patient or family.
3. Undue pessimism that people can change a particular problem behavior.
4. Insistence that a patient must change a particular problem behavior.
5. Prescribing the same treatment or "educating" a patient over and over again despite the fact that it is not working.
6. Confusion about why your treatment is not working with this particular patient when it typically works with others.
7. Boredom, anger, or sadness with a patient or family out of proportion to the patient's problem.

Family Life

Warning signs of *overinvolvement* with your own family's medical concerns:

1. When you counsel or advise family members about some serious health issue without referring them to their clinician.
   a. When you repeatedly give advice about a family member's significant health concern and learn that the relative does not go to his or her physician about the problem.
   b. When you repeatedly try to get a family member to adopt a more healthy lifestyle and change behaviors (e.g., diet, smoking, and exercise).
2. When you, and only you, take care of family health matters.
   a. When you are the only person who speaks to your family member's specialist.
   b. When you (rather than the primary care clinician) are the person who coordinates the care of the family member among the specialists.
3. When you, instead of an independent physician, evaluate a family member's serious illness.
   a. When you do a physical exam of a family member.
   b. When you order tests for a family member.
   c. When you write a referral letter to have a family member evaluated further.
4. When you treat a family member for a serious illness for which most people see a physician.

   a. When you write a prescription for medication for a family member's serious illness.

   b. When you assist in the surgery of a family member (deliver a baby, etc.).

Warning signs of *underinvolvement* with your own family's medical concerns:

1. When you do not want to hear anything about a family member's symptoms.
2. When you never comment on or discuss the medical issues of a family member.
3. When you do not provide support or sympathy for the everyday symptoms or aches and pains of family members.
4. When you avoid contact or conversation with the ill family member.

Index

510

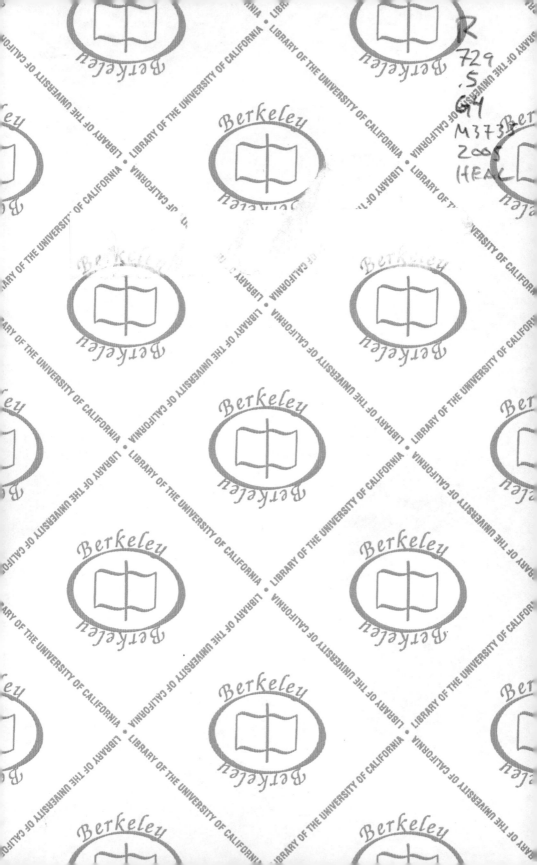